THE TERMINOLOGY OF HEALTH AND MEDICINE

Second Edition

THE TERMINOLOGY OF HEALTH AND MEDICINE

A Self-Instructional Program

JANE RICE, RN, CMA-C

Former Medical Assistant Program Director
Coosa Valley Technical College
Rome, Georgia

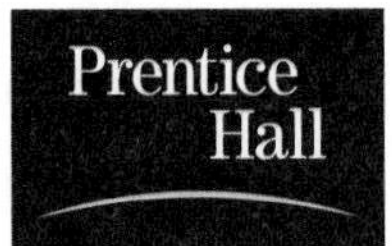

Upper Saddle River, New Jersey 07458

ISBN 0-13-042333-5

Publisher: Julie Levin Alexander
Executive Assistant & Supervisor: Regina Bruno
Senior Acquisitions Editor: Mark Cohen
Assistant Editor: Melissa Kerian
Editorial Assistant: Mary Ellen Ruttenberg
Marketing Manager: Nicole Benson
Production Managing Editor: Patrick Walsh
Director of Manufacturing and Production: Bruce Johnson
Production Editor: Lisa Garboski, Bookworks
Interior Design: Donna Wickes
Production Liaison: Alex Ivchenko
Manufacturing Manager: Ilene Sanford
Media Production Manager: Amy Pettier
Media Project Manager: Stephen Hartner
Manufacturing Buyer: Pat Brown
Creative Director: Cheryl Asherman
Senior Design Coordinator: Maria Guglielmo-Walsh
Formatting: Pine Tree Composition, Inc.
Illustrator: Barbara Cousins
Printer/Binder: Von Hoffmann Press
Copy Editor: Barbara Liguori
Proofreader: Terry Andrews
Cover Design: Joseph DePinho
Cover Printer: Phoenix Color

Pearson Education LTD.
Pearson Education Australia PTY, Limited
Pearson Education Singapore, Pte. Ltd
Pearson Education North Asia Ltd
Pearson Education Canada, Ltd.
Pearson Educación de Mexico, S.A. de C.V.
Pearson Education —Japan
Pearson Education Malaysia, Pte. Ltd

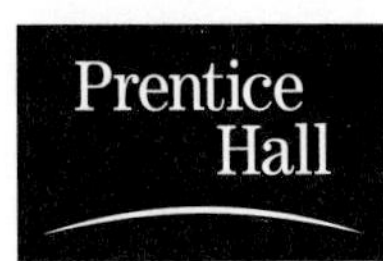

10 9 8 7 6 5 4 3 2
ISBN 0-13-042333-5

Dedicated to Charles Larry Rice,
husband, partner, and best friend

CONTENTS

Preface ix
Note to the Learner xv
How to Work the Program xvii

CHAPTER 1 INTRODUCTION TO MEDICAL TERMINOLOGY 2
CHAPTER 2 ORGANIZATION OF THE BODY 20
CHAPTER 3 THE INTEGUMENTARY SYSTEM 40
Dermatology
CHAPTER 4 THE SKELETAL SYSTEM 70
Orthopedics
CHAPTER 5 THE MUSCULAR SYSTEM 98
Rheumatology and Orthopedics
CHAPTER 6 THE NERVOUS SYSTEM 122
Neurology and Neurosurgery
CHAPTER 7 SPECIAL SENSES 148
Otorhinolaryngology and Ophthalmology
CHAPTER 8 THE ENDOCRINE SYSTEM 174
Endocrinology
CHAPTER 9 THE CARDIOVASCULAR SYSTEM 198
Cardiology
CHAPTER 10 BLOOD, LYMPH, AND THE IMMUNE SYSTEM 226
Hematology and Immunology
CHAPTER 11 THE DIGESTIVE SYSTEM 250
Gastroenterology
CHAPTER 12 THE RESPIRATORY SYSTEM 274
Pulmonary Medicine
CHAPTER 13 THE URINARY SYSTEM 294
Urology

CHAPTER 14 THE FEMALE REPRODUCTIVE SYSTEM 314
Gynecology and Obstetrics

CHAPTER 15 THE MALE REPRODUCTIVE SYSTEM 344
Urology

Appendix A Answer Key for the Review Exercises 367

Appendix B Glossary of Word Elements 383

Appendix C Abbreviations 395

Appendix D List of Tables and Figures 405

Index 409

PREFACE

The Terminology of Health and Medicine is a learner-oriented, self-study, programmed text. It is organized into distinct frames that require the individual to actively participate in his or her learning by writing in and confirming answers. The text is arranged by body systems and medical/surgical speciality areas. The medical terminology selected for this text is based upon the *International Classification of Diseases, Clinical Modification (ICD-9-CM) Diagnostic Code, Current Procedural Terminology (CPT), Diagnosis Related Groups (DRGs), and Nursing Diagnoses.*

KEY FEATURES

- **Unit Objectives:** The unit objectives state the expected learning outcomes.
- **Unit Openings:** Serving as an introduction, the unit opener gives the learning concepts for the unit. It is followed by a brief overview with appropriate tables and figures.
- **Primary Word Elements:** Following the unit opener are primary word elements. These word elements are used throughout the unit and the learner is encouraged to master their meanings. New to this edition is a **Glossary of Word Elements** of approximately 900 entries.
- **Full-Color Art and New Design:** To assist the learner in better understanding the concepts being presented, full color illustrations are appropriately placed throughout the text. New to this edition are tables of each body system with an overview of the system, its organs, and functions. Also added are numerous photographs of diseases, disorders, and x-rays. To enhance learning, a colorful, new design has been developed for the text.
- **Explanation Frames:** These frames describe and explain a selected learning concept that relates to the body system being studied, its organs and functions, the terminology associated with the unit, medical/surgical specialty area, diseases and disorders, selected drugs, and abbreviations.
- **Essential Terminology with Pronunciation Key, Word Elements, and Word Division:** Medical terms are an integral part of each unit. As a word element is introduced, selected terminology that directly relates to the word element is given, along with its pronunciation key, word division, and meaning. Where appropriate each medial term is divided into its word elements. The primary word elements are included in the text while all other word elements may be found in the **Glossary of Word Elements.**

For example:

ANSWER COLUMN

8.3 The combining form **aden / o** and the root **aden** mean gland. Medical terms that begin with these word elements are:

___________	pain in a gland, SYN: adenodynia	adenalgia (ad eh **NAL** jee ah)
___________	surgical excision of a gland	adenectomy (ad eh **NEK** toh mee)
___________	a tumor of a gland	adenoma (ad eh **NOH** mah)
___________	a softening of a gland	adenomalacia (ad eh noh mah **LAY** shee ah)
___________	a condition of hardening of a gland	adenosclerosis (ad eh noh skleh **ROH** sis)
___________	any disease condition of a gland	adenosis ad eh **NOH** sis)

- **For Review Frames:** To enable the learner to review word elements that are commonly used in medical terminology review frames are provided throughout the text.
- **Diseases and Disorders:** Common diseases, disorders, and/or conditions are included in each unit.
- **Drugs Used for Diseases and Disorders:** Selected classifications of drugs and examples are included in each unit as they relate to the body system or medical/surgical specialty area being studied.
- **Abbreviations:** Selected abbreviations with their meanings are included in each unit. These abbreviations are in current use and directly associated with the subject of the unit.
- **In the Spotlight:** This is a new feature that presents a current finding in medicine or an interesting topic that relates to the subject of the unit.
- **Case Studies:** A synopsis of a selected disease and/or disorder is provided and includes present history, signs and symptoms, diagnosis, treatment, prevention, and risk factors. The questions that follow are directly related to the case study. *Answers are provided at the end of the activity.*
- **Review Exercises:** A variety of review exercises are provided to help the learner assess his or her level of understanding of the concepts presented in the unit. Approximately 700 review items are included in the text.
- **Review A: Word Elements**
  This review allows the learner to check his or her knowledge of some of the word elements presented in the unit. Medical words are divided into their word parts with each word element identified as **Prefix (P), Word Root (R), Combining Form (CF),** and/or **Suffix (S).** The learner provides the meaning of the word element.

PRIMARY WORD ELEMENTS

The following are selected prefixes and their meanings that you will use as you build medical terms. Please commit these to memory.

PREFIXES THAT PERTAIN TO POSITION OR PLACEMENT

ab away from
ad toward
ana up
ante before
cata down
circum, peri around
endo within
epi upon, above
ex out, away from
extra outside, beyond
hyper above, excessive
hypo below, deficient
infra below
inter between
intra within
meso middle
para beside
retro backward
sub below, under
supra above, beyond

PREFIXES THAT PERTAIN TO NUMBERS AND AMOUNTS

ambi both
bi two, double
centi a hundred
deca ten
dipl double
di (s) two
milli one-thousandth
multi many, much
nulli none
poly many
primi first
quadri four
quint five
semi, hemi half
tetra four
tri three
uni one

PREFIXES THAT ARE DESCRIPTIVE AND ARE USED IN GENERAL

a, an without, lack of
anti, contra against
auto self
brachy short
brady slow
cac, mal bad
dia through
dys bad, difficult
eu good, normal
hetero different
homeo similar, same
hydro water
mega large, great
micro small
oligo scanty, little
pan all
pseudo false
sym, syn together

		ANSWER COLUMN
1.7	___________ means pertaining to away from the rule or norm.	**abnormal** (ab **NOR** mal)
	The word elements of the word **ab / norm / al** are:	
	___________ prefix that means away from	**ab**
	___________ root that means rule or norm	**norm**
	___________ suffix that means pertaining to	**-al**
1.8	___________ means (through knowledge) determining the cause and nature of a disease.	**diagnosis** (dye ag **NOH** sis)
	The word elements of the word **dia / gnosis** are:	
	___________ prefix that means through	**dia**
	___________ suffix that means knowledge	**-gnosis**

ANSWER COLUMN

continued

1.9 Some medical terms that include ____________ and measures prefixes and/or combining forms are: centimeter, kilogram, microgram, milligram, and milliliter.

weights

1.10 A ____________ is one-hundredth of a meter. **Centi** is a prefix that means a hundred. The suffix **-meter** means instrument to measure, measure. The meter is the fundamental unit of length in the metric system. It is equal to 39.37 inches, which is slightly more than a yard, or 3.28 feet.

centimeter
(SEN tih mee ter)

1.11 A ____________ is 1000 grams. It is a unit of weight or mass in the metric system. The combining form **kil / o** means ____________.

kilogram (KILL oh gram)
thousand

1.12 The combining form **kil / o** means thousand.
In the term kilogram the suffix ____________ means weight or mass.

-gram

1.13 A microgram is one-thousandth of a milligram. A milligram is one-thousandth of a gram. A milliliter is one-thousandth of a liter. The prefix ____________ means one-thousandth.

milli

1.14 A ____________ is 0.001 milligram. It is a unit of weight or mass in the metric system.
The word elements of the word **micro / gram** are:
____________ prefix that means small
____________ suffix that means a weight

microgram
(MY kroh gram)
micro
-gram

1.15 **True or False.** Some common weights and measures prefixes and combining forms are: centi, kil / o, micro, and milli.

true

FOR REVIEW

centi is a prefix that means a hundred.
kil / o is a combining form that means thousand.
micro is a prefix that means small.
milli is a prefix that means one-thousandth.

ANSWER COLUMN

1.16 The foundation of a word is called a __________ __________.

word root

EXPLANATION FRAME

A **root** is a word or word element from which other words are formed. It is the foundation of the word. The root conveys the central meaning of the word and forms the base to which prefixes and suffixes are attached for word modification. For example: using the prefix (anti), the **root (pyret),** and the suffix (-ic) you build the medical term: anti / **pyret** / ic.

1.17 The term __________ means pertaining to an agent that works against fever. Aspirin is an antipyretic agent.

antipyretic (an tih pye **RET** ik)

1.18 The word elements that make up the term **anti / pyret / ic** are:

__________ prefix that means against

__________ root that means fever

__________ suffix that means pertaining to

Note that the central meaning is conveyed by the word root.

anti
pyret
-ic

1.19 The term __________ means the condition of being self-governed (law).

autonomy (aw **TON** noh mee)

1.20 The word elements that make up the term **auto / nom / y** are:

__________ prefix that means self

__________ root that means law

__________ suffix that means condition of

auto
nom
-y

1.21 The term __________ means an agent that works against coughing.

antitussive (an tih **TUSS** iv)

1.22 The word elements that make up the term **anti / tuss / ive** are:

__________ prefix that means against

__________ root that means cough

__________ suffix that means nature of, quality of

anti
tuss
-ive

ANSWER COLUMN

continued

1.23 Underline the word root in the following terms:
abnormal
antipyretic
autonomy
antitussive

abnormal
antipyretic
autonomy
antitussive

1.24 A word root to which a vowel has been added to join the root to a second root or a suffix is called a ____________ ____________.

combining form

EXPLANATION FRAME

Combining forms may be found at the beginning of a word or within the word. The vowel "o" is used more often than any other to make combining forms. In this text a slash (/) is used to designate the vowel of the combining form.

1.25 The combining form ____________ means tumor.

onc / o

EXPLANATION FRAME

Tumors of various types are the focus of study by an oncologist.
The field of oncology is a medical specialty that studies tumors.
Tumors can be classified as benign or malignant.
Benign means that the tumor is not cancerous.
Malignant means that the tumor is cancerous.

1.26 An ____________ is one who specializes in the study of tumors.

oncologist
(ong **KALL** oh jist)

1.27 The word elements that make up the term **onc / o / log / ist** are:
____________ combining form that means tumor
____________ root that means study of
____________ suffix that means one who specializes

onc / o
log
-ist

1.28 A syllable or group of syllables united with or placed at the end of a word in order to alter or modify its meaning is called a ____________.

suffix

PRIMARY WORD ELEMENTS

The following are selected suffixes and their meanings that you will use as you build medical terms. Please commit these to memory.

SUFFIXES THAT PERTAIN TO PATHOLOGIC CONDITIONS

-algia, -dynia pain
-cele hernia, tumor, swelling
-emesis vomiting
-itis inflammation
-lith stone
-lysis destruction, separation
-malacia softening
-megaly enlargement, large
-oid resemble
-oma tumor
-osis condition of
-pathy disease
-penia deficiency
-phobia fear
-plegia paralysis, stroke
-ptosis drooping
-ptysis spitting
-rrhage bursting forth
-rrhagia bursting forth
-rrhea flow, discharge
-rrhexis rupture

SUFFIXES USED IN DIAGNOSTIC AND SURGICAL PROCEDURES

-centesis surgical puncture
-desis binding
-ectomy surgical excision
-gram a weight, mark, record
-graph to write, record
-meter measure
-opsy to view
-pexy surgical fixation
-plasty surgical repair
-rrhaphy suture
-scope instrument
-scopy to view
-stasis control, stopping
-stomy new opening
-tome instrument to cut
-tomy incision

SUFFIXES THAT ARE USED IN GENERAL

-blast immature cell, germ cell
-cyte cell
-ist one who specializes, agent
-logy study of
-phagia to eat
-phasia to speak
-philia attraction
-phraxis to obstruct
-physis growth
-plasia formation, produce
-pnea breathing
-poiesis formation
-therapy treatment
-trophy nourishment, development
-uria urine

	ANSWER COLUMN
1.29 The term suffix means to fasten on beneath or ___________.	**under**
1.30 A suffix, when attached to the end of a word, will ___________ or modify the meaning of the word or create a new word.	**alter**
1.31 The suffix ___________ means the study of.	**-logy**

EXPLANATION FRAME

-Logy is a common suffix in health and medicine. It is used to describe things studied. **Dermatology** is the study of the skin. **Biology** is the study of life. **Oncology** is the study of tumors. **Hematology** is the study of blood.

ANSWER COLUMN

continued

1.32 The suffix **-y** is one of a group of suffixes that have more than a single meaning. The meanings of the suffix **-y** are:

____

__________ ________

__________ ________

process
pertaining to
condition of

1.33 Anytime that a suffix is given alone, it will be preceded with a hyphen, as in **-ac** and the other suffixes that are listed in this frame and elsewhere in the text.

There are ten suffixes that mean pertaining to. It will be much easier for you to remember these suffixes if you learn them here. These ten suffixes are:

____
____
____
____
____
____
____
____
____
____

-ac
-al
-ar
-ary
-ic
-in
-ine
-ous
-us
-y

1.34 Underline the suffixes in the following medical words.

ili / ac
ab / norm / al
clavicul / ar
axill / ary
anti / pyret / ic
hepat / o / tox / in
intra / uter / ine
heter / o / gene / ous
poly / my / o / clon / us
cardi / o / pulmonar / y

ili / ac
ab / norm / al
clavicul / ar
axill / ary
anti / pyret / ic
hepat / o / tox / in
intra / uter / ine
heter / o / gene / ous
poly / my / o / clon / us
cardi / o / pulmonar / y

Answer Column

1.35 There are eight suffixes that mean condition of. They are:
__________ **-hexia**
__________ **-ia**
__________ **-iasis**
__________ **-ism**
__________ **-ity**
__________ **-osis**
__________ **-sis**
__________ **-y**

1.36 Underline the suffixes in the following medical words.

	Answer
cac / hexia	**cac / hexia**
dys / ton / ia	**dys / ton / ia**
micro / organ / ism	**micro / organ / ism**
spastic / ity	**spastic / ity**
necr / osis	**necr / osis**
di / ure / sis	**di / ure / sis**
auto / nom / y	**auto / nom / y**

1.37 The term __________ literally means a bad condition. — **cachexia** (kah **KEK** see ah)

1.38 The word elements of the word **cac / hexia** are:
__________ prefix that means bad — **cac**
__________ suffix that means condition of — **-hexia**

FOR REVIEW

The fundamental elements in medical terminology are the component parts that are used to build medical words. Dividing a word into its prefix, word root, combining form, and suffix will allow you to discover the word's definition.

1.39 Medical terms of __________ origin are often difficult to __________ because many of them begin with a silent letter or have a silent __________ within the word. — **Greek spell letter**

Answer Column

continued

1.40 In the term knuckle the __________ is silent.

k

1.41 In the term phlegm the __________ is silent.

g

1.42 Correct spelling is extremely __________ in medical terminology as the addition or omission of a __________ letter may change the meaning of a term to something entirely __________. For example: **ab**duct and **ad**duct.

important
single
different

1.43 To lead **away** from the middle is called __________.

abduct (ab DUKT)

1.44 To lead **toward** the middle is called __________.

adduct (ah DUKT)

1.45 The prefix that means **away** from is __________.

ab

1.46 The prefix that means **toward** is __________.

ad

1.47 In both medical words abduct and adduct, duct is a __________ that means to lead.

root

1.48 To form plural endings of medical words you change **a** as in burs**a** to __________ as in burs**ae. Ax** as in thor**ax** to **aces** as in thor**aces** or to __________ as in thorax**es.**

ae
es

1.49 **En** as in foram**en** to __________ as in foram**ina.**
Is as in cris**is** to __________ as in cris**es. Is** as in ir**is** to **ides** as in ir**ides.**
Is as in femor**is** to __________ as in femor**a.**
Ix as in append**ix** to __________ as in append**ices.**
Nx as in phala**nx** to __________ as in phala**nges.**
On as in spermatozo**on** to **a** as in __________.
Um as in ov**um** to __________ as in ov**a.**

ina
es
a
ices
ges
spermatozoa
a

Answer Column

continued

Us as in ___________ to **i** as in nucle**i**. — nucleus

Y as in arter**y** to **i** and add **es** as in ___________. — arteries

---

1.50 Write the plural form of each of the following medical words. The word ending that is to be changed is underlined.

SINGULAR FORM	PLURAL FORM	Answer
gingiva	___________	gingivae
serum	___________	sera
thrombus	___________	thrombi
ovum	___________	ova
spermatozoon	___________	spermatozoa
fungus	___________	fungi
vertebra	___________	vertebrae
phalanx	___________	phalanges
diagnosis	___________	diagnoses
ganglion	___________	ganglia

1.51 Pronunciation of medical words is often difficult for anyone who is learning medical terminology. When applicable, a pronunciation guide for the medical word will be provided for you.

___________ letters in boldface type are used to indicate the syllable that has the strongest stress. Syllables are spelled out as they ___________. — capital, sound

---

1.52 The following guidelines are provided to help you with the ___________ and spelling of medical terms: — identification

1. If the suffix begins with a ___________, drop the combining vowel from the combining form and add the suffix. — vowel

   For example: hemat / **o** plus -oma becomes hematoma. -Oma is a ___________ that starts with a vowel and it means tumor. — suffix

2. If the suffix begins with a consonant, keep the combining vowel and add the suffix to the ___________ form. — combining

   For example: kil / **o** plus gram becomes kilogram. -Gram is a suffix that means a ___________, mark, or record. — weight

3. Keep the combining vowel between two or more ___________ in a term. — roots

   For example: electr / **o** plus cardi / **o** plus -gram becomes electrocardiogram.

ANSWER COLUMN

EXPLANATION FRAME

Example word: **gastr / o / enter / o / logy** (study of the stomach and intestines). When building and defining medical words you:

1. Start with the suffix and write the definition: **-logy** (study of),
2. Next define the beginning of the word: **gastr / o** (stomach).
3. If there is a middle element define it last: **enter / o** (intestine)

1.53 This frame is designed so that you may practice using the three guidelines for identifying and spelling medical terms.

1. The suffix begins with a vowel (**-osis**) and the combining form is **necr / o**. Build the correct medical term ____________. — **necrosis** (neh **KROH** sis)
2. The suffix begins with a consonant (**-logy**) and the combining form is **onc / o**. Build the correct medical term ____________. — **oncology** (ong **KALL** oh jee)
3. **Gastr / o** means stomach. **Enter / o** means intestine. The suffix **-logy** means the study of. Build the correct medical term that means the study of the stomach and intestines ____________. — **gastroenterology** (gas troh en ter **ALL** oh jee)

1.54 Word Elements That Pertain to Color

ELEMENT(S)	MEANING	EXAMPLE WORD(S)	Answer
chrom / o	____________	chromosome	**color**
albin; leuk / o	____________	albinism; leukocyte	**white**
chlor / o	____________	chlorophyll	**green**
cirrh / o	____________	cirrhosis	**orange-yellow**
cyan / o	____________	cyanosis	**blue**
erythr / o; rube / o	____________	erythrocyte; rubeola	**red**
melan / o	____________	melanoma	**black**
poli / o	____________	poliomyelitis	**gray**
purpura	____________	purpura	**purple**
xanth / o	____________	xanthoderma	**yellow**

1.55 ____________ is defined as the microscopic bodies that carry the genes that determine hereditary characteristics, such as the color of the hair, eyes, and skin. Give the word element that means color. ____________ — **chromosome** (**KROH** moh sohm) **chrom / o**

Answer Column

	Question	Answer
1.56	___________ is defined as absence of pigment in the skin, hair, and eyes. Give the word element from this word that means white. ___________	**albinism** (**AL** bin izm) **albin**
1.57	A ___________ is a white blood cell. Give the word element from this word that means white. ___________	**leukocyte** (**LOO** koh sight) **leuk / o**
1.58	___________ is defined as the green pigment in plants that accomplishes photosynthesis. Give the word element that means green. ___________	**chlorophyll** (**KLOR** oh fill) **chlor / o**
1.59	Give the meaning of the following word elements: cyan / o ___________ erythr / o ___________ melan / o ___________ poli / o ___________ xanth / o ___________ cirrh / o ___________ rube / o ___________	 **blue** **red** **black** **gray** **yellow** **orange-yellow** **red**

REVIEW A: PREFIXES

Medical words are built using **prefixes (P), word roots (R), combining forms (CF),** and **suffixes (S).** Knowing the meanings associated with some of the more common of these word elements will enable you to determine the general meaning of many, if not most, medical words. In this review, the medical word and its definition are provided, so that you may reinforce the learning concepts associated with medical terminology.

This review allows you to familiarize yourself with some of the more common prefixes and their meanings. In the spaces provided, write the prefix and its meaning.

MEDICAL WORD	*DEFINITION*	*PREFIX*	*MEANING*
1. abnormal	pertaining to away from the norm	________	__________
2. abduct	to lead away from the middle	________	__________
3. adduct	to lead toward the middle	________	__________
4. antipyretic	pertaining to an agent that works against fever	________	__________
5. antitussive	an agent that works against coughing	________	__________
6. autonomy	the condition of being self-governed	________	__________
7. cachexia	a bad condition	________	__________
8. centimeter	one-hundredth of a meter	________	__________
9. diagnosis	through knowledge determining the cause and nature of a disease	________	__________
10. microgram	a small measurement of weight	________	__________
11. milligram	one-thousandth of a gram	________	__________

REVIEW B: WORD ROOTS AND COMBINING FORMS

This review allows you to familiarize yourself with some of the more common word roots/combining forms and their meanings. In the spaces provided, write the word root/combining form and its meaning.

MEDICAL WORD	*DEFINITION*	*ROOT/CF*	*MEANING*
1. abnormal	pertaining to away from the norm	________	____________
2. antipyretic	pertaining to an agent that works against fever	________	____________
3. antitussive	an agent that works against coughing	________	____________
4. autonomy	the condition of being self-governed	________	____________
5. gastroenterology	the study of the stomach and intestines	________	____________
6. kilogram	1000 grams	________	____________
7. oncologist	one who specializes in the study of tumors	________	____________

REVIEW C: SUFFIXES

This review allows you to familiarize yourself with some of the more common suffixes and their meanings. In the spaces provided, write the suffix and its meaning.

MEDICAL WORD	*DEFINITION*	*SUFFIX*	*MEANING*
1. abnormal	pertaining to away from the norm	________	____________
2. antipyretic	pertaining to an agent that works against fever	________	____________
3. antitussive	an agent that works against coughing	________	____________
4. autonomy	the condition of being self-governed	________	____________

MEDICAL WORD	DEFINITION	SUFFIX	MEANING
5. cachexia	a bad condition	______	______
6. centimeter	one-hundredth of a meter	______	______
7. diagnosis	through knowledge determining the cause and nature of a disease	______	______
8. gastroenterology	the study of the stomach and intestines	______	______
9. kilogram	1000 grams	______	______
10. microgram	a small measurement of weight	______	______
11. milligram	one-thousandth of a gram	______	______
12. oncologist	one who specializes in the study of tumors	______	______

REVIEW D: WORD ELEMENTS THAT PERTAIN TO COLOR

Give the word element(s) for the following colors.

COLOR	WORD ELEMENT(S)
1. white	______ or ______
2. green	______
3. orange-yellow	______
4. blue	______
5. red	______ or ______
6. black	______
7. gray	______
8. purple	______
9. yellow	______

REVIEW E: FORMING PLURAL ENDINGS OF MEDICAL WORDS

Write the plural form of each of the following medical words.

SINGULAR FORM	*PLURAL FORM*
1. ganglion	____________
2. gingiva	____________
3. diagnosis	____________
4. serum	____________
5. phalanx	____________
6. vertebra	____________
7. thrombus	____________
8. fungus	____________
9. spermatozoon	____________
10. ovum	____________

2 ORGANIZATION OF THE BODY

LEARNING CONCEPTS

- the human body
- levels of organization
- homeostasis
- essential terminology
- pronunciation guide
- word elements
- explanation frames
- directional terminology
- planes of the body
- body cavities
- nine regions of the abdominopelvic cavity
- the four regions of the abdomen
- in the spotlight: water
- review exercises

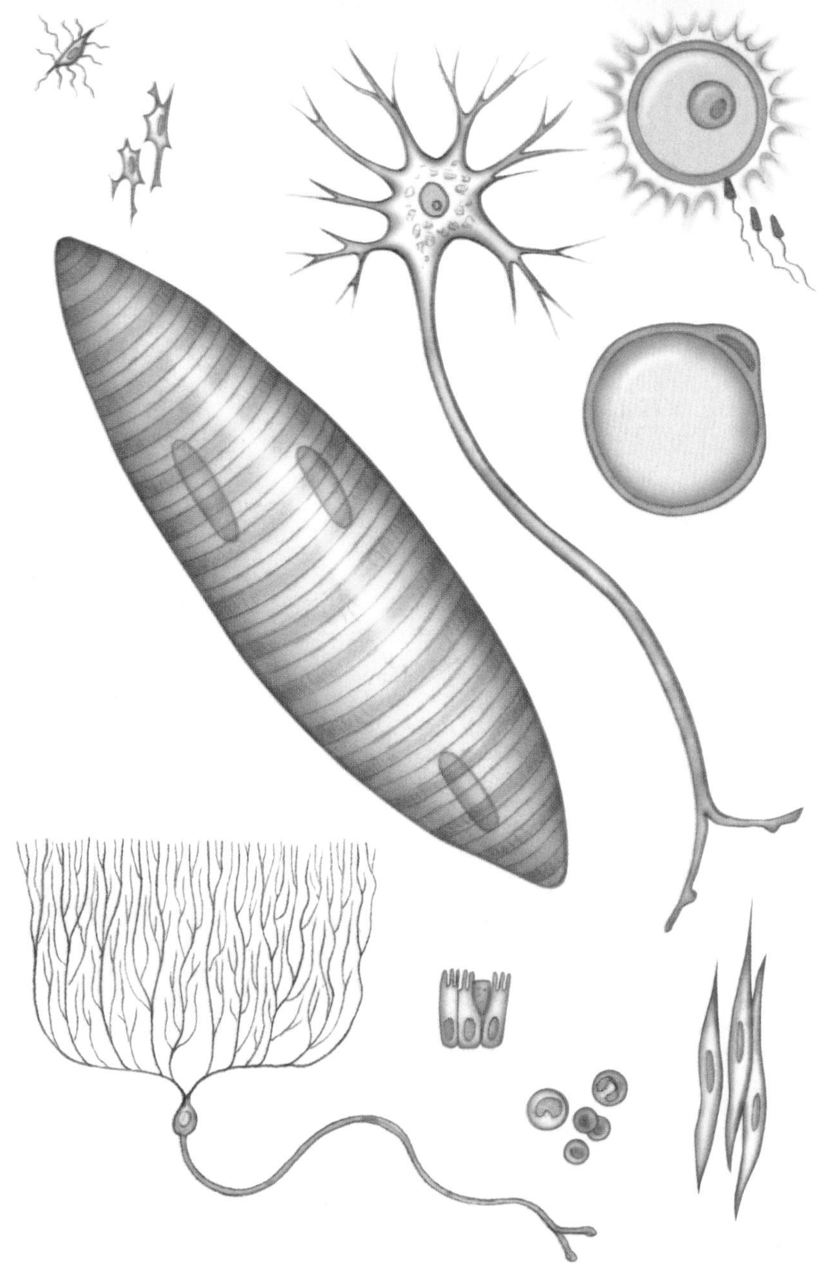

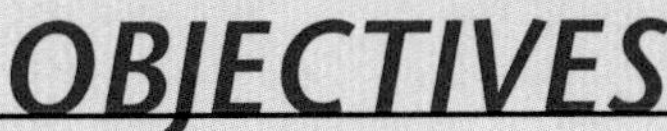

OBJECTIVES

ON COMPLETION OF THIS UNIT, YOU SHOULD BE ABLE TO:

- ▶ Briefly describe the amazing human body.
- ▶ Identify selected Head-To-Toe Assessment body parts and their word elements.
- ▶ Define terms that describe the body and its structural units.
- ▶ Describe the major functions of the various organ systems of the body.
- ▶ Define terms that are used to describe direction, planes, and cavities of the body.
- ▶ List the nine regions of the abdominopelvic cavity.
- ▶ Identify the four regions of the abdomen that are referred to as quadrants.
- ▶ Describe water as the most important constituent of the body.
- ▶ Analyze, build, spell, and pronounce selected medical words.
- ▶ Successfully complete the review section.

TECH LINK

CD-ROM Use the CD-ROM enclosed with your textbook to gain additional reinforcement through interactive word building exercises, spelling games, labeling activities, and additional quizzes.

www.prenhall.com/rice Use the above address to access the free, interactive Companion Web-site created specifically for this textbook. Get hints, instant feedback, and textbook references to chapter-related multiple choice and true/false questions, fill-in-the-blank, and labeling exercises. In addition, you will find an audio glossary, and essay questions.

THE AMAZING HUMAN BODY

Thirty trillion cells make up a baby. There are 206 bones and 600 muscles in the body; 42% of a person's body weight is made up of muscles and 18% is made up of the skeleton (bones). An average adult has approximately 5 liters of blood with 25,000 miles of blood vessels. A new outer skin layer occurs every 27 days. If the alveoli in the lungs were flattened out they would cover about one-half of a tennis court. If the tubules in the kidney were stretched out and untangled there would be about 70 miles of them.

The largest single cell in the human body is the ovum (the female sex cell) and the smallest single cell is the sperm (male sex cell). An average female's ovaries contain about 500,000 ova cells, but only around 400 mature and are capable of being fertilized. The average male's testes produce approximately 200 million sperm per day. An ejaculation of 2 mL contains about 120 to 300 million sperm.

The human body is made up of atoms, molecules, organelles, cells, tissues, organs, and systems. See Figure 2–1. An **atom** is the smallest chemical unit of matter. Chemical elements are made up of atoms. In chemistry, an element is a substance that cannot be separated into substances different from itself by ordinary chemical means. It is the basic component of which all matter is composed. There are at least 105 different chemical elements that have been identified. Elements found in the human body include aluminum, carbon, calcium, chlorine, cobalt, copper, fluorine, hydrogen, iodine, iron, manganese, magnesium, nitrogen, oxygen, phosphorus, potassium, sodium, sulfur, and zinc. See Table 2–1.

A **molecule** is a chemical combination of two or more atoms that form a specific chemical compound. An **organelle** is a specialized part of a cell

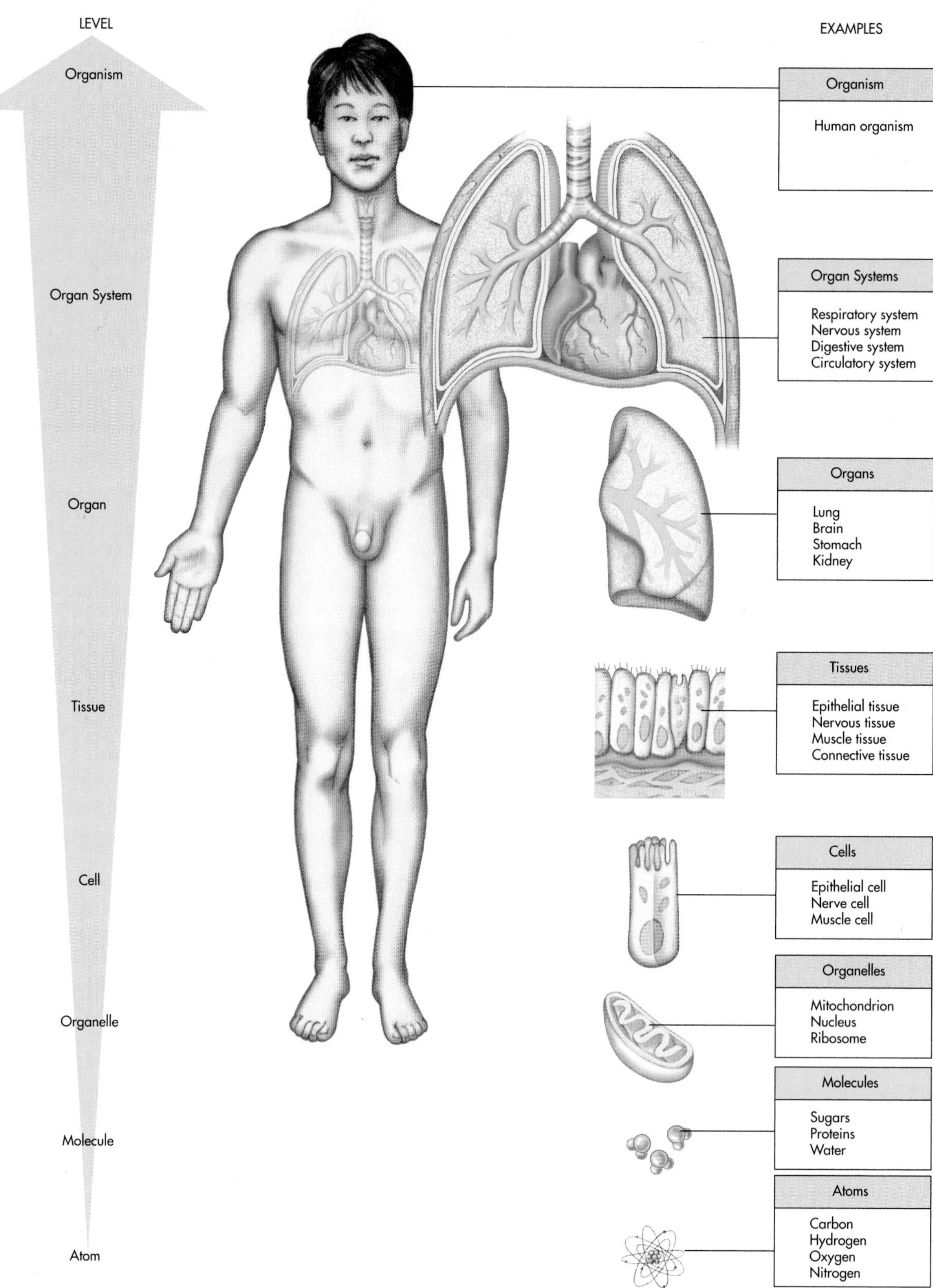

LEVEL
Organism
Organ System
Organ
Tissue
Cell
Organelle
Molecule
Atom
EXAMPLES
Organism
Human organism
Organ Systems
Respiratory system
Nervous system
Digestive system
Circulatory system
Organs
Lung
Brain
Stomach
Kidney
Tissues
Epithelial tissue
Nervous tissue
Muscle tissue
Connective tissue
Cells
Epithelial cell
Nerve cell
Muscle cell
Organelles
Mitochondrion
Nucleus
Ribosome
Molecules
Sugars
Proteins
Water
Atoms
Carbon
Hydrogen
Oxygen
Nitrogen

FIGURE 2–1
The human body: levels of organization.

TABLE 2–1 ELEMENTS FOUND IN THE HUMAN BODY

Symbol	Element	Atomic Weight
Al	aluminum	13
C	carbon	6
Ca	calcium	20
Cl	chlorine	17
Co	cobalt	27
Cu	copper	29
F	fluorine	9
H	hydrogen	1
I	iodine	53
Fe	iron	26
Mn	manganese	25
Mg	magnesium	12
N	nitrogen	7
O	oxygen	8
P	phosphorus	15
K	potassium	19
Na	sodium	11
S	sulfur	16
Zn	zinc	30

that performs a distinctive function. **Cells** are the basic building blocks for the various structures that together make up the human being. A **tissue** is a grouping of similar cells that together perform specialized functions. An **organ** is a group of tissues serving a common purpose or function. A group of organs functioning together for a common purpose is called a **system.**

Unit 2 provides some of the essential ingredients that will enable you to understand basic concepts concerning the amazing human body and relate these concepts to the terminology of health and medicine.

PRIMARY WORD ELEMENTS

HEAD-TO-TOE ASSESSMENT

Enrich your understanding of the human body by learning the following selected body parts and their word elements. An example medical term is provided with the word element in italics.

BODY PART	WORD ELEMENT	EXAMPLE MEDICAL TERM
abdomen	abdomin, celi	*abdomin*al, *celi*ac
ankle	ankyl	*ankyl*osis
arm	brach / i, brachi / o	*brachi*algia, *brachi*ocrural
armpit	axill	*axill*ary

(continued)

BODY PART	WORD ELEMENT	EXAMPLE MEDICAL TERM
bladder	cyst / o, vesic	*cystocele, vesical*
body	somat	psycho*somatic*
bone	oste	*osteoma*
cheek	bucc	*buccal*
chest	thorac, pector, steth / o	*thoracic, pectoral, stethoscope*
ear	ot, aur	*otitis, aural*
elbow	cubit	ante*cubital*
eye	ophthalm / o, ocul, opt	*ophthalmology, ocular, optic*
eyelid	blephar	*blepharitis*
finger and/or toe	dactyl / o	*dactylospasm*
foot	illus	*illus*
great (big) toe	hallux	*hallux*
gums	gingiv	*gingivitis*
hair	trich / o, pil /o	*trichomycosis, pilomotor*
hand	manus	*manus*
head	cephal	*cephalalgia*
heart	cardi / o	*cardiologist*
heel	calcane	*calcaneal*
joint	arthr / o	*arthroscope*
kidney	ren, nephr	*renal, nephritis*
kneecap, patella	patell	*patellar*
leg	crur	*crural*
lip	cheil	*cheilosis*
liver	hepat	*hepatitis*
lung	pneum / o, pulm / o	*pneumonia, pulmonary*
mouth	or, stomat	oral, *stomatitis*
muscle	muscul / o, my / o	*musculoskeletal, myofibroma*
nail	onych, onych / o, ungu	*onychitis, onychomycosis,* sub*ungual*
navel	umbilic	*umbilical*
neck	cervic	*cervical*
nerve	neur	*neuritis*
nose	nas / o, rhin / o	*nasopharyngeal, rhinorrhea*
rib	cost	sub*costal*
skin	derm / a, dermat / o	*dermatome, dermatology*
skull	crani / o	*craniotomy*
spine	rachi, spin	*rachialgia, spine*
stomach	gastr / o	*gastrodynia*
tailbone	coccyg / o	*coccygodynia*
teeth	dent	*dentist*
temples	tempor	*temporal*
throat, pharynx	pharyng	*pharyngitis*
thumb	pollex	*pollex*
tongue	lingu, gloss / o	sub*lingual, glossotomy*
voice box, larynx	laryng / o	otorhino*laryngology*
wrist	carp	*carpal*

ANSWER COLUMN

2.1 ____________ literally means to cut up. It is the study of the structure of an organism such as humans.

anatomy (ah **NATT** oh mee)

Answer Column

2.2 The word elements that make up the term **ana / tomy** are:
ana ______ prefix that means up — **ana**
tomy ______ suffix that means incision — **-tomy**

2.3 Physiology ______ is the study of the nature of an organism. — **physiology** (fiz ee **ALL** oh je)

2.4 The word elements that make up the term **physi / o / logy** are:
______ combining form that means nature — **physi / o**
______ suffix that means the study of — **-logy**

2.5 An ______ is the smallest chemical unit of matter. — **atom (AT** om)

2.6 An atom consists of a ______ that contains protons and neutrons and is surrounded by electrons. The nucleus is at the center of the atom and a ______ is a positively charged particle, while a ______ is without an electrical charge. The ______ is a negatively charged particle that revolves about the nucleus. — **nucleus (NOO** klee us) **proton (PROH** ton) **neutron (NOO** tron) **electron** (ee **LEK** tron)

2.7 A ______ is a chemical combination of two or more ______ that form a specific chemical compound. — **molecule (MOLL** eh kyool) **atoms (AT** oms)

EXPLANATION FRAME

Water is the most important constituent of all body fluids, secretions, and excretions. It makes up 65% of a male's body weight and 55% of a female's body weight. It is an ideal transportation medium for inorganic and organic compounds.

2.8 In a ______ molecule oxygen forms polar covalent bonds with two hydrogen atoms (H_2O). — **water** (**WAW** ter)

2.9 ______ may be described as the basic building blocks of the human body. See Figure 2–2. — **cells** (**SELLS**)

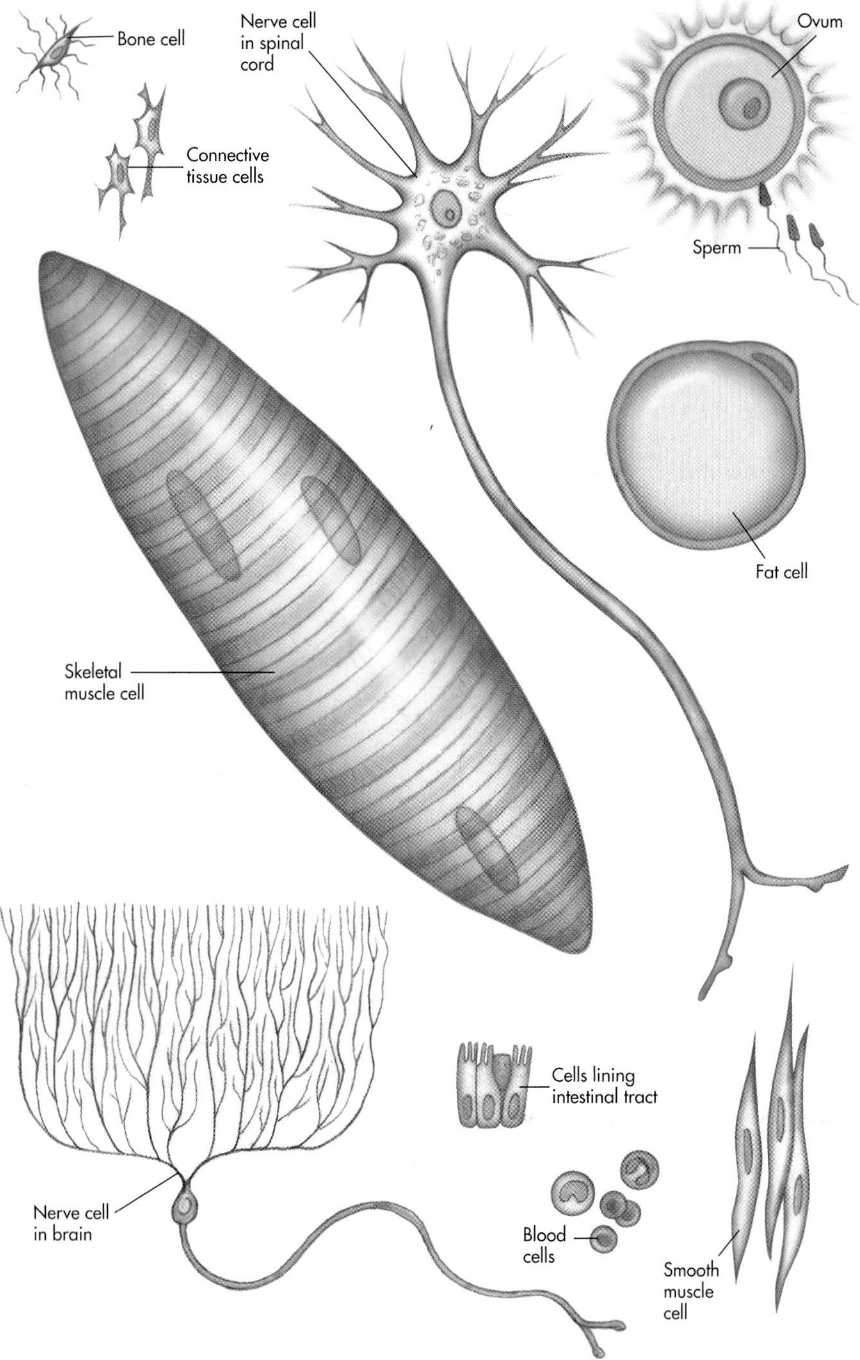

FIGURE 2–2

Cells may be described as the basic building blocks of the human body. They have many different shapes and vary in size and function. These examples show the range of forms and sizes with the dimensions they would have if magnified approximately 500 times.

ANSWER COLUMN

2.10 The outer covering of a cell is called the cell __________ or plasma membrane.

membrane (**MEM** brane)

EXPLANATION FRAME

The cell membrane has the capability of allowing some substances to pass into and out of the cell while denying passage to other substances. This selectivity allows cells to receive nutrition and dispose of waste, just as the human being eats food and disposes of waste.

2.11 The substance within the cell membrane is called __________. It is the essential matter of a living cell and the word elements of the word **proto / plasm** are:

__________ prefix that means first

__________ suffix that means a thing formed, plasma

protoplasm (**PROH** toh plazm)

proto

-plasm

2.12 A __________ is a grouping of similar cells that together perform specialized functions.

tissue (**TISH** oo)

2.13 There are four basic types of tissue in the body: __________, __________, muscle, and nerve. Each of the four basic tissues has several subtypes named for their shape, appearance, arrangement, or function.

epithelial (ep ih **THEE** lee al)
connective (con **NEK** tiv)

EXPLANATION FRAME

Connective tissue is the most widespread and abundant of the body tissues. Connective tissue forms the supporting network for the organs of the body, sheaths the muscles, connects muscles to bones, and connects bones to form joints. Bone is a dense form of connective tissue.

2.14 __________ tissue is the most widespread and abundant of the four body tissues.

connective (con **NEK** tiv)

EXPLANATION FRAME

Histology is the study of tissue, and a **histologist** is one who specializes in studying tissues. The suffix **-logy** means study of and the suffix **-ist** means one who specializes.

ANSWER COLUMN

continued

2.15 The study of tissue is known as ____________.

histology (hiss **TALL** oh jee)

2.16 The word elements that make up the term **hist / o / logy** are:
____________ combining form that means tissue
____________ suffix that means study of

hist / o
-logy

2.17 Fatty tissue throughout the body is called ____________.
The term **adip / ose** is composed of a root and a suffix. The ____________ **adip** means fat and the suffix **-ose** means like. Together they form a word that describes fatlike tissue.

adipose (**ADD** ih pohs)
root

2.18 Tissues serving a common purpose or function make up structures called ____________.

organs
(**OR** gans)

EXPLANATION FRAME

The organ systems of the body are the integumentary, skeletal, muscular, nervous, endocrine, cardiovascular, blood and the lymphatic, respiratory, digestive, urinary, and reproductive.

2.19 Organs are specialized components of the body. Examples include the brain, the heart, and the largest organ, the ____________.

skin
(**SKIN**)

2.20 A group of organs functioning together for a common purpose is called a ____________. See Figure 2–3.

system
(**SIS** tem)

2.21 As long as the body is in a state of balance known as ____________ it is able to perform at its maximum potential.

homeostasis
(hoh mee oh **STAY** sis)

2.22 The word elements that make up the term **homeo / stasis** are:
____________ prefix that means similar, same
____________ suffix that means control, stopping

homeo
-stasis

EXPLANATION FRAME

Four primary reference systems have been adopted to provide uniformity to the anatomic description of the body. These reference systems are direction, planes, cavities, and structural units. The standard anatomic position for the body is erect, head facing forward, arms by the sides with palms to the front.

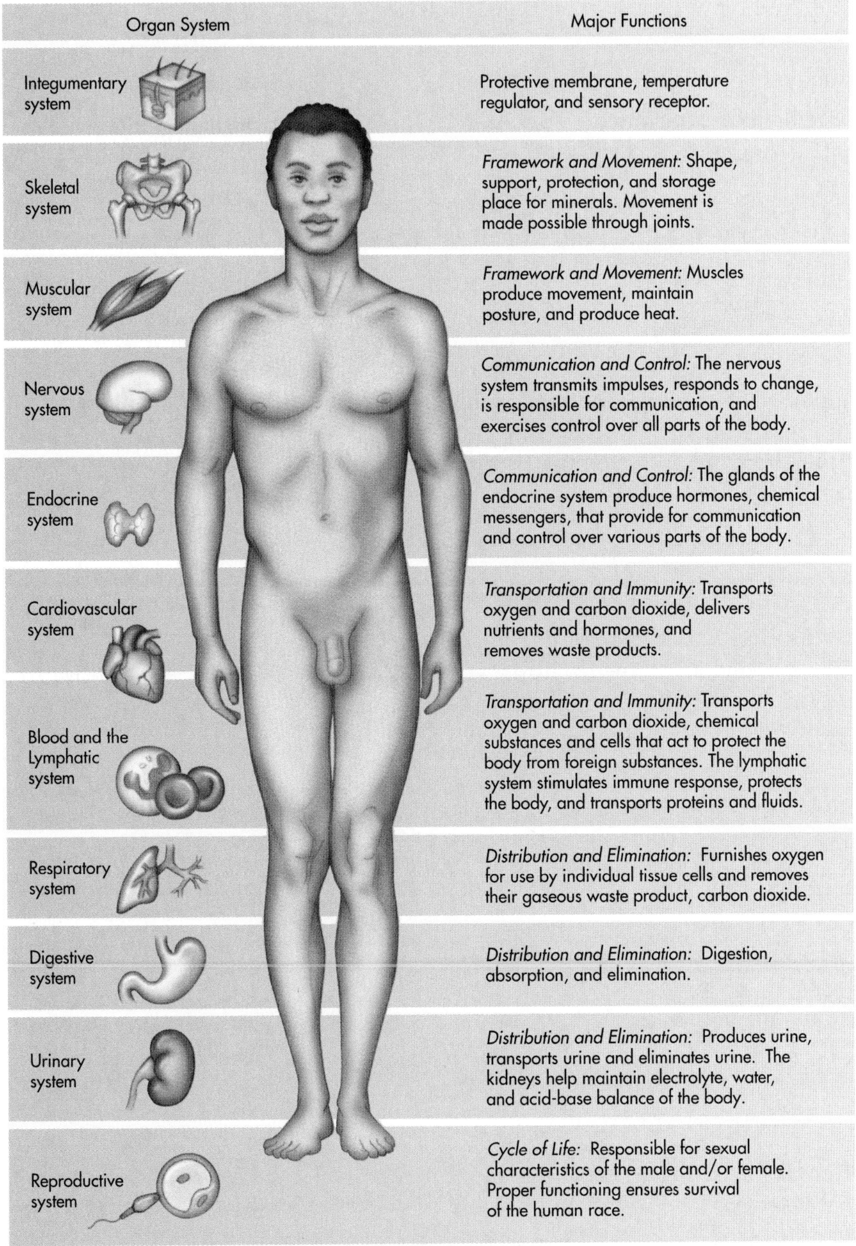

Organ System
Major Functions
Integumentary system
Protective membrane, temperature regulator, and sensory receptor.
Skeletal system
Framework and Movement: Shape, support, protection, and storage place for minerals. Movement is made possible through joints.
Muscular system
Framework and Movement: Muscles produce movement, maintain posture, and produce heat.
Nervous system
Communication and Control: The nervous system transmits impulses, responds to change, is responsible for communication, and exercises control over all parts of the body.
Endocrine system
Communication and Control: The glands of the endocrine system produce hormones, chemical messengers, that provide for communication and control over various parts of the body.
Cardiovascular system
Transportation and Immunity: Transports oxygen and carbon dioxide, delivers nutrients and hormones, and removes waste products.
Blood and the Lymphatic system
Transportation and Immunity: Transports oxygen and carbon dioxide, chemical substances and cells that act to protect the body from foreign substances. The lymphatic system stimulates immune response, protects the body, and transports proteins and fluids.
Respiratory system
Distribution and Elimination: Furnishes oxygen for use by individual tissue cells and removes their gaseous waste product, carbon dioxide.
Digestive system
Distribution and Elimination: Digestion, absorption, and elimination.
Urinary system
Distribution and Elimination: Produces urine, transports urine and eliminates urine. The kidneys help maintain electrolyte, water, and acid-base balance of the body.
Reproductive system
Cycle of Life: Responsible for sexual characteristics of the male and/or female. Proper functioning ensures survival of the human race.

FIGURE 2–3
Organ systems of the body with major functions.

Answer Column

continued

2.23 Terms that describe direction are:

		Answer
__________	above, in an upward direction	**superior** (soo **PEE** ree or)
__________	below, in a downward direction	**inferior** (in **FEE** ree or)
__________	in front of or before	**anterior** (an **TEE** ree or)
__________	toward the back	**posterior** (poss **TEE** ree or)
__________	toward the head	**cephalad (SEF** ah lad)
__________	pertaining to the skull	**cranial (KRAY** nee al)
__________	toward the midline	**medial (MEE** dee al)
__________	to the side	**lateral (LAT** er al)
__________	nearest the point of attachment	**proximal (PROK** sim al)
__________	away from the point of attachment	**distal (DISS** tal)
__________	the same as anterior, the front side	**ventral (VEN** tral)
__________	the same as posterior, the backside	**dorsal (DOR** sal)
__________	toward the surface	**superficial** (soo per **FISH** al)
__________	far down from the surface	**deep (DEEP)**
__________	the top or highest point	**vertex (VER** teks)
__________	the pointed end of a cone-shaped structure	**apex (AY** peks)
__________	pertaining to the tail	**caudal (KAWD** al)
__________	the body is lying face *upward*	**supine** (soo **PINE)**
__________	the body is lying face downward	**prone (PROHN)**

EXPLANATION FRAME

There are certain terms that are used to describe the imaginary planes that pass through the body and divide it into various sections. These planes are the sagittal, the transverse or horizontal, and the coronal or frontal. See Figure 2–4.

2.24 The __________ plane vertically divides the body as it passes through the midline to form right and left sides.

sagittal
(SAJ ih tal)

2.25 A __________ or horizontal plane divides the body into __________ and inferior portions.

transverse (trans **VERS)**
superior (soo **PEE** ree or)

2.26 A __________ or frontal plane divides the body into anterior and __________ portions.

coronal (kah **RON** al)
posterior (poss **TEE** ree or)

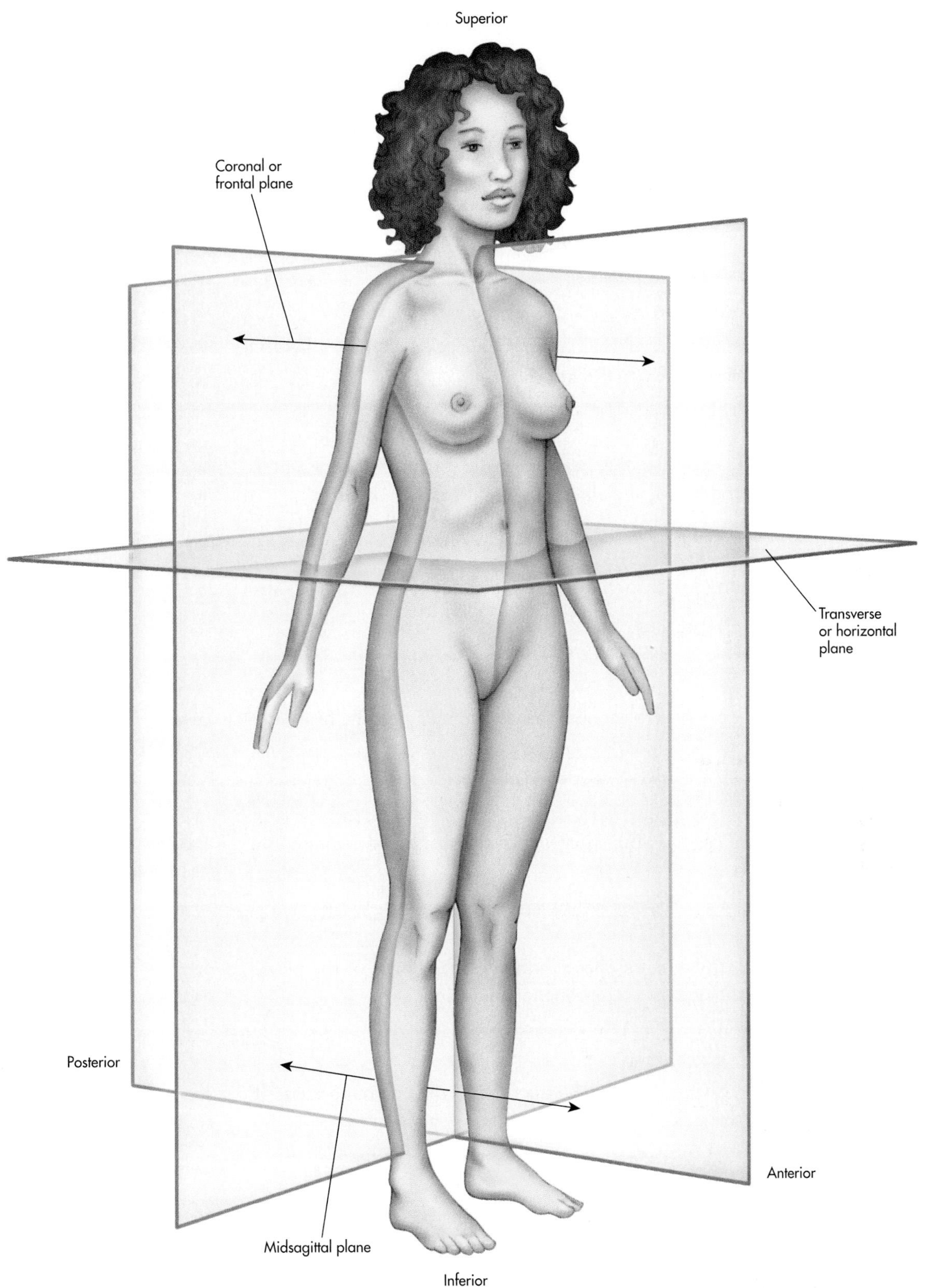

FIGURE 2–4
Planes of the body: coronal or frontal, transverse, and midsagittal.

Answer Column

EXPLANATION FRAME

A cavity is a hollow space containing body organs. Body cavities are classified into two groups according to their location. On the front is the ventral or anterior cavity and on the back is the dorsal or posterior cavity. See Figure 2–5.

2.27 The ____________ cavity is the hollow portion of the human torso extending from the neck to the pelvis.

ventral (VEN tral)

2.28 The ventral cavity contains the heart and the organs of respiration, ____________ reproduction, and elimination.

digestion
(dye **JEST** shun)

EXPLANATION FRAME

The ventral cavity can be subdivided into three distinct areas: thoracic, abdominal, and pelvic.

2.29 The ____________ cavity is the area of the chest containing the heart and the lungs.

thoracic
(tho **RASS** ik)

2.30 The ____________ cavity is the space below the diaphragm, commonly referred to as the belly.

abdominal
(ab **DOM** ih nal)

2.31 The ____________ cavity is the space formed by the bones of the pelvic area and contains the organs of reproduction and elimination.

pelvic
(**PELL** vik)

2.32 The ____________ cavity contains the structures of the nervous system. It is subdivided into the ____________ cavity and the spinal cavity.

dorsal (DOR sal)
cranial (KRAY nee al)

2.33 The cranial cavity is the space in the skull containing the ____________.

brain (BRAIN)

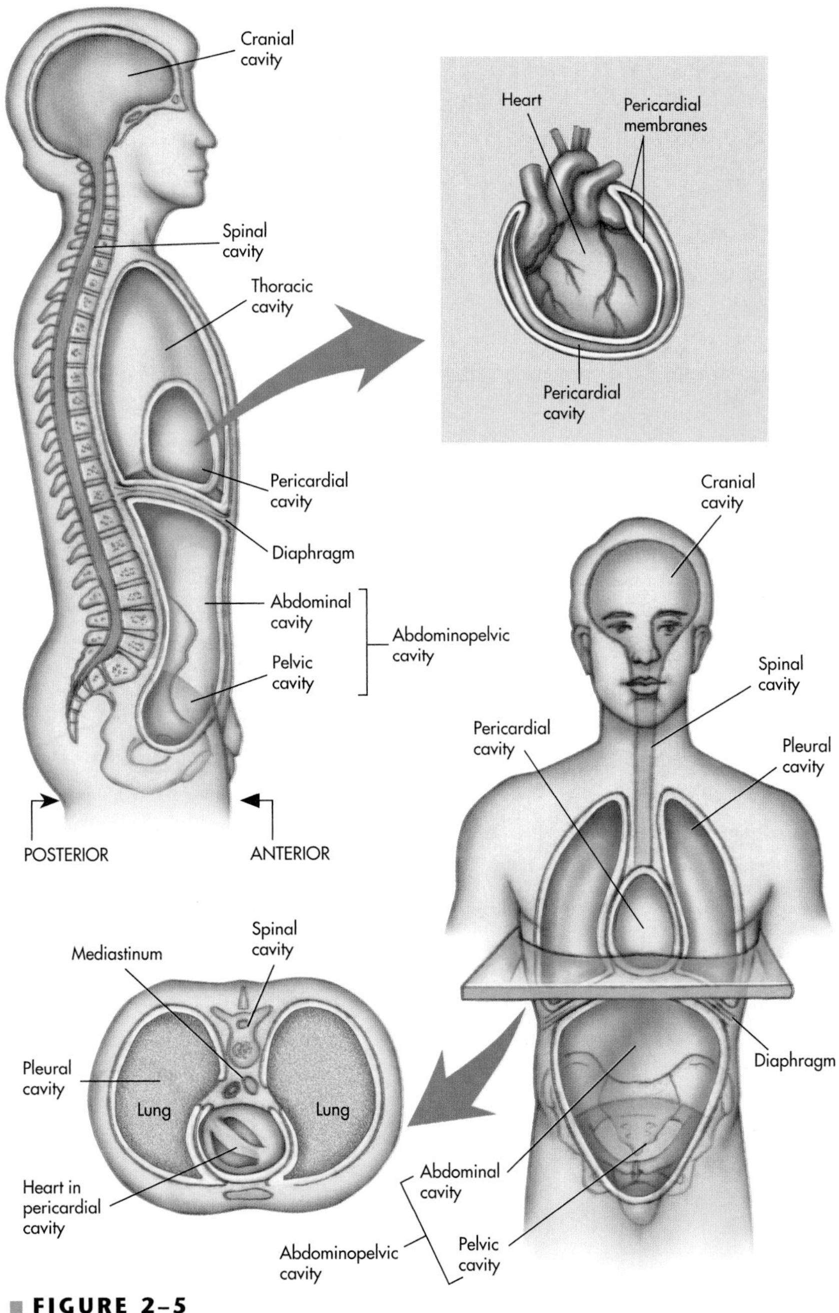

FIGURE 2–5
Body cavities.

ANSWER COLUMN

2.34 The spinal cavity is the space within the bony spinal column that contains the ____________ ____________ and spinal fluid.

spinal cord (SPYE nal KORD)

ANSWER COLUMN

continued

2.35 The ____________ cavity is the combination of the abdominal and pelvic cavities.

abdominopelvic (ab dom ih noh **PELL** vik)

2.36 The abdominopelvic cavity is divided into nine regions. See Figure 2–6. Using a tic-tac-toe pattern drawn across the abdominopelvic cavity these regions are:

____________ ____________ upper right region at the level of the ninth rib cartilage

____________ ____________ upper left region at the level of the ninth rib cartilage

____________ region over the stomach

____________ ____________ right middle lateral region

____________ ____________ left middle lateral region

____________ at the navel

____________ ____________ or ____________ right lower lateral region

____________ ____________ or ____________ left lower lateral region

____________ lower middle region below the navel

right hypochondriac (high poh **KON** dree ak)

left hypochondriac (high poh **KON** dree ak)

epigastric (epih **GAS** trik)

right lumbar (**LUM** bar)

left lumbar (**LUM** bar)

umbilical (um **BILL** ih kal)

right iliac / inguinal (**ILL** ee ak / **ING** gwih nal)

left iliac / inguinal (**ILL** ee ak / **ING** gwih nal)

hypogastric (high poh **GAS** trik)

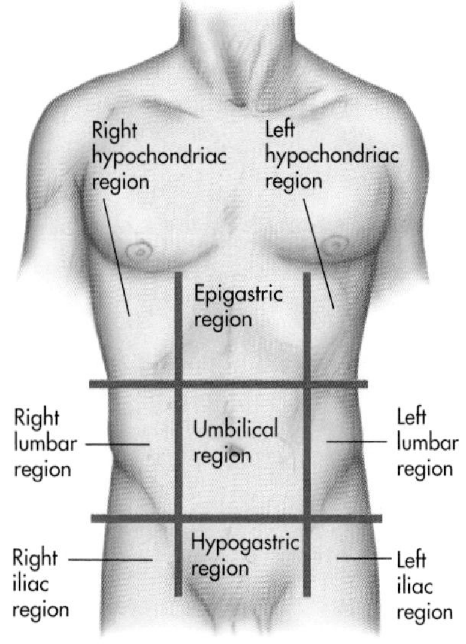

FIGURE 2–6
The nine regions of the abdominopelvic cavity.

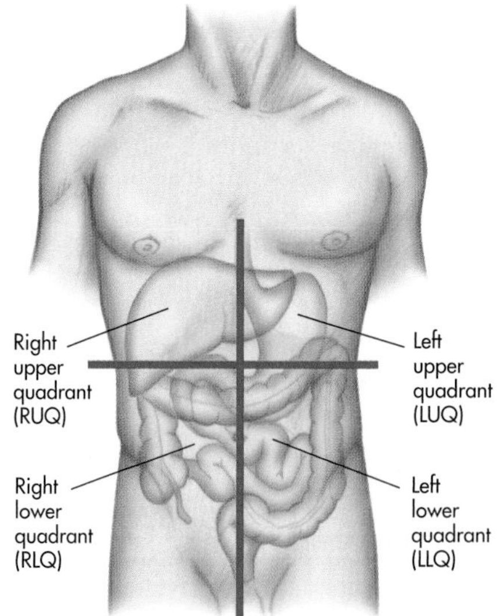

FIGURE 2–7
The four regions of the abdomen that are referred to as quadrants.

IN THE SPOTLIGHT

WATER—THE MOST IMPORTANT CONSTITUENT OF THE BODY

Water is the most important constituent of the human body and is essential to every body process. Bones depend on water intake to provide adequate blood for delivery and removal of calcium. The intestines and kidneys use water to remove waste. Muscles need water to remove acids that would otherwise build up, causing cramps and diminishing muscle action. Nerve function depends on the presence of certain minerals, which are kept in balance by water levels in the body. The immune system depends on sufficient water to ensure blood flow for delivery of immune cells and removal of diseased cells. Water in saliva and the stomach aids digestion and absorption of nutrients.

It is recommended that the average healthy adult drink eight 8-ounce glasses of water per day. One may need more than eight glasses of water per day before, during, and after exercise; in warm weather (especially if doing any type of out-of-door activity); during and after drinking alcohol or caffeine; when breast-feeding; during illness (especially diarrhea, fever, and/or prolonged vomiting); with certain medication (especially diuretics); after surgery; and/or after severe burns or bleeding. It is estimated that one may lose up to a pint of water during every hour of air travel. It is recommended that drinking ample water before and during a flight will decrease the risk of dehydration. Dehydration increases the risk of developing clots in the leg veins while flying.

To maintain homeostasis it is essential that the body be supplied with adequate fluids. The following is a description of an average daily input and daily output of fluids. Naturally, if one consumes more or less than these averages, the daily input and output will be affected.

Water Balance

Daily Input		Daily Output	
Moist foods	1000 mL	Urine	1000 mL
Ingested fluids	1000 mL	Skin (evaporation)	750 mL
Cell metabolism	300 mL	Lung (evaporation	400 mL
		Feces	150 mL
Total	2300 mL		2300 mL

ANSWER COLUMN

2.37 The __________ is divided into four corresponding regions that are used for descriptive and diagnostic purposes.

abdomen
(**AB** doh men)

2.38 The four regions of the abdomen are referred to as __________. See Figure 2–7.

quadrants
(**KWOD** rants)

ANSWER COLUMN

continued

2.39 The quadrants and their abbreviations are identified as:

____

____

____

____

right upper quadrant (RUQ) (**KWOD** rant)

left upper quadrant (LUQ) (**KWOD** rant)

right lower quadrant (RLQ) (**KWOD** rant)

left lower quadrant (LLQ) (**KWOD** rant)

REVIEW A: ORGANIZATION OF THE BODY

Please provide the correct answer for each of the following statements.

1. ____________ is the study of the structure of an organism such as humans.
2. ____________ is the study of the nature of an organism.
3. The smallest chemical unit of matter is called an ____________.
4. An ____________ is a negatively charged particle that revolves about the nucleus.
5. A ____________ is a positively charged particle.
6. A chemical combination of two or more atoms that form a specific chemical compound is called a ____________.
7. The basic building blocks of the human body are called ____________.
8. The essential matter of a living cell is called ____________.
9. A grouping of similar cells that together perform specialized functions is called a ____________.
10. A group of organs functioning together for a common purpose is called a ____________.

REVIEW B: TERMS USED TO DESCRIBE DIRECTION

Please place the correct letter from column II on the appropriate line of column I.

COLUMN I		*COLUMN II*
________	1. superior	A. toward the head
________	2. inferior	B. toward the back
________	3. anterior	C. away from the point of attachment
________	4. posterior	D. to the side
________	5. cephalad	E. above, in an upward direction
________	6. cranial	F. in front of or before
________	7. medial	G. nearest the point of attachment
________	8. lateral	H. pertaining to the skull
________	9. proximal	I. toward the midline
________	10. distal	J. below, in a downward direction

REVIEW C: TERMS USED TO DESCRIBE PLANES OF THE BODY & BODY CAVITIES

Please provide the correct answer for each of the following statements.

1. The ____________ plane vertically divides the body as it passes through the midline to form a right and left half.
2. A ____________ or horizontal plane divides the body into superior and inferior portions.
3. A ____________ or frontal plane divides the body into anterior and posterior portions.
4. The ____________ cavity is the hollow portion of the human torso extending from the neck to the pelvis.
5. The ____________ cavity is the area of the chest containing the heart and the lungs.
6. The ____________ cavity is the space below the diaphragm, commonly referred to as the belly.
7. The ____________ cavity is the space formed by the bones of the pelvic area and contains the organs of reproduction and elimination.
8. The ____________ cavity contains the structures of the nervous system.
9. The ____________ cavity is the space in the skull containing the brain.
10. The ____________ cavity is the combination of the abdominal and pelvic cavities.

REVIEW D: TERMS USED TO DESCRIBE THE NINE REGIONS OF THE ABDOMEN

Please provide the correct answer for each of the following.

The abdominopelvic cavity is divided into nine regions.

Using a tic-tac-toe pattern drawn across the abdominopelvic cavity these regions are:

1. ____________ ____________ upper right region at the level of the ninth rib cartilage
2. ____________ ____________ upper left region at the level of the ninth rib cartilage
3. ____________ region over the stomach
4. ____________ ____________ right middle lateral region
5. ____________ ____________ left middle lateral region
6. ____________ at the navel
7. ____________ ____________ or ____________ right lower lateral region
8. ____________ ____________ or ____________ left lower lateral region
9. ____________ lower middle region below the navel

REVIEW E: WORD ELEMENTS

This review allows you to check your knowledge of some of the word elements presented in this unit. In the spaces provided, write the word element and its meaning. See the example given in number 1.

MEDICAL WORD	*DEFINITION*	*ELEMENT*	*MEANING*
1. anatomy	means to cut up; study of the structure of an organism	ana (P) -tomy (S)	up incision
2. physiology	the study of the nature of an organism	__________ __________	__________ __________
3. protoplasm	the substance within the cell membrane	__________ __________	__________ __________
4. histology	the study of tissue	__________ __________	__________ __________
5. adipose	fatty tissue throughout the body	__________ __________	__________ __________
6. homeostasis	a state of balance	__________ __________	__________ __________

3 THE INTEGUMENTARY SYSTEM: DERMATOLOGY

LEARNING CONCEPTS

- the skin and its accessory structures
- essential terminology
- pronunciation guide
- word elements
- explanation frames
- the ABCDs of melanoma
- skin signs
- selected diseases and disorders
- drugs used for the integumentary system
- abbreviations
- in the spotlight: skin cancer
- case study: contact dermatitis
- review exercises

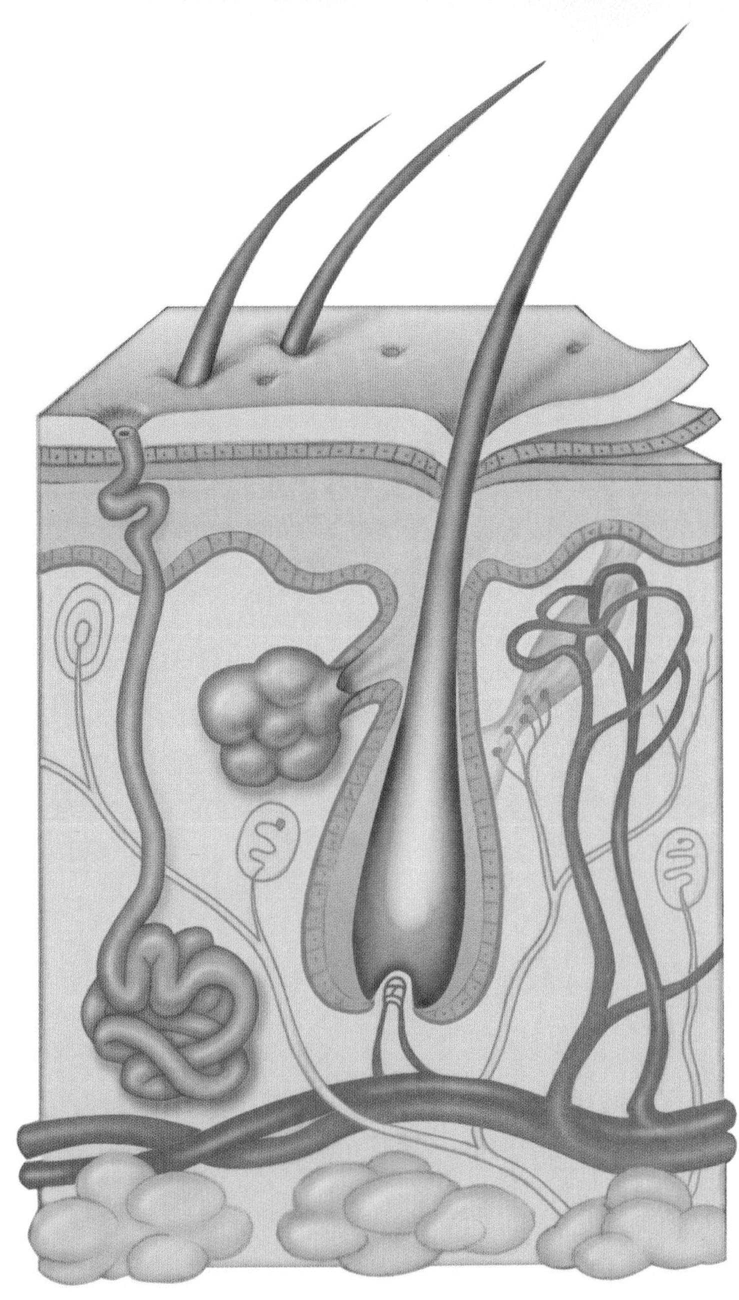

OBJECTIVES

ON COMPLETION OF THIS UNIT, YOU SHOULD BE ABLE TO:

- Briefly describe the integumentary system.
- Describe the primary functions of the various organs or structures of the integumentary system.
- Identify and give the meaning of the primary word elements for this unit.
- Analyze, build, spell, and pronounce selected medical words.
- Describe the ABCDs of melanoma.
- Give the definition of various skin signs and an example of each.
- Describe selected diseases/disorders of the integumentary system.
- Describe selected drugs that are used for dermatologic diseases or disorders.
- Define selected abbreviations that pertain to the integumentary system.
- Describe skin cancer, giving the types, signs, and six steps to help reduce the risk of sunburn and developing skin cancer.
- Complete the Case Study on Contact Dermatitis: Poison Ivy.
- Successfully complete the review section.

TECH LINK

CD-ROM Use the CD-ROM enclosed with your textbook to gain additional reinforcement through interactive word building exercises, spelling games, labeling activities, and additional quizzes.

www.prenhall.com/rice Use the above address to access the free, interactive Companion Website created specifically for this textbook. Get hints, instant feedback, and textbook references to chapter-related multiple choice and true/false questions, fill-in-the-blank, and labeling exercises. In addition, you will find an audio glossary, and essay questions.

The integumentary system is composed of the skin and its accessory structures: the hair, nails, sebaceous glands, and sweat glands. The skin is the largest organ in the human body. In an average adult it covers more than 3000 square inches of surface area and weighs more than 6 pounds. In a lifetime, a person may lose 40 pounds of skin, as colonies of cells die off on a regular basis. These cells are washed away or sloughed off.

The skin is well supplied with blood vessels and nerves and has four main functions: protection, regulation, sensation, and secretion.

Protection

The skin serves as a protective membrane against invasion by bacteria and other potentially harmful agents that might try to penetrate to deeper tissues. It also protects against mechanical injury of delicate cells located beneath its epidermis or outer covering. The skin also serves to inhibit loss of water and electrolytes and provides a reservoir for food and water storage. The skin guards the body against excessive exposure to the sun's ultraviolet rays by producing a protective pigmentation, and it helps to produce the body's supply of vitamin D.

Regulation

The skin serves to raise or lower body temperature as necessary. When the body needs to lose heat, the blood vessels in the skin dilate, bringing more blood to the surface for cooling by radiation. At the same time, the sweat glands are secreting more sweat for cooling by means of evaporation. Conversely, when the body needs to conserve heat, the reflex action of the nervous system causes constriction of the skin's blood vessels, thereby allowing more heat-carrying blood to circulate to the muscles and vital organs.

Sensation

The skin contains millions of microscopic nerve endings that act as sensory receptors for pain, touch, heat, cold, and pressure. When stimulation occurs, nerve impulses are sent to the cerebral cortex of the brain. The nerve endings in the skin are specialized according to the type of sensory information transmitted and, once this information reaches the brain, any necessary response is triggered. For example, touching a hot surface with the hand causes the brain to recognize the senses of touch, heat, and pain and results in the immediate removal of the hand from the hot surface.

Secretion

The skin contains million of sweat glands, which secrete perspiration or sweat, and sebaceous glands, which secrete oil for lubrication. Perspiration is largely water with a small amount of salt and other chemical compounds. This secretion, when left to accumulate, causes body odor, especially where it is trapped among hairs in the axillary region. Sebaceous glands produce sebum, which acts to protect the body from dehydration and possible absorption of harmful substances.

TABLE 3-1 THE INTEGUMENTARY SYSTEM

Organ/Structure	Primary Functions
Skin	Protection, regulation, sensation, and secretion
The Epidermis	The outer layer of the skin. It is divided into four strata:
Stratum corneum	Forms protective covering for the body
Stratum lucidum	Translucent layer that is frequently absent and not seen in thinner skin
Stratum granulosum	Active in the keratinization process, its cells become hard or horny
Stratum germinativum	Responsible for the regeneration of the epidermis
The Dermis	Nourishes the epidermis, provides strength, and supports blood vessels
Papillae	Produce ridges that are one's fingerprints
Subcutaneous Tissue	Supports, nourishes, insulates, and cushions the skin
Hair	Provides sensation and some protection for the head. Hair around the eyes, in the nose, and in the ears serves to filter out foreign particles.
Nails	Protects ends of fingers and toes
Sebaceous Glands	Lubricates the hair and skin
Sweat (Sudoriferous) Glands	Secretes sweat or perspiration, which helps to cool the body by evaporation. Sweat also rids the body of waste.

The skin is essentially composed of two layers, the epidermis and the dermis. The hair, nails, sebaceous glands, and sweat (sudoriferous) glands are the accessory structures of the skin. See Table 3–1.

The color of skin is its most obvious characteristic. Melanin, the pigment that gives color to the skin, is formed in the stratum germinativum—one of the strata of the epidermis. The more abundant the melanin, the darker the color of the skin. Pigment protects the skin from the sun's harmful rays and the darker the pigment, the more the protection.

PRIMARY WORD ELEMENTS

The following word elements (prefixes, roots, combining forms, and suffixes) will be used to build medical terms that relate to this unit. Please commit these to memory.

PREFIX

PREFIX	MEANING	PREFIX	MEANING
anti	against	**hypo**	below, deficient
ep, epi	upon, above	**par**	around
hyper	above, excessive	**sub**	below, under

COMBINING FORM

COMBINING FORM / ROOT	MEANING	COMBINING FORM / ROOT	MEANING
cutane	skin	**onych**	nail
derm, dermat	skin	**onych / i, onych /o**	nail
derm / o, dermat / o	skin	**pachy**	thick
erythr / o	red	**pedicul**	louse
hidr	sweat	**prurit**	itching
icter	jaundice	**rhytid**	wrinkle
integument	covering	**rhytid / o**	wrinkle
kel	tumor	**seb / o**	oil
melan	black	**trich / o, pil / o**	hair
melan / o	black	**ungu**	nail
myc	fungus	**xer / o**	dry

SUFFIX

SUFFIX	MEANING	SUFFIX	MEANING
-al, -ary, -ic, -ous	pertaining to	**-oid**	resemble
-clysis	injection	**-oma**	tumor
-derma, -dermis	skin	**-phagia**	to eat
-ia, -osis	condition of	**-plasty**	surgical repair
-ist	one who specializes	**-rrhea**	flow, discharge
-itis	inflammation	**-tome**	instrument to cut
-logy	study of	**-um**	tissue

Answer Column

3.1 The ___________ system consists of the skin and its appendages. It protects the body from environmental hazards and aids in temperature control. By breaking the medical word integumentary into its word elements you have:

___________ root that means covering and a suffix ___________ that means pertaining to

integumentary (in teg you **MEN** tah ree)

integument

-ary

3.2 The skin is essentially composed of two layers, the ___________ and the ___________. In the term **epi / dermis** the prefix ___________ means upon, above and the suffix **-dermis** means ___________. See Figure 3–1.

epidermis (ep ih **DER** mis)

dermis (**DER** mis)

epi

skin

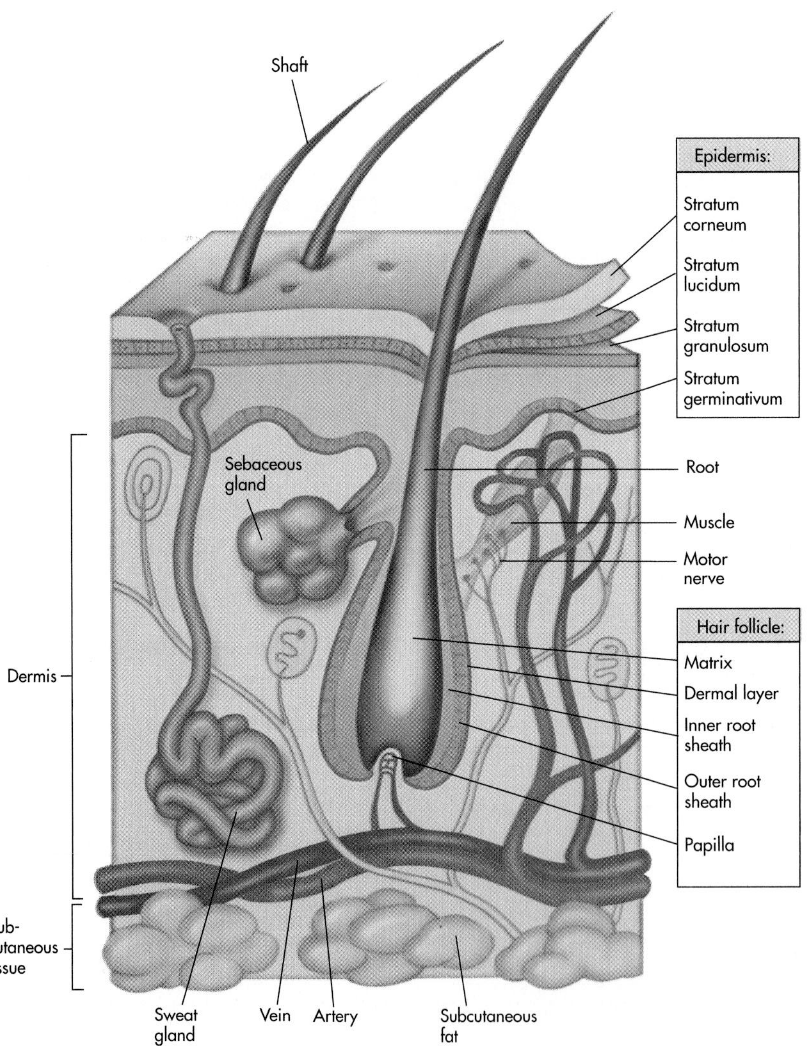

FIGURE 3–1
The integument: the epidermis, dermis, subcutaneous tissue, and its appendages.

Answer Column

		Answer Column
3.3	There are several word elements that mean skin. The word roots ___________ and ___________; the combining forms ___________ and ___________; also, the suffixes ___________ and **-dermis** are used to indicate the skin.	**derm dermat** **dermat / o derm / o** **-derma**
3.4	___________ means inflammation of the skin. The word elements used to build **dermat / itis** are: ___________ root that means skin ___________ suffix that means inflammation	**dermatitis** (der mah **TYE** tis) **dermat** **-itis**
3.5	A physician who specializes in the study of the skin is called a ___________.	**dermatologist** (der mah **TALL** oh jist)
3.6	The word elements that make up the term **dermat / o / log / ist** are: ___________ combining form that means skin ___________ root that means study ___________ suffix that means one who specializes	**dermat / o** **log** **-ist**
3.7	Using the combining form **dermat / o** and the suffix **-logy** that means study of, build a medical term that means study of the skin. ___________	**dermatology** (der mah **TALL** oh jee)
3.8	An instrument used to cut the skin for grafting is called a ___________. The combining forms **derm / a** and ___________ mean skin. The suffix ___________ means instrument to cut; therefore, a dermatome is an instrument used to cut the skin for grafting. In anatomy, a **dermatome** is a delineated area of skin innervated by a spinal cord segment. Each cord segment has a representative skin area: Cervical (C), Thoracic (T), Lumbar (L), and Sacral (S).	**dermatome** (**DER** mah tohm) **dermat / o** **-tome**
3.9	___________ is an abnormal redness of the skin, usually pertaining to widespread areas of *erythema*. Erythroderma is also called *erythrodermia*. The word elements that are used to build **erythr / o / derma** are: ___________ combining form that means red ___________ suffix that means skin	**erythroderma** (eh rith roh **DER** mah) **erythr / o** **-derma**

	ANSWER COLUMN
continued	
3.10 ____________ is a form of *macula* showing diffused redness over the skin.	**erythema** (er ih **THEE** mah)
3.11 The combining form **xer / o** means ____________.	**dry**
3.12 Using the combining form **xer / o** and the suffix **-derma,** build a medical word that means dry skin: ____________.	**xeroderma** (zee roh **DER** mah)
3.13 The ____________ membrane or skin is the largest organ in the human body. In most individuals it makes up approximately 16% of the body weight.	**cutaneous** (kew **TAY** nee us)
The word elements that make up **cutane / ous** are:	
____________ root that means skin	**cutane**
____________ suffix that means pertaining to	**-ous**
3.14 ____________ means pertaining to below the skin. Subcutaneous tissue is actually a layer of fat tissue to which the dermis is attached. The prefix **sub** means below, the root **cutane** means skin, and the suffix **-ous** means pertaining to.	**subcutaneous** (sub kew **TAY** nee us)
3.15 **Hypo** and **hyper** are common prefixes that can easily be confused with one another. ____________ means under, beneath, below, or indicates less than. ____________ means over, above, excessive, or beyond.	**hypo** **hyper**
3.16 A hypodermic injection would be given ____________ ____________ ____________. SYN: subcutaneous injection.	**under the skin**
3.17 The word elements that make up the term **hypo / derm / ic** are:	
____________ prefix that means under, beneath, below, less than	**hypo**
____________ root that means skin	**derm**
____________ suffix that means pertaining to	**-ic**

ANSWER COLUMN

EXPLANATION FRAME

Injection of fluids under the skin to supply the body with a quick replacement of fluids is called hypodermoclysis. Remember that the prefix **hypo** means under, beneath, below and the combining form **derm / o** means skin. The suffix -**clysis** means injection.

3.18 The suffix **-clysis** means ___________.

injection (in **JEK** shun)

3.19 ___________ and **dermomycosis, dermatomycosis** are medical terms that mean a fungus condition of the skin.

tinea (**TIN** ee ah)

EXPLANATION FRAME

Tinea, a Latin word for worm, is the medical term for a skin disease commonly known as ringworm. Tinea or ringworm is not caused by a worm. Actually, ringworm is one of several contagious skin diseases affecting both humans and domestic animals, caused by certain fungi, and marked by the localized appearance of discolored, scaly patches on the skin. Examples: Tinea Cruris (leg) and Tinea Capitis (scalp).

3.20 ___________ (SYN: dermatomycosis) is a skin condition caused by a fungus.

Now look at the word elements that are used to build this term.

___________ combining form that means skin

___________ root that means fungus

___________ suffix that means condition of

dermomycosis (der moh my **KOH** sis)

derm / o

myc

-osis

3.21 A pigment that gives color to the skin is called ___________.

melanin (MEL an in)

3.22 ___________ is a cancerous tumor that has black pigmentation.

Now look at the word elements that are used to build this term.

___________ combining form that means black

___________ root that means cancer

___________ suffix that means tumor

melanocarcinoma (mel ah noh kar sih **NOH** mah)

melan / o

carcin

-oma

Answer Column

EXPLANATION FRAME

Cancer that develops in the pigment cells is called melanoma. Often the first sign of melanoma is change in the size, shape, or color of a mole. The ABCDs of melanoma describe the changes that can occur in a mole using the letters:

A	Asymmetry—the shape of one half does not match the other.
B	Border—the edges are ragged, notched, or blurred.
C	Color—is uneven. Shades of black, brown, or tan are present. Areas of white, red, or blue may be seen.
D	Diameter—there is a change in size.

See Figures 3–2 and 3–3.

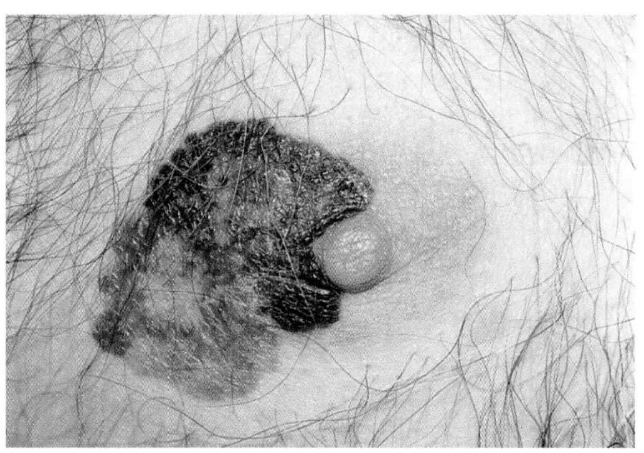

FIGURE 3–2
Melanoma.
(Courtesy of Jason L. Smith, MD.)

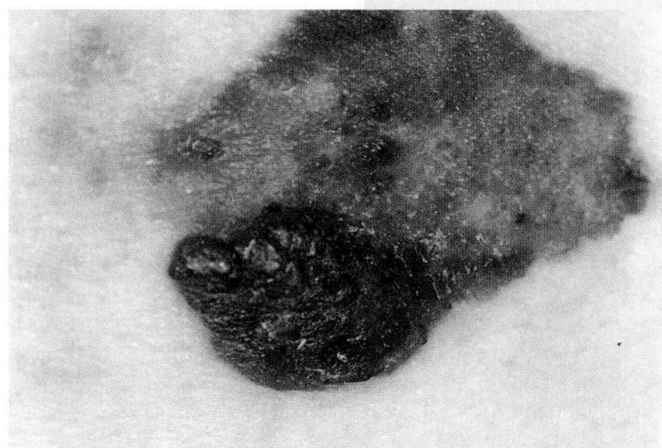

FIGURE 3–3
Melanoma, forearm.
(Courtesy of Jason L. Smith, MD.)

3.23 A __________ is a malignant black mole or tumor.
The word elements used to build **melan / oma** are:
__________ root that means black
__________ suffix that means tumor

melanoma
(mel ah **NOH** mah)
melan
-oma

3.24 **True or False.** Often the first sign of melanoma is change in size, shape, or color of a mole.

true

ANSWER COLUMN

EXPLANATION FRAME

Finger- and toenails are horny cell structures of the epidermis and are composed of hard keratin. A nail consists of a body, a root, and a matrix or nailbed. The crescent-shaped white area of the nail is the lunula. See Figure 3–4. Average nail growth is 1 mm per week. A lost fingernail usually regenerates in 3½ to 5½ months. A lost toenail may require 6 to 8 months for regeneration.

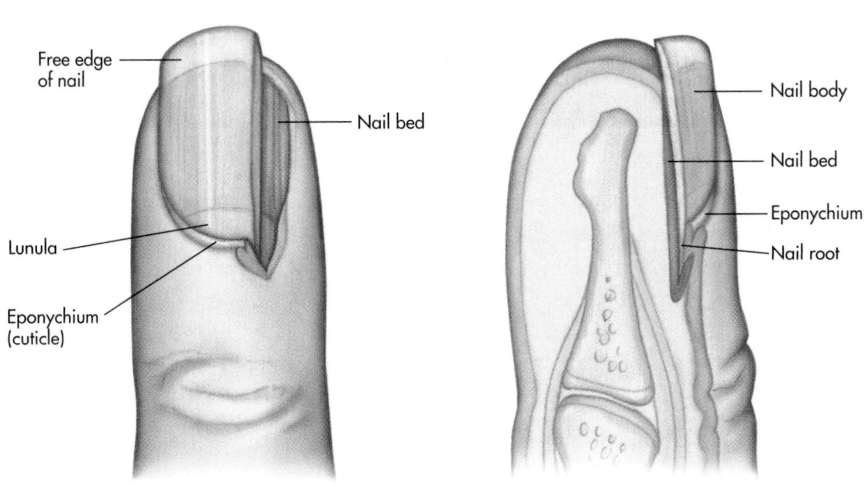

FIGURE 3–4
The fingernail, an appendage of the integument.

3.25 __________ is a tough protein substance in hair, nails, and horny tissue. — **keratin** (**KAIR** ah tin)

3.26 __________ is the horny embryonic tissue from which the nail develops. — **eponychium** (ep oh **NICK** ee um)

The word elements that are used to build this term are:

__________ prefix that means upon — **ep**

__________ combining form that means nail — **onych / i**

__________ suffix that means tissue — **-um**

Answer Column

continued

3.27 An infectious condition of the marginal structures around the nail is called ____________.

The word elements used to build **par / onych / ia** are:

____________ prefix that means around
____________ root that means nail
____________ suffix that means condition of

paronychia
(pair oh **NICK** ee ah)

par
onych
-ia

3.28 The medical term for nail biting is called ____________.
The word elements that are used to build **onych / o / phagia** are:

____________ combining form that means nail
____________ suffix that means to eat

onychophagia
(on ih koh **FAY** jee ah)
onych / o
-phagia

3.29 ____________ is a disease of the nails that is caused by a fungus. *A fungus is a plantlike organism that subsists on organic matter. Fungi are a division of plantlike organisms that includes molds and yeasts.* See Figure 3-5.

onychomycosis
(on ih koh my **KOH** sis)

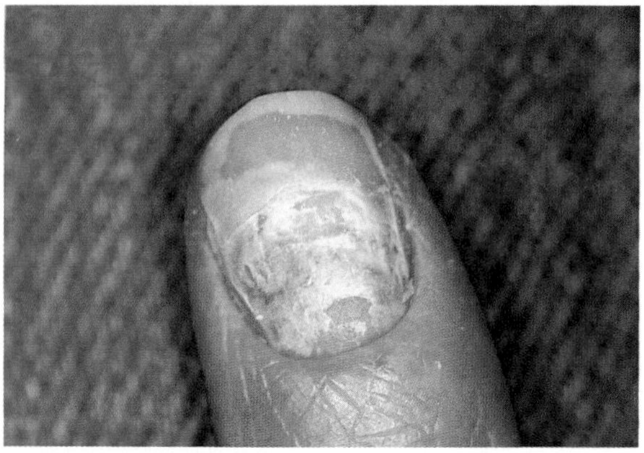

FIGURE 3–5
Onychomycosis.
(Courtesy of Jason L. Smith, MD.)

3.30 The word elements that are used to build **onych / o / myc / osis** are:

____________ combining form that means nail
____________ root that means fungus
____________ suffix that means condition of

onych / o
myc
-osis

Answer Column

3.31 The term __________ means pertaining to below the nail. The prefix __________ means below, the root **ungu** means nail, and the suffix __________ means pertaining to.

subungual (sub **UNG** gwall)
sub
-al

EXPLANATION FRAME

The skin contains millions of sweat glands and sebaceous glands. Sweat glands produce sweat or perspiration, which is largely water and, when left to accumulate, causes body odor. See Figure 3–1. Sebaceous glands secrete oil for lubrication. Sebum, the product of sebaceous glands, acts to protect the body from dehydration and possible absorption of harmful substances.

3.32 The word root __________ means sweat. Two examples of using **hidr** as a root are: __________ (the inflammation of the sweat glands) and __________ (a condition of excessive sweating). See Figure 3–6.
In the term **hidr / aden / itis** the word root **hidr** means __________. __________ is a root that means gland and **-itis** is a suffix that means __________. In the term **hyper / hidr / osis** the prefix __________ means excessive, the root **hidr** means sweat, and the suffix __________ means condition of.

hidr
hidradenitis
(high drad eh **NYE** tis)
hyperhidrosis
(high per high **DROH** sis)
sweat **aden**
inflammation **hyper**
-osis

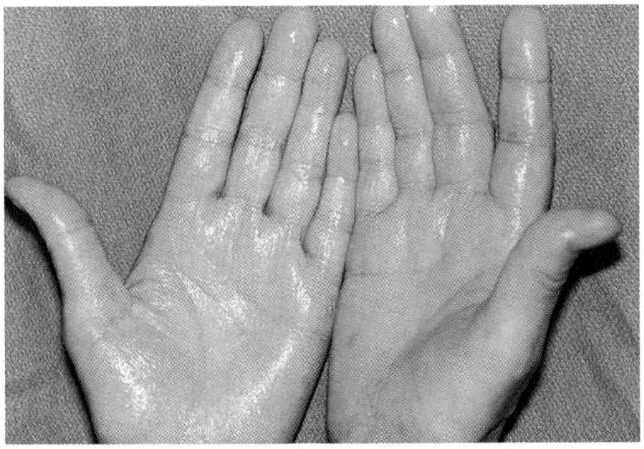

■ **FIGURE 3–6**
Hyperhidrosis.
(Courtesy of Jason L. Smith, MD.)

3.33 The suffix **-rrhea** means __________, __________. This suffix is found often in medicine and is one of several that begin with the letters **"rrh."** It means flow, discharge. When this suffix is linked to the combining form **seb / o**, which means oil, we get a word describing the excessive flow or discharge of oil from the sebaceous glands: __________.

flow, discharge

seborrhea
(seb or **EE** ah)

ANSWER COLUMN

continued

3.34 ____________ is an inflammatory condition of the sebaceous glands and the hair follicles of the skin. *It is characterized by comedos, papules, and pustules. Cysts and nodules may develop and scarring is common. It is usually associated with seborrhea.* See Figure 3-7.

acne (**ACK** nee)

EXPLANATION FRAME

Hair is an accessory organ of the skin. It is a thin, threadlike structure formed by a group of cells that develop within a hair follicle or socket. Hair is distributed over the whole body with the exception of the palms of the hands and the soles of the feet. Hair grows at a rate of approximately ½ inch a month.

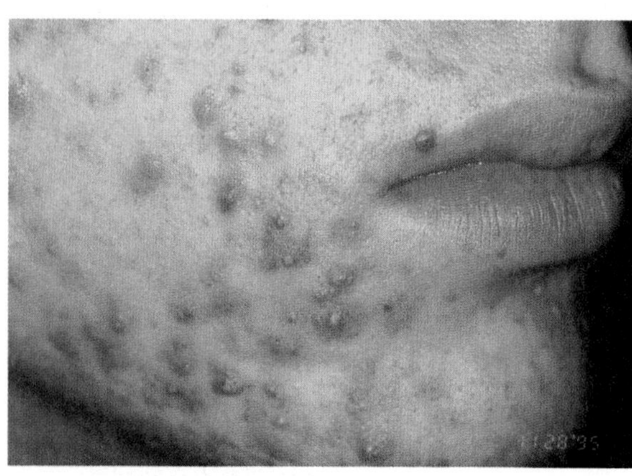

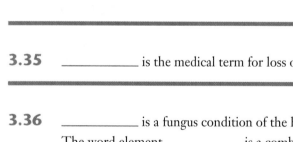

FIGURE 3–7
Acne.
(Courtesy of Jason L. Smith, MD.)

3.35 ____________ is the medical term for loss of hair.

alopecia (al oh **PEE** she ah)

3.36 ____________ is a fungus condition of the hair.
The word element ____________ is a combining form meaning hair. In the term **trich / o / myc / osis,** ____________ is a suffix that means condition of. The word root **myc** means ____________.

trichomycosis
(trik oh my **KOH** sis)
trich / o **-osis**
fungus

3.37 ____________ is a condition characterized by excessive growth of hair or the presence of hair in unusual places, especially in women.

hirsutism (**HER** soot izm)

ANSWER COLUMN

3.38 ____________ is another combining form that means hair.
Medical terms that are built using this word element are:
____________ means hairy, downy
____________ pertaining to the hair and sebaceous glands
____________ ____________ is a cyst (a closed sac or pouch) in the sacrococcygeal area where epithelial tissue and hair are trapped below the skin.

pil / o

pilose (PYE lohs)

pilosebaceous (pye loh see **BAY** shus)

pilonidal cyst (pye loh **NYE** dal **SIST**)

3.39 Skin signs are objective evidence of an illness or disorder. They can be seen, measured, or felt. See Figure 3–8.
Types of skin signs with examples are:
____________ is a discolored spot on the skin; example: *freckle.*
____________ is a solid, circumscribed, elevated area on the skin; example: *pimple.*
____________ is a small, fluid filled sac; example: *blister.* A *bulla* is a large vesicle.
____________ is a dry, serous or seropurulent, brown, yellow, red, or green exudation that is seen in secondary lesions; example: *eczema.*
____________ is a thin, dry flake of cornified epithelial cells; example: *psoriasis.*
____________ is a localized, evanescent elevation of the skin that is often accompanied by itching; example: *urticaria.*
____________ is a larger papule; example: *acne.*
____________ is a small, elevated, circumscribed lesion of the skin that is filled with pus; example: *varicella (chickenpox).*
____________ or ____________ is an eating or gnawing away of tissue; examples: *an open sore, decubitus ulcer.*
____________ is a cracklike sore or slit that extends through the epidermis into the dermis; example: *athlete's foot.*

macule (MACK yool)

papule (PAP yool)

vesicle (VESS ih kl)

crust (KRUST)

scale (SKAL)

wheal (WEEL)

nodule (NOD yool)

pustule (PUS tyool)

erosion, ulcer (ee **ROH** zhun, **ULL** ser)

fissure (FISH er)

3.40 ____________ is the former name for the genus of fungi now called *Candida*.

monilia (moh **NIL** ee ah)

3.41 ____________ is an infection of the skin or mucous membranes by yeastlike fungi. *It is usually localized in skin, nails, mouth, vagina, bronchi, or lungs and it is also known as* ***candidiasis.***

moniliasis (mon ih **LYE** ah sis)

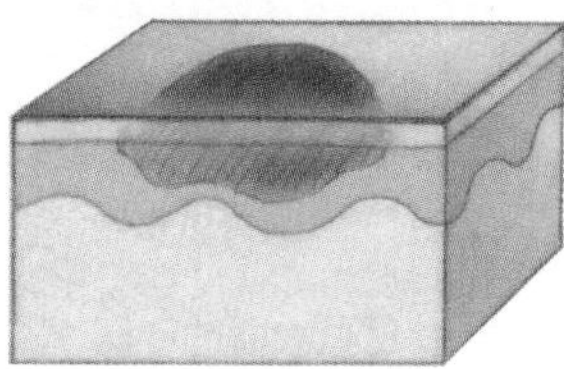

A macule is a discolored spot on the skin; freckle

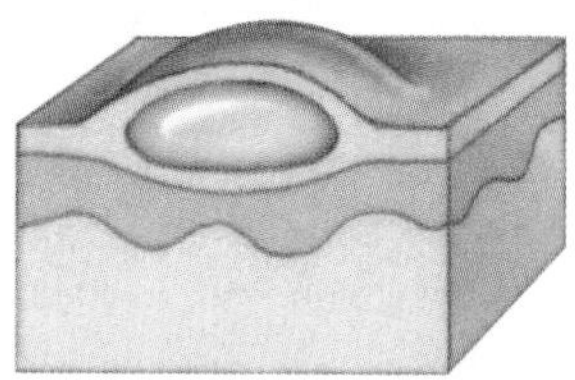

A wheal is a localized, evanescent elevation of the skin that is often accompanied by itching; urticaria

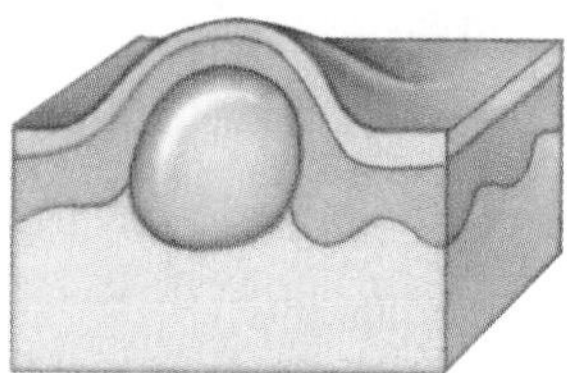

A papule is a solid, circumscribed, elevated area on the skin; pimple

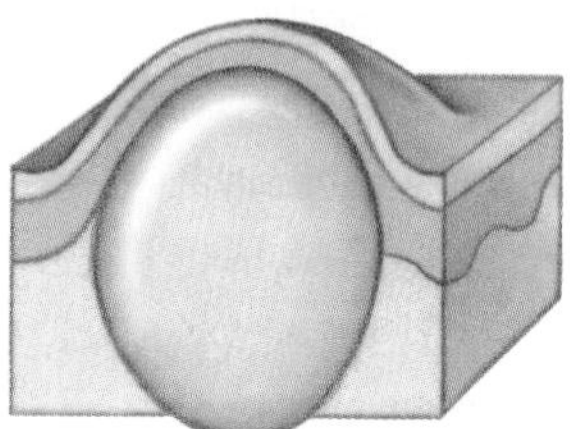

A nodule is a larger papule; acne vulgaris

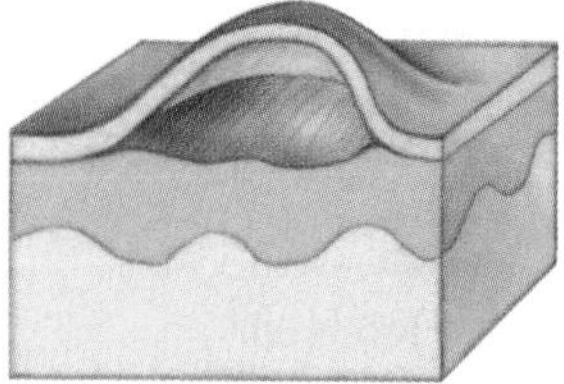

A vesicle is a small fluid filled sac; blister. A bulla is a large vesicle.

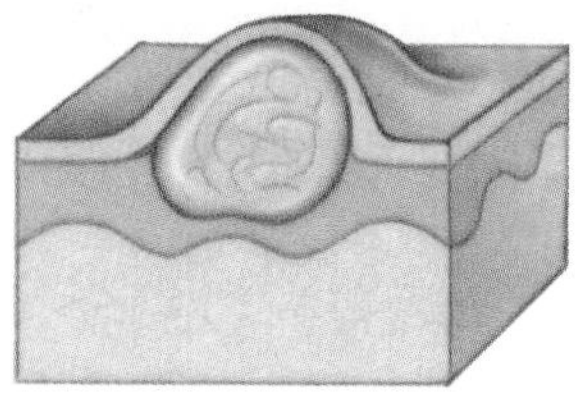

A pustule is a small, elevated, circumscribed lesion of the skin that is filled with pus; varicella (chickenpox)

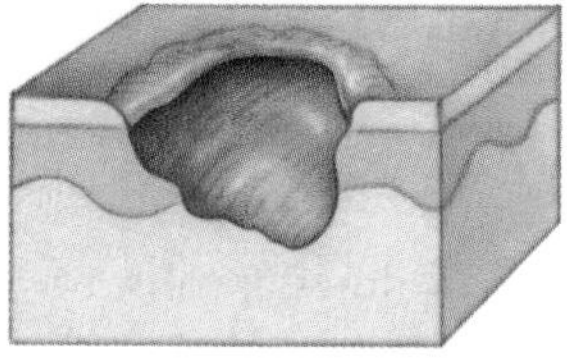

An erosion or ulcer is an eating or gnawing away of tissue; decubitus ulcer

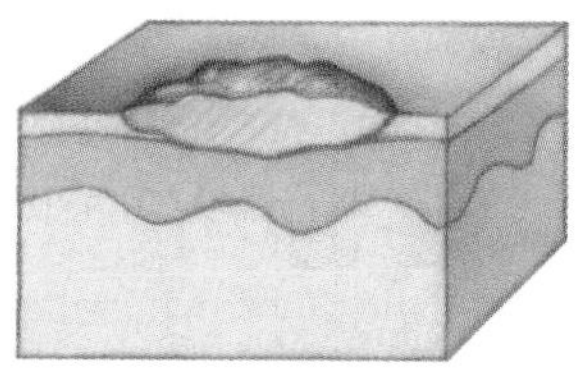

A crust is a dry, serous or seropurulent, brown, yellow, red, or green exudation that is seen in secondary lesions; eczema

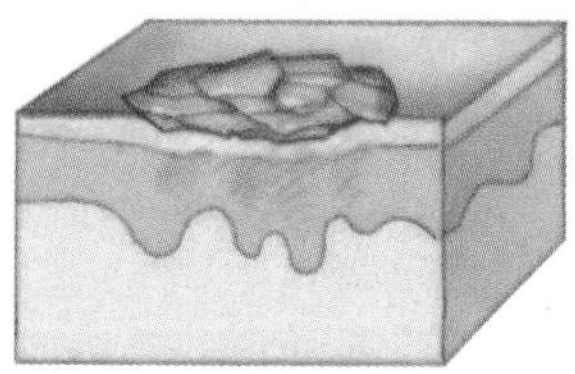

A scale is a thin, dry flake of cornified epithelial cells; psoriasis

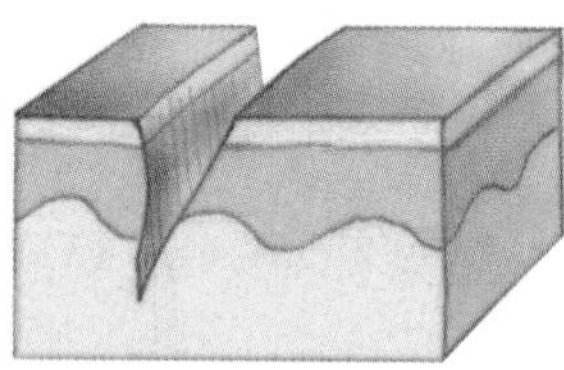

A fissure is a crack-like sore or slit that extends through the epidermis into the dermis; athlete's foot

FIGURE 3–8

Skin signs are objective evidence of an illness or disorder. They can be seen, measured, or felt.

ANSWER COLUMN

3.42 ____________ is a condition of infestation with lice. This infestation may involve different areas of the body:

the head: pediculosis capitis. See Figure 3–9.

the body: pediculosis corporis

the eyebrows and eyelashes: pediculosis palpebrarum

the pubis: pediculosis pubis

The word elements of the term **pedicul / osis** are:

____________ root that means a louse

____________ suffix that means condition of

pediculosis
(pee dik you **LOH** sis)

pedicul

-osis

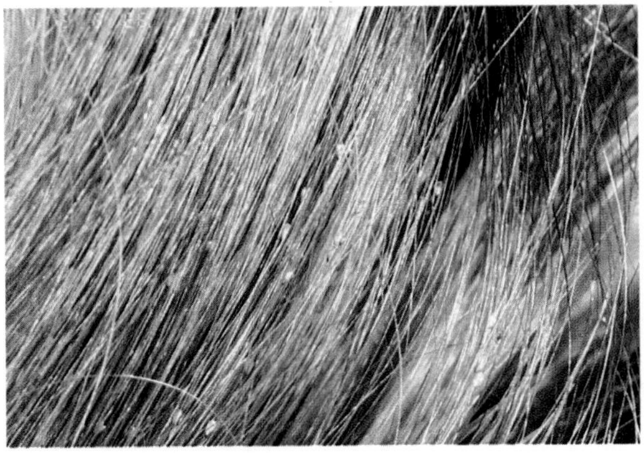

■ **FIGURE 3–9**
Pediculosis capitis.
(Courtesy of Jason L. Smith, MD.)

3.43 The medical term for a bedsore is known as ____________.
Decubitus literally means lying down; a bedsore.

decubitus
(dee **KYOO** bih tus)

3.44 ____________ is a medical term that literally means "an itching." *It is a chronic disease characterized by pink or dull-red lesions (erythematous papules), and as the disease progresses and if untreated, a silvery, yellow-white scale develops.* See Figure 3–10.

psoriasis
(soh **RYE** ah sis)

3.45 ____________ is the medical term for freckle. *Freckles are small brown macules or yellow-brown pigmented areas on the skin that may be caused by exposure to the sun and weather.*

lentigo
(len **TYE** goh)

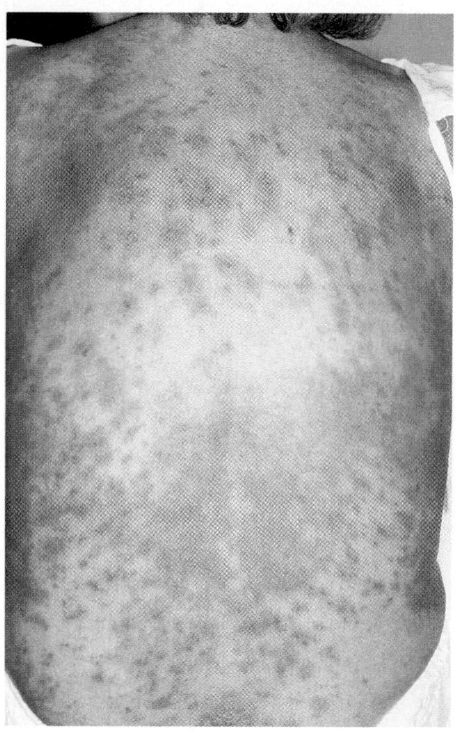

FIGURE 3–10
Psoriasis, back.
(Courtesy of Jason L. Smith, MD.)

ANSWER COLUMN

continued

3.46 __________ is an acute or chronic inflammatory skin disease, often referred to as dermatitis. *The symptoms may include erythema, papules, vesicles, pustules, scales, crusts, or scabs alone or in combination.*

eczema
(EK zeh ma)

3.47 __________ is an inflammatory skin disease marked by isolated pustules that become crusted and rupture. *The contagious form of impetigo is especially seen in children. It is generally caused by the staphylococci or streptococci bacteria.*

impetigo
(im peh **TYE** goh)

EXPLANATION FRAME

Varicella, or chickenpox, is a contagious viral disease characterized by fever, headache, and a crop of red spots that become macules, papules, vesicles, and crusts.

3.48 __________ is also known as chickenpox. See Figure 3–11.

varicella
(var ih **SELL** ah)

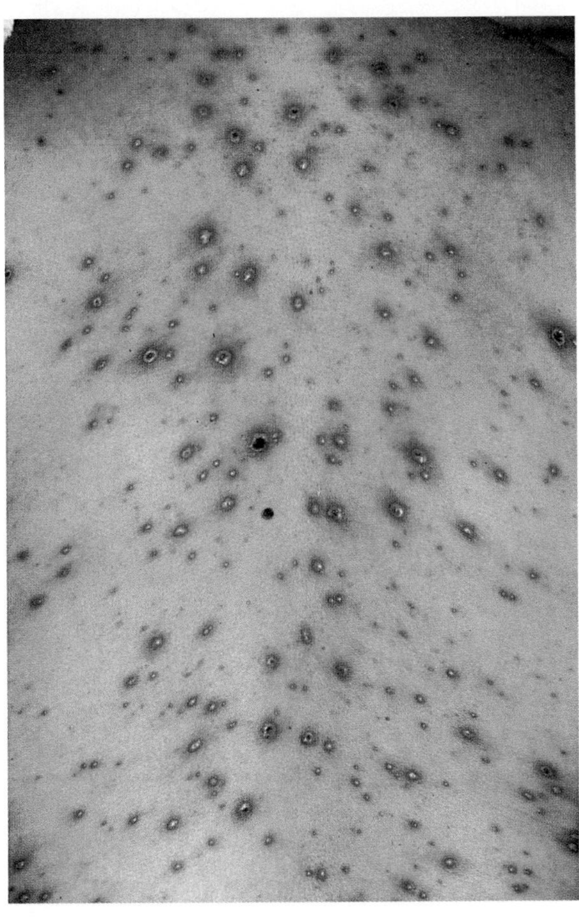

■ **FIGURE 3–11**
Varicella (chickenpox).
(Courtesy of Jason L. Smith, MD.)

ANSWER COLUMN

3.49 __________ __________ is an acute infectious disease caused by the varicella-zoster virus. *The virus that causes reactivation of herpes zoster is the same as that which causes chickenpox. Herpes zoster is commonly called "shingles."*

herpes zoster
(**HER** peez **ZOS** ter)

EXPLANATION FRAME

Cicatrix is a Latin term that means scar. Cicatricial tissue is less elastic than normal tissue; therefore, it usually presents a contracted appearance.

3.50 A physician may refer to a scar left after the healing of a wound as a __________.

cicatrix
(**SIK** ah triks)

3.51 Overgrowth of scar tissue due to excessive collagen formation is called a __________. See Figure 3–12.

keloid
(**KEE** loyd)

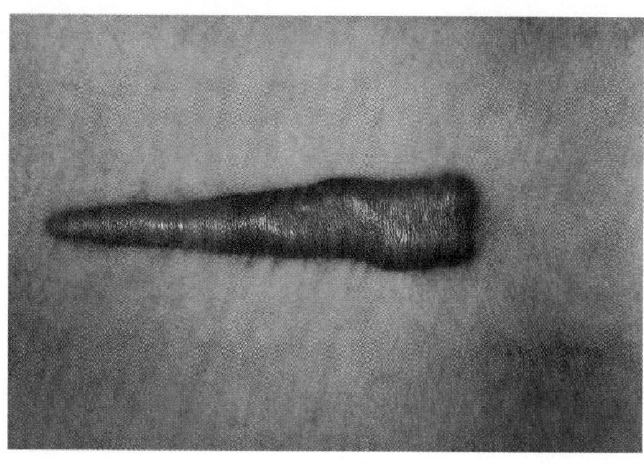

■ **FIGURE 3–12**
Keloid.
(Courtesy of Jason L. Smith, MD.)

ANSWER COLUMN

continued

3.52 The term **kel / oid** consists of two word elements.
__________ a root meaning tumor plus **-oid**, a suffix that means __________. *The combination of these meanings describes the overgrowth of scar tissue seen in certain individuals with a predisposition to form keloids after an injury.*

kel
resemble

EXPLANATION FRAME

A pachyderm is a thick-skinned mammal such as an elephant, hippopotamus, or rhinoceros. An unusual thickness of the skin in a person is called pachyderma. **Pachy** is a Greek word root that means thick.

3.53 The word root **pachy** means __________.

thick

3.54 The word root **icter** means __________.
The medical term that means pertaining to jaundice is called __________.
The word elements that are used to build this term are:
__________ root that means jaundice
__________ suffix that means pertaining to

jaundice (**JAWN** diss)
icteric (ick **TER** ik)
icter
-ic

3.55 A plastic surgeon may perform a __________ to remove wrinkles.
The word root __________ and the combining form **rhytid / o** mean wrinkle. The suffix __________ means surgical repair.
Plastic surgery for the removal of wrinkles is called rhytidoplasty, which is commonly called a "face lift."

rhytidoplasty
(**RIT** ih doh plas tee)
rhytid
-plasty

Answer Column

3.56 __________ is another medical term that may be used to indicate the removal of wrinkles. The suffix **-ectomy** means surgical excision.

rhytidectomy (rit eh **DECK** toh mee)

EXPLANATION FRAME

Petechiae are small, pinpoint, purplish hemorrhagic spots on the skin. They may appear in certain severe fevers, such as typhus, and may be caused by abnormalities in a person's blood-clotting mechanism.

3.57 Small, pinpoint, purplish hemorrhagic spots on the skin are called __________.

petechiae (pee **TEE** kee ee)

3.58 The medical name for severe itching is called __________.

pruritus (proo **RIGH** tus)

3.59 The separation or bursting open of a surgical wound is called __________. See Figure 3–13.

dehiscence (dee **HIS** sens)

3.60 A __________ is commonly called a blackhead.

comedo (**KOM** ee doh)

3.61 A __________ is a pigmented, elevated spot above the surface of the skin. It is commonly called a mole. See Figure 3–14.

nevus (**NEV** us)

FIGURE 3–13
Wound dehiscence, back.
(Courtesy of Jason L. Smith, MD.)

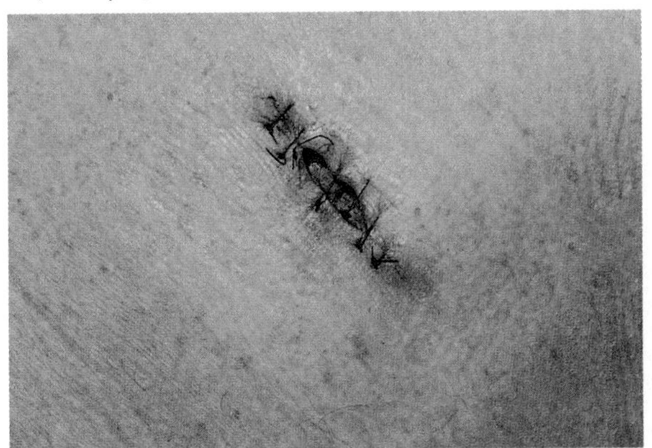

FIGURE 3–14
Nevus (mole).
(Courtesy of Jason L. Smith, MD.)

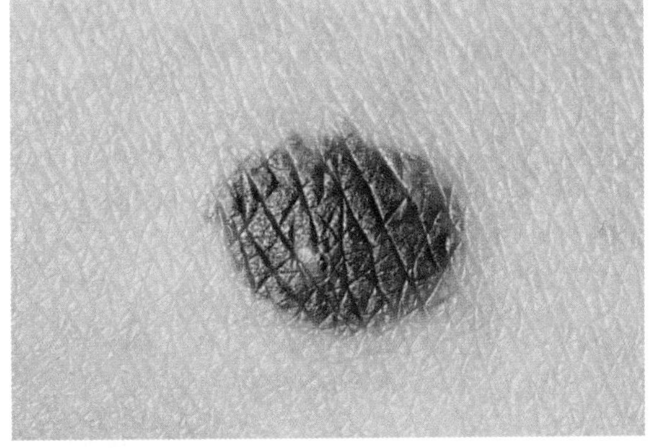

Answer Column

continued

3.62 A __________ is an acute, painful nodule formed in the subcutaneous layers of the skin, a gland, or a hair follicle. *It is most often caused by staphylococci and it is also referred to as a furuncle. A carbuncle is a cluster of boils.* See Figure 3–15.

boil
(BOYL)

3.63 __________ is the medical term for a wart. *A wart is a tumor of the epidermis and produces a circumscribed elevated area. It is caused by the papilloma virus.* See Figure 3–16.

verruca
(ver **ROO** kah)

3.64 An __________ is a scraping away of skin or mucous membrane. It is a result of injury or caused by mechanical means.

abrasion
(ah **BRAY** zhun)

3.65 __________ means without decay, *sterile,* free from all living microorganisms.

asepsis
(ay **SEP** sis)

3.66 __________ is the forcible tearing away of a body part or structure, such as a finger, toe, foot, or hand.

avulsion
(ah **VUL** shun)

3.67 A __________ is an injury in which the skin is not broken but becomes discolored due to escape of fluid into subcutaneous tissue. *SYN: contusion. Symptoms include pain, swelling, tenderness, and discoloration.*

bruise
(BROOZ)

FIGURE 3–15
Carbuncles.
(Courtesy of Jason L. Smith, MD.)

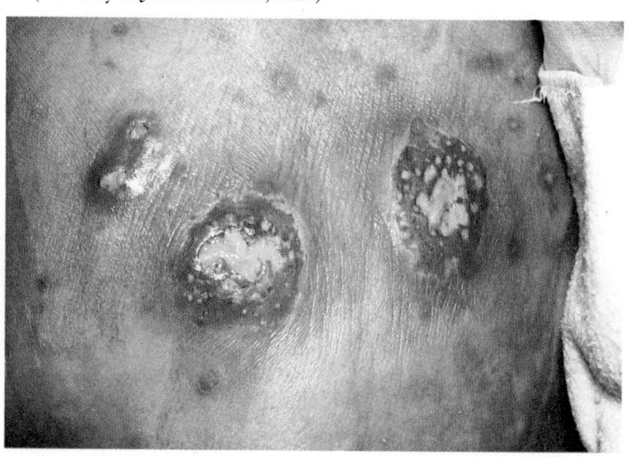

FIGURE 3–16
Verrucae (warts).
(Courtesy of Jason L. Smith, MD.)

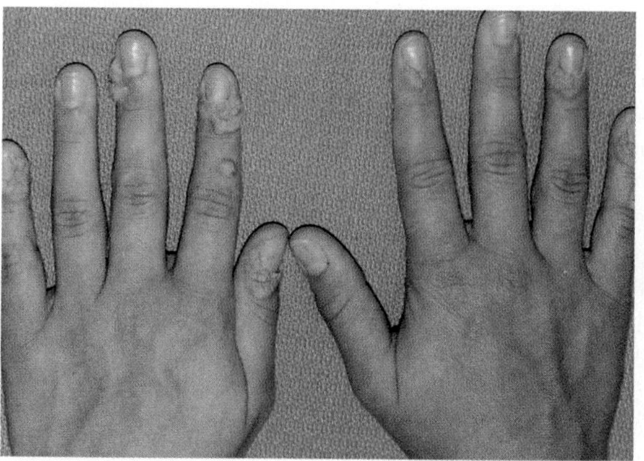

Answer Column

3.68 __________ is the removal of foreign material, dead or damaged tissue from a wound, especially from a severe burn.

debridement (day breed **MON**)

3.69 __________ is an irregular tearing of a surface, especially the skin.

laceration (lass er **AY** shun)

EXPLANATION FRAME

Herpes simplex is an inflammatory skin disease caused by a herpes virus (type I). It may be called a cold sore or fever blister.

3.70 **True or False.** Herpes simplex may be called a cold sore or fever blister.

true

3.71 __________ is the medical term for measles. *Rubeola is a contagious disease characterized by fever, inflammation of the mucous membranes, and rose-colored spots on the skin. It is commonly called measles.*

rubeola (roo bee **OH** lah)

3.72 __________ is the medical term that means eruption of itching and burning swellings of the skin; hives. See Figure 3–17.

urticaria (er tih **KAY** ree ah)

3.73 A __________ is an injury to tissue caused by heat, fire, chemical agents, electricity, lightning, or radiation. Burns are classified according to degree or depth of skin damage. See Figure 3–18.

burn (**BURN**)

FIGURE 3–17
Urticaria (hives).
(Courtesy of Jason L. Smith, MD.)

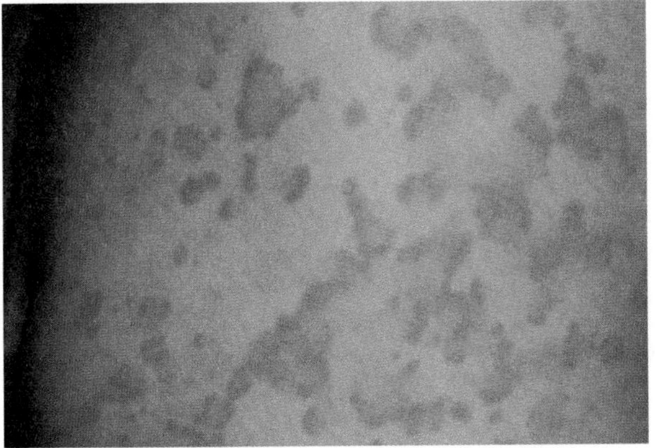

FIGURE 3–18
Burn, second degree.
(Courtesy of Jason L. Smith, MD.)

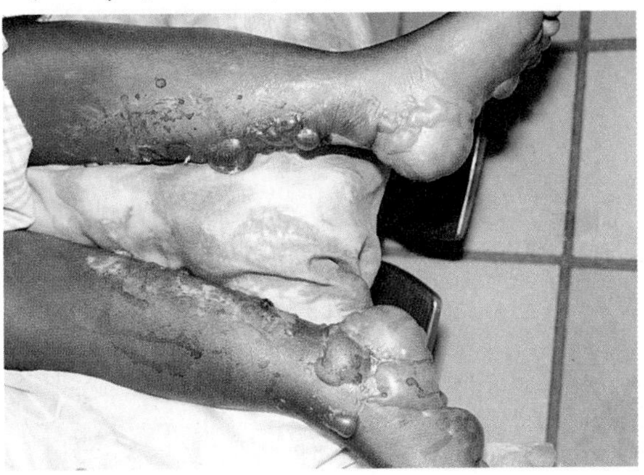

EXPLANATION FRAME

Drugs that are used for dermatologic diseases or disorders include emollients, keratolytics, local anesthetic, antipruritic, antibiotic, antifungal, antiviral, anti-inflammatory, and antiseptic agents. Other drugs include Retin-A and Rogaine.

3.74 Emollients are substances that are generally ____________ in nature. They are used for dry skin caused by aging, excessive bathing, and **psoriasis.**

oily

3.75 ____________ are agents that cause or promote loosening of horny (keratin) layers of the skin. These agents may be used for acne, warts, psoriasis, corns, calluses, and fungal infections.

keratolytics
(kair ah toh **LIT** iks)

3.76 ____________ agents prevent or relieve itching.
The word elements used to build this term are:
____________ prefix that means against
____________ root that means severe itching
____________ suffix that means pertaining to

antipruritic
(an tih proo **RIT** ik)
anti
prurit
-ic

3.77 ____________ agents are used to destroy or inhibit the growth of fungi and yeast. These agents are used to treat fungus and/or yeast infection of the skin, nails, and scalp.

antifungal
(an tih **FUNG** gal)

3.78 ____________ agents combat specific viral diseases.
____________ (acyclovir) is an antiviral medication that may be used in the treatment of herpes simplex types 1 and 2, varicella-zoster, Epstein-Barr, and cytomegalovirus.

antiviral (an tih **VYE** ral)
zovirax (**ZOH** vir aks)

3.79 ____________ agents are used to relieve the swelling, tenderness, redness, and pain of inflammation. Topically applied corticosteroids are used in the treatment of dermatitis and psoriasis.

anti-inflammatory
(an tee in **FLAM** mah toh ree)

ANSWER COLUMN

3.80 ____________ agents prevent or inhibit the growth of pathogens. Antiseptics are generally applied to the surface of living tissue.

antiseptic
(an tih **SEP** tik)

3.81 Retin-A (tretinoin) is used in the treatment of acne ____________.
Vulgaris means ordinary, common.

vulgaris
(vul **GAY** ris)

3.82 Rogaine (minoxidil) is available as a topical solution to stimulate hair growth. It was first approved as a treatment of male pattern baldness. Baldness is the lack of or partial loss of hair on the head. It is also known as ____________. See Figure 3–19.

alopecia
(al oh **PEE** she ah)

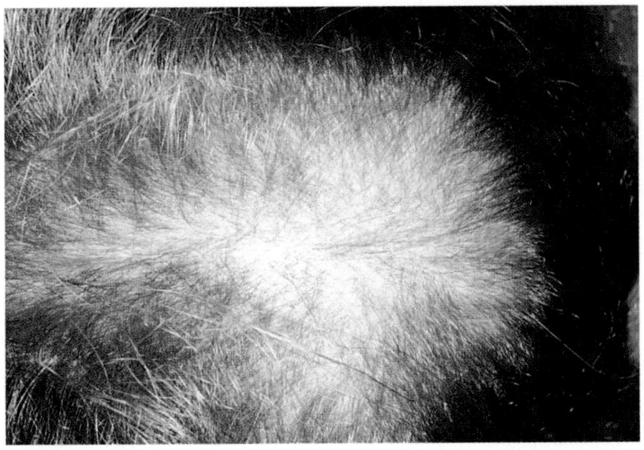

FIGURE 3–19
Male pattern alopecia.
(Courtesy of Jason L. Smith, MD.)

3.83 Abbreviations
Write in the correct abbreviation for the following:

____________	chief complaint	**CC**
____________	decubitus	**decub**
____________	dermatology	**derm**
____________	diagnosis	**Dx**
____________	hypodermic	**H**
____________	history	**Hx**
____________	past history	**PH**
____________	symptom	**Sx**
____________	treatment	**Tx**

IN THE SPOTLIGHT

SKIN CANCER

Skin cancer is a disease in which malignant cells are found in the epidermis. The epidermis contains three kinds of cells: flat, scaly cells on the surface called squamous cells; round cells called basal cells; and cells, called melanocytes, that give the skin its color.

The most common types of skin cancer are basal cell cancer and squamous cell cancer. Skin cancer is more common in persons with light-colored skin who have spent a lot of time in the sunlight. Skin cancer can occur anywhere on the body, but it is most common in places that have been exposed to more sunlight, such as the face, neck, hands, and arms.

The most common sign of skin cancer is a change on the skin, such as a growth or a sore that will not heal. Sometimes there may be a small lump. This lump can be smooth, shiny, and waxy looking, or it can be red or reddish brown. Skin cancer may also appear as a flat red spot that is rough or scaly. Not all changes in the skin are cancer, but it is very important to have a dermatologist evaluate any change that occurs in one's skin. It is recommended that one check his or her skin on a regular basis and have a skin examination every 3 years if between the ages of 20 and 40 and every year after age 40.

Cancer that develops in the pigment cells is called melanoma. It usually occurs in adults, but may occasionally be found in children and adolescents. Melanoma strikes more than 50,000 Americans annually and causes an estimated 7800 deaths.

Scientists have pinpointed a genetic marker that may serve as an early indicator for melanoma. Protein produced by the gene, known as Id1, was found in tissue samples of early-stage melanoma. If this research holds up, then a physician can biopsy a mole and if it is positive for Id1, it can be surgically removed. This is very important because the disease is curable if caught early, but is usually fatal if not.

Melanoma is a more serious type of cancer than basal cell or squamous cell cancers. Like most cancers, melanoma is best treated when it is found early. Melanoma can metastasize quickly to other parts of the body through the lymph system or through the blood.

The American Academy of Dermatology and the Skin Cancer Foundation recommend the following six steps to help reduce the risk of sunburn and developing skin cancer:

1. Minimize exposure to the sun at midday between the hours of 10:00 A.M. and 3:00 P.M.
2. Apply sunscreen with at least a SPF-15 or higher to all areas of the body that are exposed to the sun.
3. Reapply sunscreen every two hours, even on cloudy days. Reapply after swimming or perspiring.
4. Wear clothing that covers the body and shades the face. Hats should provide shade for both the face and the back of the neck.
5. Avoid exposure to UV radiation from sunlamps or tanning parlors.
6. Protect children: Keep them from excessive sun exposure when the sun is strongest (10:00 A.M.–3:00 P.M.). Apply sunscreen liberally and frequently to children 6 months of age and older. Do not use sunscreen on children under 6 months of age. Children under 6 months of age should have their exposure to the sun severely limited.

CASE STUDY

Please read the following case study and then work frames 3.84–3.91. Write in your answer in the answer column. Check your responses with the answers provided at the end of frame 3.91.

A 42-year-old female was seen by a dermatologist and the following is a synopsis of her visit.

PRESENT HISTORY: The patient states that she apparently came into contact with poison oak or poison ivy while she was working in her yard.

SIGNS AND SYMPTOMS: Chief Complaint: moderate itching at first and then severe (pruritus); small blisters (vesicles) on right side of the neck extending up and into the hairline; redness of skin (erythroderma) with moderate swelling (edema) of surrounding tissue.

DIAGNOSIS: Contact Dermatitis Poison Ivy.

TREATMENT: Antipruritic agent—Hydroxyzine HCl 25 mg Tab; corticosteroid therapy—Temovate 0.05% cream—apply twice a day to affected area; and Sterapred 12-day unipak—take as directed.

PREVENTION: Stay away from poison oak and/or poison ivy. When working outside in the yard, wear clothing that covers arms and legs. After working in the yard, immediately take a bath or shower to remove any possible contamination of skin with poison oak or poison ivy.

3.84 What is the medical term that means severe itching? ___________

3.85 What is the medical term that means a papule with a fluid core; blister? ___________

3.86 A person who is sensitive to poison oak or poison ivy may develop ___________.

3.87 An antipruritic agent is used to help relieve ___________.

3.88 Temovate 0.05% cream is a form of ___________ therapy.

3.89 Prevention is a key concept in today's health care delivery system. List three preventive measures that the patient with contact dermatitis may use to help and/or prevent her condition.

1. ___________
2. ___________
3. ___________

3.90 The medical term for redness of the skin is ___________.

3.91 The medical term for swelling is ___________.

CASE STUDY ANSWERS

3.84 pruritus

3.85 vesicle

3.86 contact dermatitis

3.87 itching

3.88 corticosteroid

3.89
1. Stay away from poison oak and/or poison ivy.
2. When working outside, wear clothing that covers arms and legs.
3. After working in the yard, immediately take a bath or shower to remove any possible contamination of skin with poison oak or poison ivy.

3.90 erythroderma

3.91 edema

REVIEW A: WORD ELEMENTS

This review allows you to check your knowledge of some of the word elements presented in this unit. In the spaces provided, write the meaning of the word elements that are identified as **Prefix (P), Word Root (R), Combining Form (CF), and/or Suffix (S).**

MEDICAL WORD	*WORD ELEMENT*	*MEANING*
1. integumentary	integument (R)	____________
	-ary (S)	____________
2. epidermis	epi (P)	____________
	-dermis (S)	____________
3. dermatitis	dermat (R)	____________
	-itis (S)	____________
4. dermatologist	dermat / o (CF)	____________
	log (R)	____________
	-ist (S)	____________
5. dermatology	dermat / o (CF)	____________
	-logy (S)	____________
6. dermatome	derm / a (CF)	____________
	-tome (S)	____________
7. erythroderma	erythr / o (CF)	____________
	-derma (S)	____________
8. cutaneous	cutane (R)	____________
	-ous (S)	____________
9. melanocarcinoma	melan / o (CF)	____________
	carcin (R)	____________
	-oma (S)	____________
10. melanoma	melan (R)	____________
	-oma (S)	____________
11. onychophagia	onych / o (CF)	____________
	-phagia (S)	____________
12. eponychium	ep (P)	____________
	onychi (CF)	____________
	-um (S)	____________

REVIEW B: MEDICAL TERMS

Please place the correct letter from column II on the appropriate line of column I.

COLUMN I		COLUMN II
___________	1. melanin	A. infestation with lice
___________	2. varicella	B. bedsore
___________	3. cicatrix	C. ringworm
___________	4. decubitus	D. jaundice
___________	5. alopecia	E. gives color to the skin
___________	6. pediculosis	F. small, pinpoint, purplish hemorrhagic spots
___________	7. urticaria	G. chickenpox
___________	8. tinea	H. scar
___________	9. icteric	I. loss of hair
___________	10. petechiae	J. hives

REVIEW C: SKIN SIGNS

Please provide the correct type of skin sign for each of the following descriptions.

1. ___________ is a discolored spot on the skin; *freckle.*
2. ___________ is a solid, circumscribed, elevated area on the skin; *pimple.*
3. ___________ is a small, fluid filled sac; *blister.*
4. ___________ is a dry, serous or seropurulent, brown, yellow, red, or green exudation that is seen in secondary lesions; *eczema.*
5. ___________ is a thin, dry flake of cornified epithelial cells; *psoriasis.*

REVIEW D: UNSCRAMBLE THE WORDS

Unscramble the following medical terms and place the correct term on the line directly across from the scrambled word.

1. echtaepei ___________
2. rtuspuri ___________
3. sihedcence ___________
4. domeco ___________
5. usven ___________
6. loib ___________
7. ealwh ___________
8. eolabur ___________

REVIEW E: DRUGS USED FOR THE INTEGUMENTARY SYSTEM

Please provide the correct answer for each of the following descriptions.

1. ____________ are agents that cause or promote loosening of horny (keratin) layers of the skin.
2. ____________ are substances that are generally oily in nature.
3. ____________ agents prevent or relieve itching.
4. ____________ is an antiviral medication that may be used in the treatment of herpes simplex types 1 and 2.

REVIEW F: ABBREVIATIONS

Please provide the correct abbreviation and/or meaning for the abbreviation.

1. ____________ chief complaint
2. Dx ____________
3. ____________ treatment
4. Hx ____________
5. ____________ symptom
6. ____________ past history

4 THE SKELETAL SYSTEM: ORTHOPEDICS

LEARNING CONCEPTS

- the skeletal system
- essential terminology
- pronunciation guide
- word elements
- explanation frames
- features of long bones
- classification of joints
- types of body movements
- abnormal curvatures of the spine
- types of fractures
- the curvatures of the spine
- differences in the male and female pelvis
- selected diseases and disorders
- drugs used for the skeletal system
- abbreviations
- in the spotlight: aging - changes in the bones, joints, and muscles
- case study: osteoporosis
- review exercises

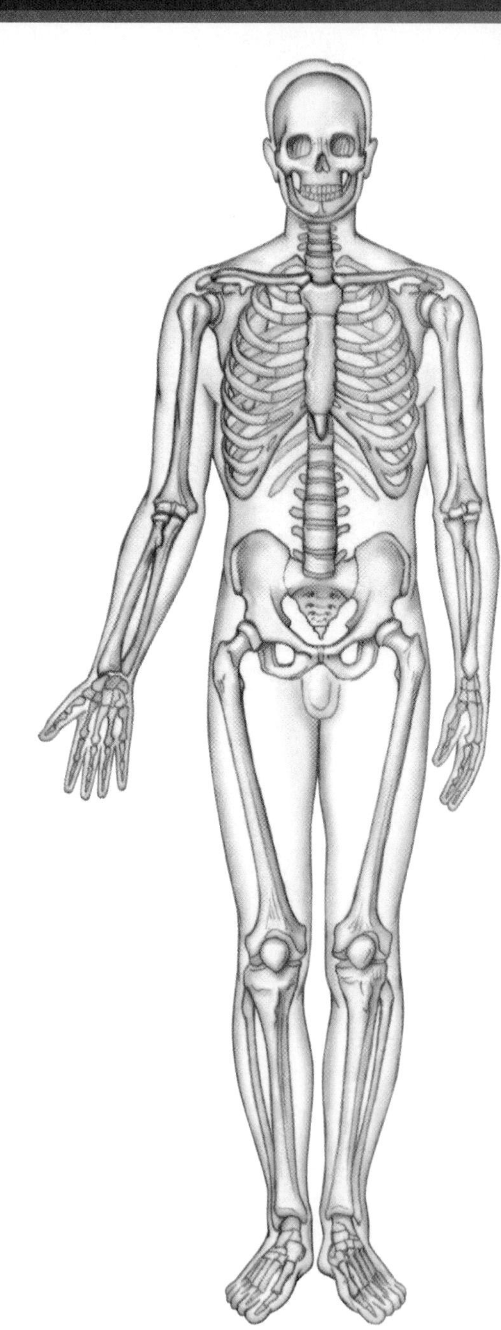

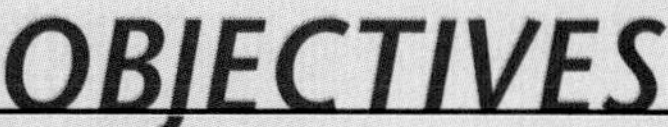

OBJECTIVES

ON COMPLETION OF THIS UNIT, YOU SHOULD BE ABLE TO:

- Briefly describe the skeletal system.
- Describe the primary functions of the various organs or structures of the skeletal system.
- Identify and give the meaning of the primary word elements for this unit.
- Analyze, build, spell, and pronounce selected medical words.
- Describe the parts of bones.
- Give and define the commonly used terms that describe the markings of bones.
- Describe the types of body movements that occur at the diarthrotic joints.
- Identify abnormal curvatures of the spine.
- Define selected types of fractures.
- Describe the four spinal curves.
- Describe the female pelvis and the male pelvis.
- Describe selected diseases/disorders of the skeletal system.
- Describe selected drugs that are used for skeletal system diseases or disorders.
- Define selected abbreviations that pertain to the skeletal system.
- Describe some aging changes that occur in the bones, joints, and muscles.
- Complete the Case Study on Osteoporosis.
- Successfully complete the review section.

TECH LINK

CD-ROM Use the CD-ROM enclosed with your textbook to gain additional reinforcement through interactive word building exercises, spelling games, labeling activities, and additional quizzes.

www.prenhall.com/rice Use the above address to access the free, interactive Companion Website created specifically for this textbook. Get hints, instant feedback, and textbook references to chapter-related multiple choice and true/false questions, fill-in-the-blank, and labeling exercises. In addition, you will find an audio glossary, and essay questions.

Bones begin to develop during the second month of fetal life as cartilage cells enlarge, break down, disappear, and are replaced by bone-forming cells called osteoblasts. Most bones of the body are formed by this process known as endochondral ossification. In this process, the bone cells deposit organic substances in the spaces vacated by cartilage to form bone matrix. As this process proceeds, blood vessels form within the bone and deposit salts such as calcium and phosphorus that serve to harden the developing bone.

The epiphyseal plate is the center for longitudinal bone growth in children. See Figure 4–1. It is possible to determine the biological age of a child from the development of epiphyseal ossification centers as shown radiographically. About 3 years from the onset of puberty the ends of the long bones (epiphyses) knit securely to their shafts (diaphysis), and further growth can no longer take place.

The skeletal system is composed of 206 bones that, together with cartilage and ligaments, make up the framework or skeleton of the body. See

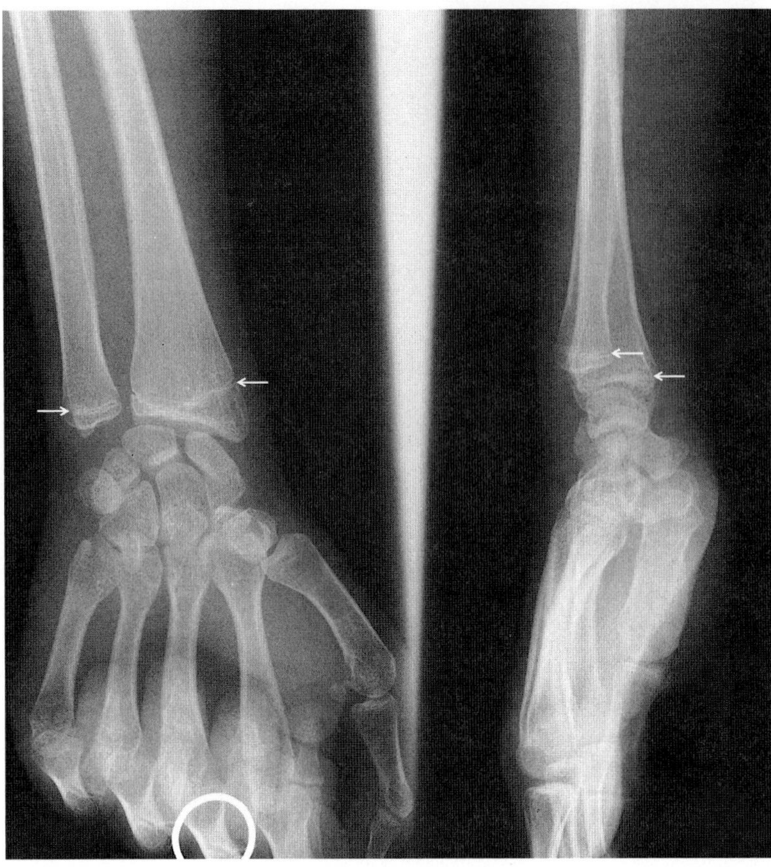

■ **FIGURE 4–1**
Epiphyseal plate (arrows).
(Courtesy of Teresa Resch.)

Table 4–1. The skeleton can be divided into two main groups of bones: the axial skeleton consisting of 80 bones and the appendicular skeleton with the remaining 126 bones. See Figure 4–2. The principal bones of the axial skeleton are the skull, spine, ribs, and sternum. The shoulder girdle, arms, and hands and the pelvic girdle, legs, and feet are the primary bones of the appendicular skeleton. See Figure 4–3.

TABLE 4–1 THE SKELETAL SYSTEM

Organ/Structure	Primary Functions
Bones	Provide shape, support, protection, and the framework of the body Serve as a storage place for mineral salts, calcium, and phosphorus Play an important role in the formation of blood cells Provide areas for the attachment of skeletal muscles Help make movement possible
Cartilages	Form the major portion of the embryonic skeleton and part of the skeleton in adults
Ligaments	Connect the articular ends of bones, binding them together and facilitating or limiting motion Connect cartilage and other structures Serve to support or attach fascia or muscles

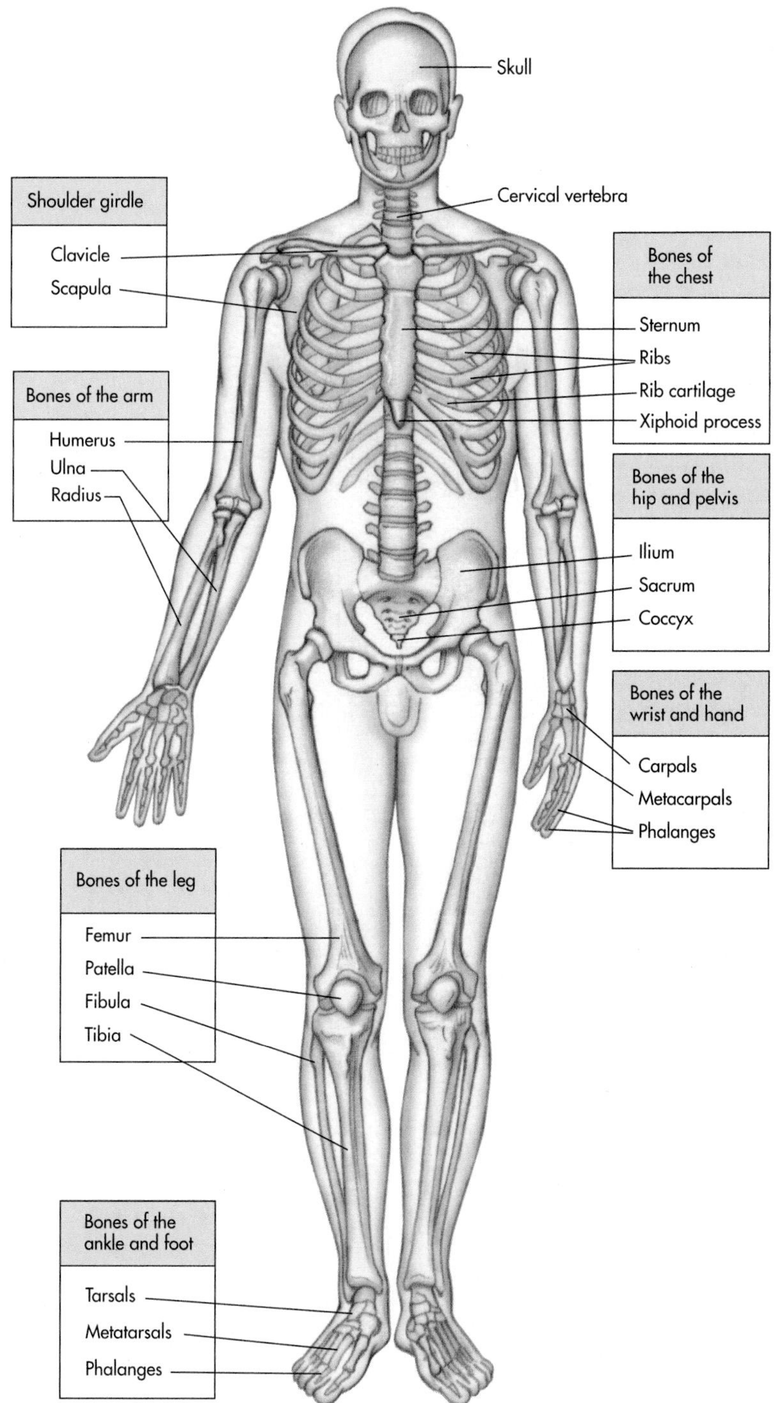

FIGURE 4–2
The skeleton can be divided into two main groups of bones: the axial and the appendicular skeleton.

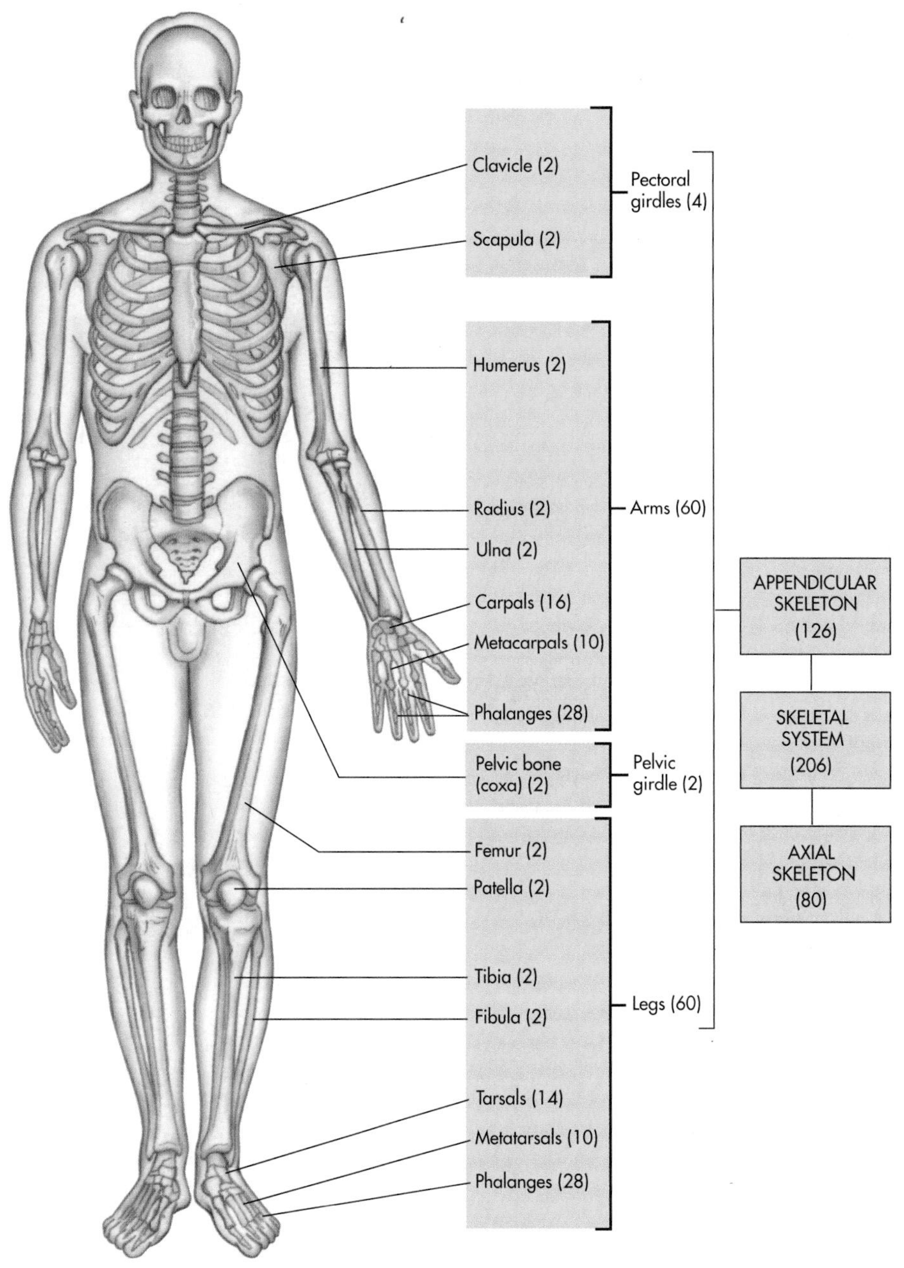

FIGURE 4–3

The principal bones of the appendicular skeleton.

The bones are the primary organs of the skeletal system and are composed of about 50% water and 50% solid matter. Bones provide shape and support, protection for internal organs, and areas for the attachment of skeletal muscles. They also serve as a storage place for mineral salts, calcium, and phosphorus. They play an important role in the formation of blood cells and help make movement possible.

The largest bone of the human body is the femur, which is located in the thigh, and the smallest bones are the ossicles (malleus, incus, and stapes), which are located in the middle ear.

PRIMARY WORD ELEMENTS

The following word elements (prefixes, roots, combining forms, and suffixes) will be used to build medical terms that relate to this unit. Please commit these to memory.

PREFIX

PREFIX	MEANING	PREFIX	MEANING
ab	away from	**peri**	around
endo	within	**poly**	many, much
epi	upon, above	**sym, syn**	together, with
meta	beyond		

COMBINING FORM

COMBINING FORM / ROOT	MEANING	COMBINING FORM / ROOT	MEANING
acr	extremity, point	**kyph**	hump
acr / o	extremity, point	**lord**	bending
arthr	joint	**myel**	bone marrow
arthr / o	joint	**orth / o**	straight
burs	a pouch	**oste / o**	bone
chondr	cartilage	**path**	disease
chondr / o	cartilage	**ped**	foot, child
cran / i, crani / o	skull	**ped / i**	foot, child
dors / i	backward	**por**	passage
duct	to lead	**scol / i**	curvature
flex	to bend		

SUFFIX

SUFFIX	MEANING	SUFFIX	MEANING
-al, -ic	pertaining to	**-itis**	inflammation
-algia	pain	**-logy**	study of
-blast	immature cell, germ cell	**-malacia**	softening
-cele	hernia, tumor, swelling	**-omion**	shoulder
-centesis	surgical puncture	**-osis**	condition of
-cytes	cells	**-pathy**	disease
-desis	surgical binding	**-plasty**	surgical repair
-ectomy	surgical excision	**-tomy**	incision
-ist	one who specializes		

ANSWER COLUMN

4.1 __________ is the medical/surgical specialty that deals with prevention and/or correction of disorders that involve locomotor structures of the body, especially the skeleton, joints, muscles, fascia, ligaments, tendons, and cartilage.

orthopedics
(or thoh **PEE** diks)

ANSWER COLUMN

continued

4.2 The word elements used to build **orth / o / ped / ics** are:

		Answer
____________	combining form that means straight	**orth / o**
____________	root that means child; foot	**ped**
____________	suffix that means pertaining to	**-ic(s)**

The Greek origin of the word was originally used to describe the straightening of a child's limb.

4.3 An ____________ is a physician who specializes in orthopedics. — **orthopedist** (or thoh **PEE** dist)

The word elements used to build this term are:

		Answer
____________	combining form that means straight	**orth / o**
____________	root that means child; foot	**ped**
____________	suffix that means one who specializes	**-ist**

4.4 A bone-forming cell is called an ____________. — **osteoblast** (**OSS** tee oh blast)

Oste / o is a combining form that means bone and **-blast** is a suffix that means immature cell or germ cell.

EXPLANATION FRAME

The combining form **oste / o** begins many of the medical terms in this unit. **Oste / o** plus **-blast** = bone-forming cell. **Osteo** plus **-genesis** = bone formation. **Oste / o** plus **-dynia** = bone pain.

4.5 The combining form **oste / o** means bone. Some medical terms that begin with this word element are:

		Answer
____________	inflammation of the bone and joint	**osteoarthritis** (oss tee oh ar **THRY** tis)
____________	cancerous tumor of a bone	**osteocarcinoma** (oss tee oh kar sih **NOH** mah)
____________	inflammation of the bone marrow	**osteomyelitis** (oss tee oh my ell **EYE** tis)
____________	softening of the bone(s)	**osteomalacia** (oss tee oh mah **LAY** she ah)
____________	instrument used for cutting bone	**osteotome** (**OSS** tee oh tohm)
____________	inflammation of the bone and cartilage	**osteochondritis** (oss tee oh kon **DRY** tis)
____________	a malignant tumor of the bone arising from connective tissue	**osteosarcoma** (oss tee oh sar **KOH** mah)

ANSWER COLUMN

4.6 **True or False**. The skeleton can be divided into two main groups of bones: the axial skeleton (80 bones) and the appendicular skeleton (126 bones).

true

EXPLANATION FRAME

The principal bones of the axial skeleton are the skull, spine, ribs, and sternum. The appendicular skeleton consists of the bones of the upper extremities: the shoulder girdle (clavicle—collar bone; scapula—shoulder blade), arms (humerus, radius, ulna), and hands (carpals, metacarpals, phalanges); and the lower extremities: the pelvic girdle (ilium, sacrum, coccyx), legs (femur, patella, fibula, tibia), and feet (tarsals, metatarsals, phalanges). See Figure 4–3.

4.7 The principal bones of the ____________ skeleton are the skull, spine, ribs, and sternum.

axial (AK see al)

4.8 The ____________ skeleton consists of the shoulder girdle, arms, and hands, and the pelvic girdle, legs, and feet.

appendicular (app en **DIK** yoo lar)

EXPLANATION FRAME

Long bones, such as the tibia, femur, humerus, and radius, have most of the parts found in bones. These parts are:

Epiphyses. The ends of a developing bone.
Diaphysis. The shaft of a long bone.
Periosteum. The membrane that forms the covering of bones except at their articular surfaces.
Compact bone. The dense, hard layer of bone tissue.
Medullary canal. A narrow space or cavity throughout the length of the diaphysis.
Endosteum. A tough, connective tissue membrane lining the medullary canal and containing the bone marrow.
Cancellous. Also called spongy bone, this is the reticular tissue making up most of the volume of bone.

See Figure 4–4.

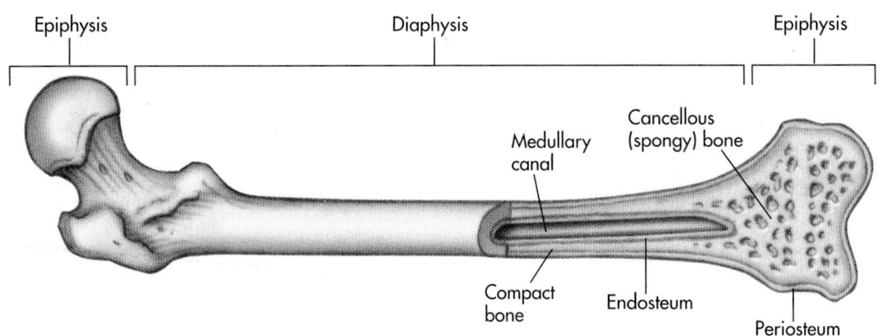

FIGURE 4–4
The parts of a long bone.

	ANSWER COLUMN
continued	
4.9 The __________ is the shaft of a long bone.	**diaphysis** (dye **AFF** ih sis)
4.10 The __________ are the ends of a developing bone.	**epiphyses** (eh **PIFF** ih seez)
4.11 The __________ is the membrane that forms the covering of bones.	**periosteum** (pair ee **AH** stee um)

EXPLANATION FRAME

There are certain commonly used terms that describe the markings of bones. These terms are described in frames 4.12–4.20.

4.12 An air cavity within certain bones is called a __________. *Sinuses develop embryologically from nasal cavities, are lined with the same type of epithelium, are filled with air, and communicate with nasal cavities through their various ostia (little openings). Air sinuses that occupy the body of the sphenoid bone and connect with the nasal cavity are called sphenoidal sinuses.*	**sinus** (**SIGH** nuss)
4.13 A __________ is an opening in the bone for blood vessels, ligaments, and nerves.	**foramen** (for **AY** men)
4.14 A __________ is a tubelike passage or canal.	**meatus** (mee **AY** tus)
4.15 A __________ is a very large process of the femur. A process is a projection or outgrowth of bone or tissue.	**trochanter** (troh **KAN** ter)

Answer Column

4.16 A __________ is a small, rounded process.

tubercle (TOO ber kl)

4.17 A __________ is a large, rounded process.

tuberosity (too ber **OSS** ih tee)

4.18 A __________ is a rounded process that enters into the formation of a joint, articulation.

condyle (KON dile)

4.19 A __________ is a ridge on a bone.

crest (KREST)

4.20 A __________ is a pointed, sharp, slender process.

spine (SPYN)

EXPLANATION FRAME

Cartilage is a specialized type of fibrous connective tissue present in adults, which forms the major portion of the embryonic skeleton.

4.21 Cartilage cells are known as __________

chondrocytes (**KON** droh sights)

4.22 The word elements of the word **chondr / o / cytes** are:

__________ combining form that means cartilage

__________ suffix that means cells

chondr / o
-cytes

4.23 In the medical term **endo / chondr / al**

the prefix **endo** means __________

the word root **chondr** means __________

and the suffix **-al** means __________ __________

within
cartilage
pertaining to

Answer Column

continued

4.24 The word root **chondr** and the combining form **chondr / o** mean cartilage. Now, build some medical terms that use these word elements plus the following suffixes: **-al, -algia, -ectomy,** and **-malacia.**

__________ pertaining to cartilage

__________ pain in or around cartilage

__________ surgical excision of a cartilage

__________ softening of cartilage

chondral (**KON** dral)
chondralgia (kon **DRAL** jee ah)
chondrectomy (kon **DREK** toh mee)
chondromalacia (kon droh mah **LAY** she ah)

4.25 __________ is the study of diseases of cartilage.

chondropathology (kon droh pah **THALL** oh jee)

EXPLANATION FRAME

The word root **arthr** means joint. The suffix **-itis** means inflammation. Both are frequently used word elements that should be remembered. Moreover, by linking the word root **arthr** with the vowel **"o"** we create the combining form **arthr / o**, which also means joint and begins many of the terms in this unit.

4.26 Inflammation of a joint is called __________.

arthritis (ar **THRY** tis)

4.27 __________ is a medical term that means joint disease.
The word elements used to build this term are:
__________ combining form that means joint
__________ suffix that means disease

arthropathy (ar **THROP** ah thee)
arthr / o
-pathy

4.28 The word root **arthr** and the combining form **arthr / o** mean joint. Now, build some medical terms that use these word elements plus the following suffixes: **-algia, -ectomy, -centesis, -desis, -plasty,** and **-scope.**

__________ pain in a joint

__________ surgical excision of a joint

__________ surgical puncture of a joint

arthralgia (ar **THRAL** jee ah)
arthrectomy (ar **THREK** toh mee)
arthrocentesis (ar throh sen **TEE** sis)

continued

ANSWER COLUMN

_________ surgical binding of a joint — **arthrodesis** (ar throh **DEE** sis)

_________ surgical repair of a joint — **arthroplasty** (**AR** throh plas tee)

_________ an instrument used to examine the interior of the knee — **arthroscope** (**AR** throh skope)

EXPLANATION FRAME

A joint is an articulation, a place where two or more bones connect. The manner in which bones connect determines the type of movement allowed at the joint. Joints are classified as:

Synarthrosis. Does not permit movement.
Amphiarthrosis. Permits very slight movement.
Diarthrosis. Allows free movement in a variety of directions. Examples of diarthrotic joints are the knee, hip, elbow, wrist, and foot.

Types of Body Movements

Frames 4.29 to 4.43 describe the types of body movements that occur at the diarthrotic joints. See Figure 4–5.

4.29 _________ is the process of bending a limb. — **flexion** (**FLEK** shun)

4.30 _________ is the process of moving a body part away from the middle. — **abduction** (ab **DUCK** shun)

4.31 The word elements of the term **ab / duct / ion** are:

_________ prefix that means away from — **ab**
_________ root that means to lead — **duct**
_________ suffix that means process — **-ion**

4.32 _________ is the process of bending a body part backward. — **dorsiflexion** (dor see **FLEK** shun)

4.33 The word elements of the word **dors / i / flex** / ion are:

_________ combining form that means backward — **dors / i**
_________ root that means to bend — **flex**
_________ suffix that means process — **-ion**

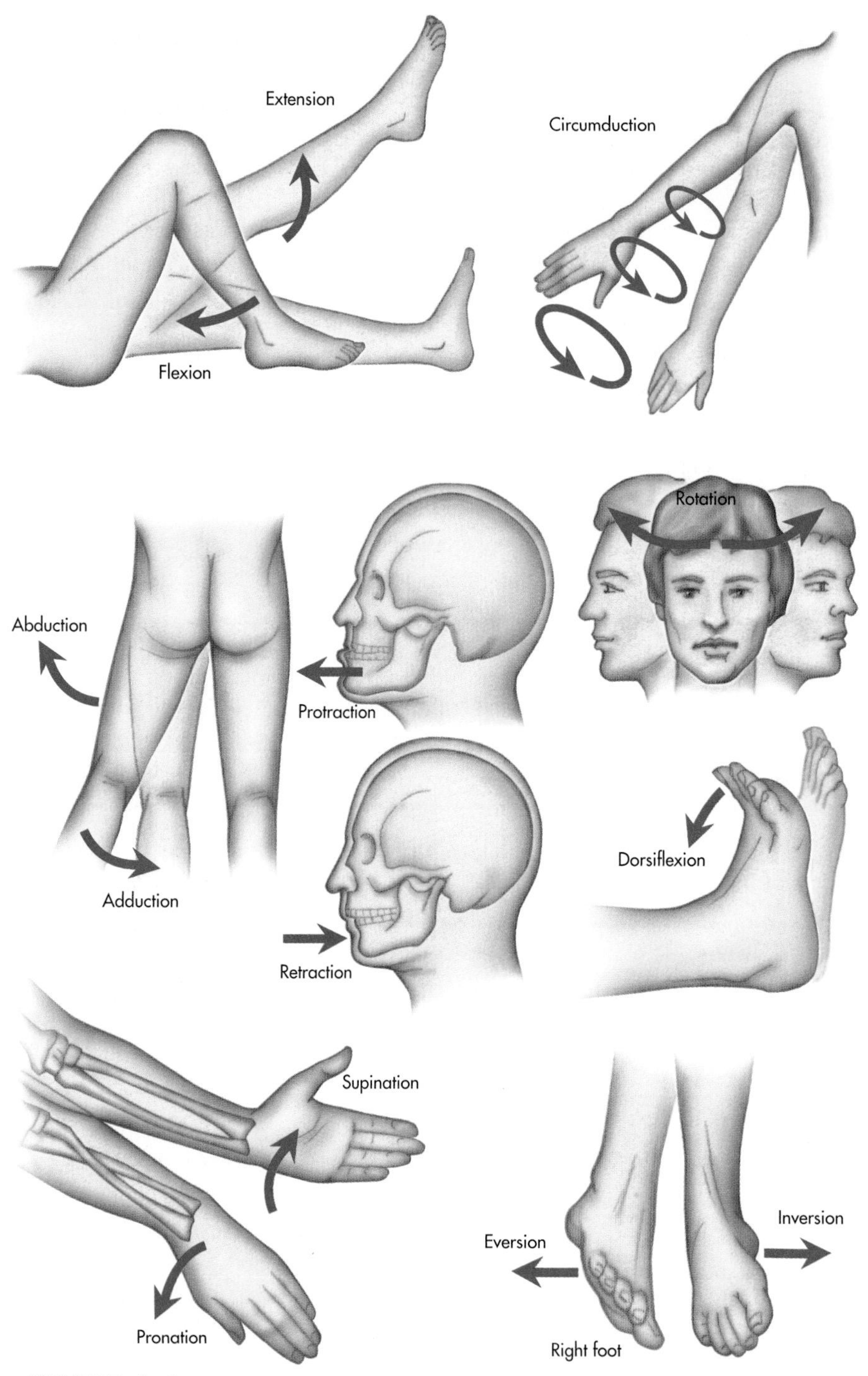

■ **FIGURE 4–5**
Types of body movements.

Answer Column

4.34 __________ is the process of moving a body part toward the middle.

adduction (ad **DUCK** shun)

4.35 __________ is the process of moving a body part in a circular motion.

circumduction (sir kum **DUCK** shun)

4.36 __________ is the process of turning outward.

eversion (ee **VER** zhun)

4.37 __________ is the process of turning inward.

inversion (in **VER** zhun)

4.38 __________ is the process of straightening a flexed limb.

extension (eks **TEN** shun)

4.39 __________ is the process of lying prone or face downward; also the process of turning the palm face downward.

pronation (proh **NAY** shun)

4.40 __________ is the process of lying s*up*ine or face *up*ward; also the process of turning the palm face *up*ward.

supination (soo pin **NAY** shun)

4.41 __________ is the process of moving a body part forward.

protraction (proh **TRAK** shun)

4.42 __________ is the process of moving a body part backward.

retraction (ree **TRAK** shun)

4.43 __________ is the process of moving a body part around a central axis.

rotation (ro **TAY** shun)

EXPLANATION FRAME

A bursa is a small space between muscles, tendons, and bones that is lined with synovial membrane and contains a fluid, synovia.

4.44 __________ is inflammation of a bursa.

Burs is a word root that means a pouch and **-itis** is a suffix that means inflammation.

bursitis (ber **SIGH** tis)

ANSWER COLUMN

EXPLANATION FRAME

In **lordosis**, there is an abnormal anterior curvature of the spine. This condition may be referred to as "swayback" as the abdomen and buttocks protrude due to an exaggerated lumbar curvature. **Scoliosis** is perhaps a better-known condition. It is characterized by an abnormal lateral curvature of the spine and usually appears in adolescence during periods of rapid growth. A third type of abnormal curvature is kyphosis. In **kyphosis**, the normal thoracic curvature becomes exaggerated, producing a "humpback" appearance. This condition may be caused by a congenital defect, a disease process, or osteoporosis. See Figure 4–6.

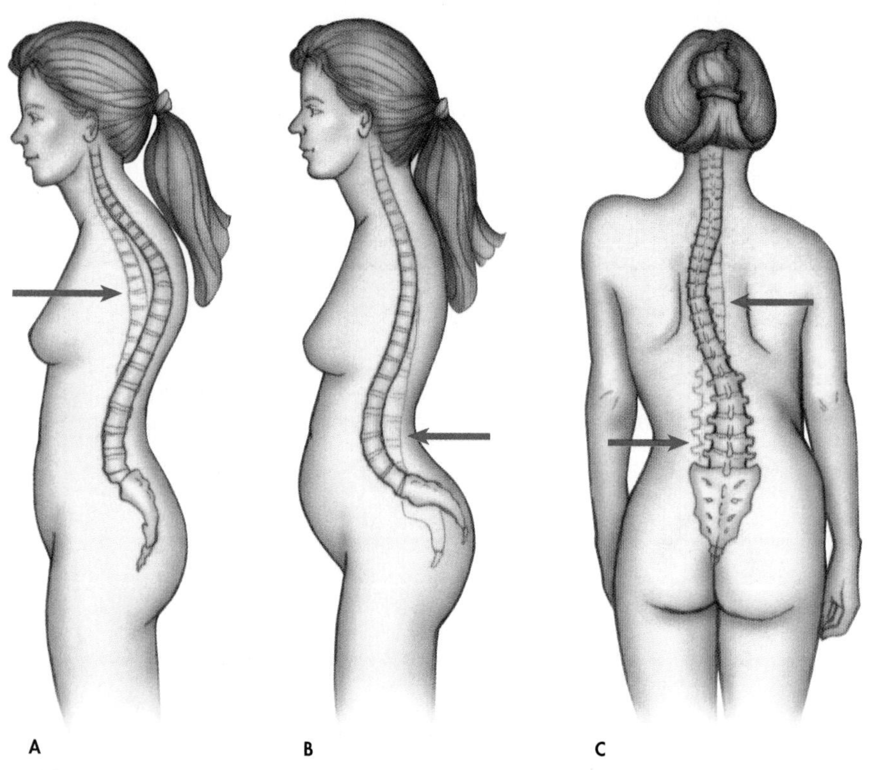

FIGURE 4–6
Abnormal curvatures of the spine: (A) kyphosis, (B) lordosis, (C) scoliosis.

4.45 Abnormal anterior curvature of the spine is called ___________. The word elements used to build this term are:

___________ root that means bending
___________ suffix that means condition

lordosis (lor **DOH** sis)

lord
-osis

ANSWER COLUMN

4.46 ___________ is characterized by an abnormal lateral curvature of the spine and usually appears in adolescence during periods of rapid growth.

The word elements used to build this term are:

___________ root that means curvature

___________ suffix that means condition

scoliosis (skoh lee **OH** sis)

scoli

-osis

4.47 In ___________ the normal thoracic curvature becomes exaggerated, producing a "humpback" appearance. This condition may be caused by a congenital defect, a disease process, or osteoporosis.

The word elements used to build this term are:

___________ root that means hump

___________ suffix that means condition of

kyphosis (kye **FOH** sis)

kyph

-osis

EXPLANATION FRAME

Fractures are classified according to their external appearance, the site of the fracture, and the nature of the crack or break in the bone. Fractures may be described as closed, or simple, and open, or compound. These generally denote external appearance. See Figure 4–7.

4.48 A ___________ fracture is one that occurs at the lower end of the fibula and medial malleolus of the tibia with dislocation of foot outward and backward. *A malleolus is the protuberance on both sides of the ankle joint, the lower extremity of the fibula being known as the lateral malleolus and the lower end of the tibia as the medial malleolus.*

Pott's (POTS)

4.49 ___________, or simple, fractures are completely internal; they do not involve a break in the skin.

closed (KLOZD)

4.50 Open, or ___________ fractures, project through the skin; they are most dangerous because of the possibility of infection or uncontrolled bleeding.

compound (KOM pownd)

4.51 ___________ fractures shatter the affected area into a multitude of bony fragments.

comminuted
(kom ih **NYOOT** ed)

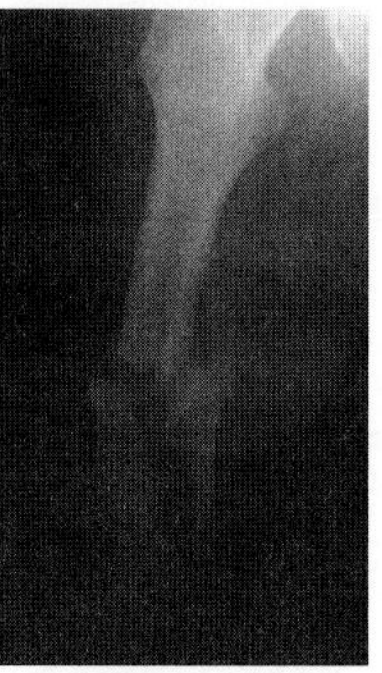

Femur, AP view, comminuted fracture

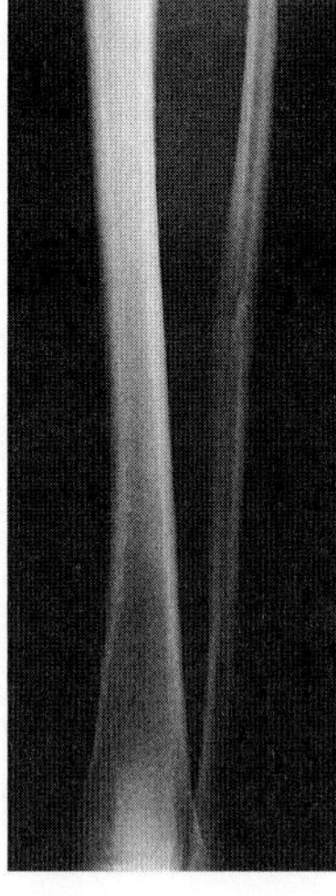

Tibia, simple, transverse fracture

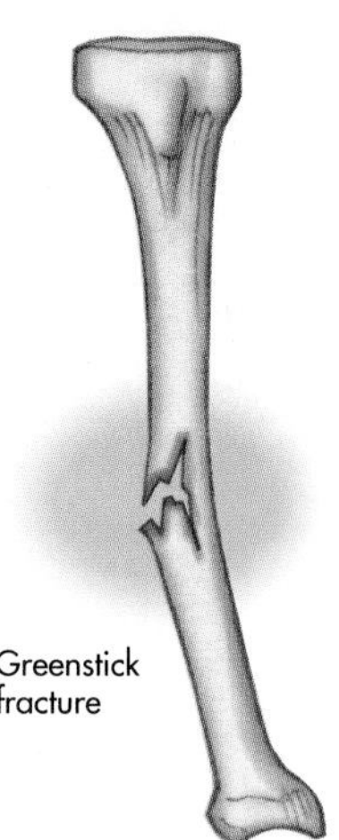

Greenstick fracture

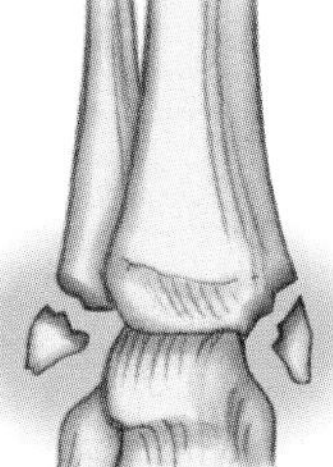

Pott's fracture–dislocation

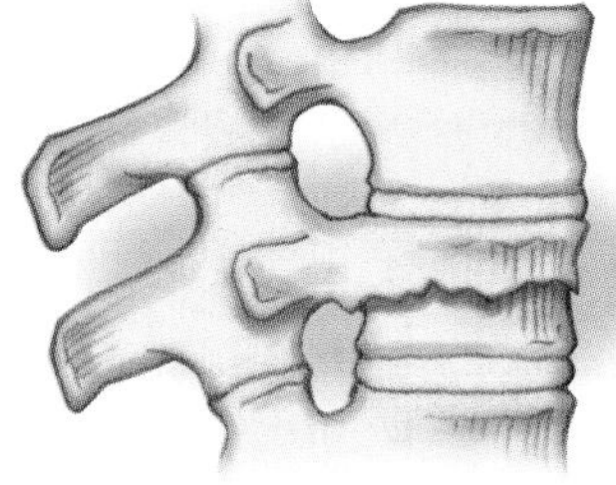

Compression fracture

Epiphyseal plate fracture

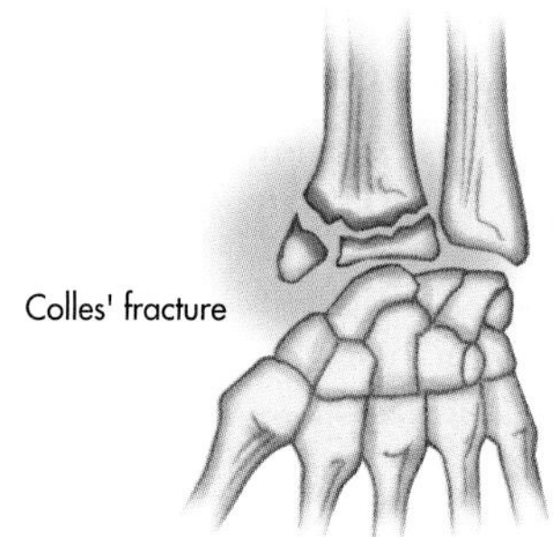

Colles' fracture

FIGURE 4–7
Various types of fractures.

ANSWER COLUMN

continued

4.52 In a ____________ fracture, only one side of the shaft is broken, and the other is bent; this usually occurs in children whose long bones have yet to fully ossify.

greenstick (GREEN stik)

4.53 A ____________ fracture is a break in the distal portion of the radius; it is often the result of reaching out to cushion a fall.

Colles' (KOL eez)

ANSWER COLUMN

EXPLANATION FRAME

The word root **acr** and the combining form **acr / o** mean extremity, point. **Acroarthritis** is inflammation of the joints of the hands or feet (extremity), and **acromion** is the projection of the spine of the scapula that forms the point of the shoulder and articulates with the clavicle.

4.54 The word root **acr** means ____________, ____________.

extremity, point

4.55 ____________ is a medical term that means inflammation of the joints of the hands or feet.

The word elements used to build this term are:

____________ combining form that means extremity

____________ root that means joint

____________ suffix that means inflammation

acroarthritis (ak roh ar **THRY** tis)

acr / o

arthr

-itis

4.56 ____________ is the projection of the spine of the scapula that forms the point at the shoulder and articulates with the clavicle.

The word elements used to build **acr / omion** are:

____________ root that means extremity, point

____________ suffix that means shoulder

acromion (ah **KROH** mee on)

acr

-omion

4.57 The ____________ are classified as irregular bones. The vertebral column is composed of a series of separate bones (vertebrae) connected in such a way as to form four spinal curves. These curves have been identified as the cervical, thoracic, lumbar, and sacral. See Figure 4–8.

The ____________ curve is the first seven vertebrae.

The ____________ curve is the next twelve vertebrae.

The ____________ curve is the next five vertebrae.

The ____________ curve consists of the sacrum and coccyx.

vertebrae (**VER** teh bray)

cervical (**SER** vih kal)

thoracic (tho **RASS** ik)

lumbar (**LUM** bar)

sacral (**SAY** kral)

4.58 Surgical repair of the skull is called ____________.

The word elements used to build this term are:

____________ combining form that means skull

____________ suffix that means surgical repair

cranioplasty (**KRAY** nee oh plas tee)

crani / o

-plasty

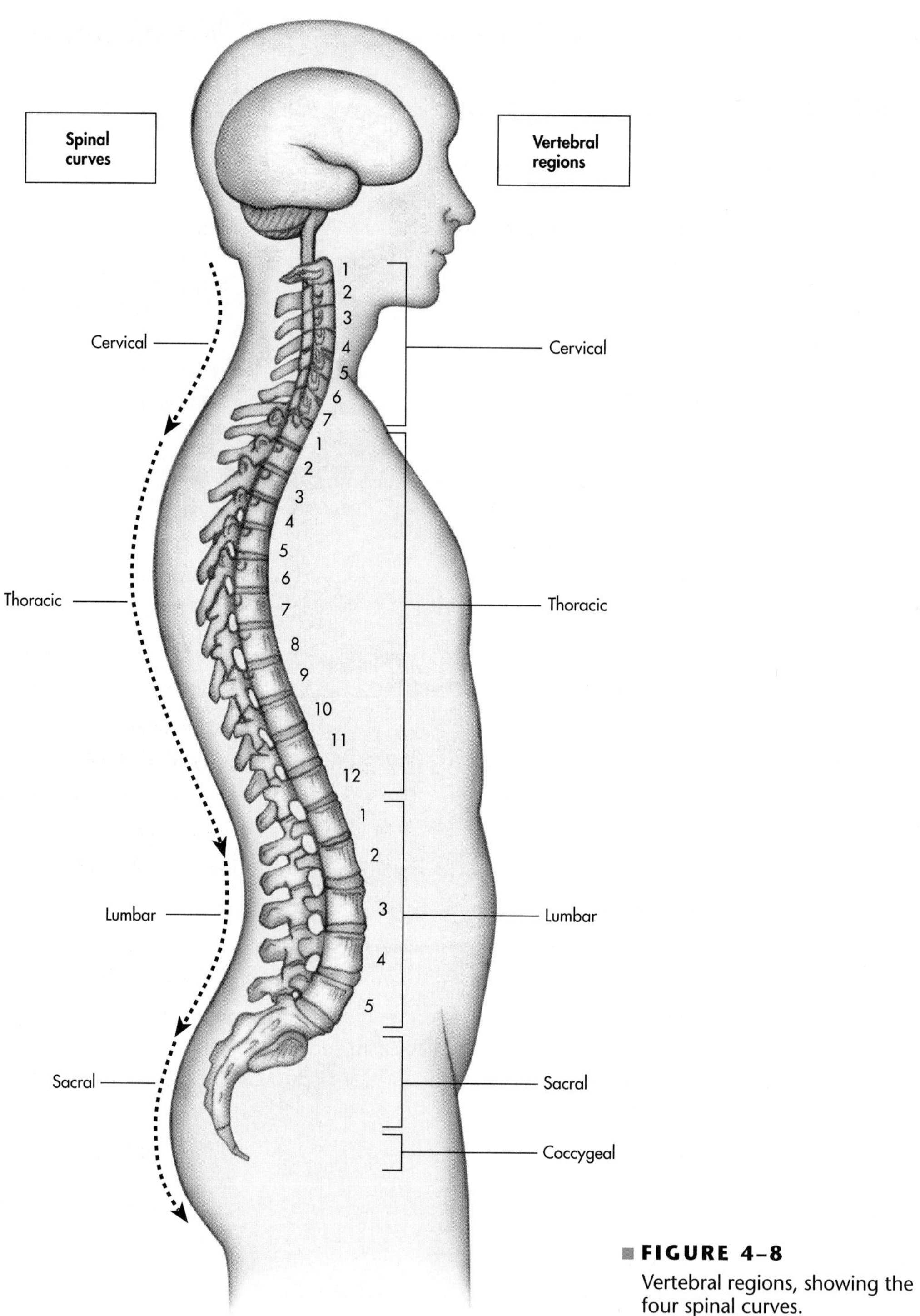

■ **FIGURE 4–8**
Vertebral regions, showing the four spinal curves.

Answer Column

4.59 The combining forms **crani / o** and **cran / i** mean skull. Now, build some medical terms that use these word elements plus the following suffixes: **-cele, -ectomy, -logy,** and **-tomy.**

____________ protrusion (herniation) of the brain from the skull — **craniocele** (**KRAY** nee oh seel)

____________ surgical excision of a portion of the skull — **craniectomy** (kray nee **EK** toh mee)

____________ the study of the skull — **craniology** (kray nee **ALL** oh jee)

____________ incision into the skull — **craniotomy** (kray nee **OTT** oh mee)

4.60 The medical term for the big toe is ____________. — **hallux** (**HAL** uks)

4.61 The medical term for pertaining to the heel bone is ____________. — **calcaneal** (kal **KAY** nee al)

4.62 The medical term for a fingerprint is ____________. — **dactylogram** (dak **TIL** oh gram)

4.63 The medical term for knock-knee is ____________ ____________. — **genu valgum** (**JEE** noo **VAL** gum)

4.64 ____________ is also known as **pes planus.** In this condition there is an abnormal flatness of the sole and arch of the foot. — **flatfoot** (**FLAT** foot)

4.65 The medical term for pertaining to a rib is ____________. — **costal** (**KOSS** tal)

EXPLANATION FRAME

The carpals are the bones of the wrist. The metacarpals are the bones of the hand. The tarsals are the bones of the ankle. The metatarsals are the bones of the foot, and the phalanges are the bones of the toes and/or fingers.

4.66 The bones of the ankle are called ____________. — **tarsals** (**TAHR** sals)

ANSWER COLUMN

EXPLANATION FRAME

The female pelvis is shaped like a basin. It may be oval to round, and it is wider than the male pelvis. The female pelvis is constructed to accommodate the fetus during pregnancy and to facilitate its downward passage through the pelvic cavity in childbirth. In general the female pelvis is broader and lighter than the male pelvis. The male pelvis is shaped like a funnel forming a narrower outlet than the female. It is heavier and stronger than the female pelvis; therefore, it is more suited for lifting and running. See Figure 4–9.

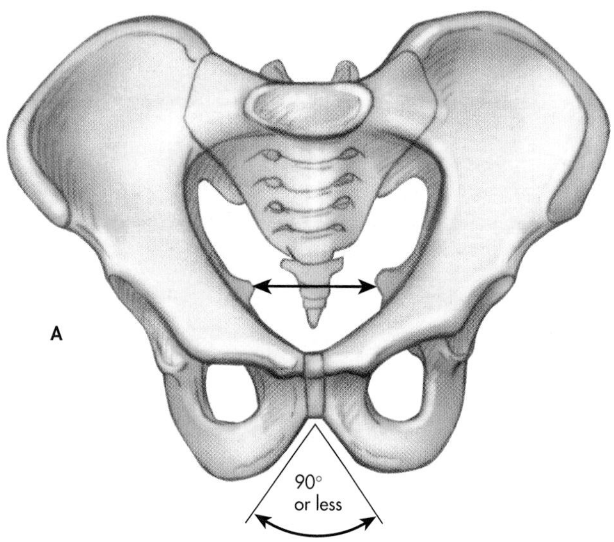

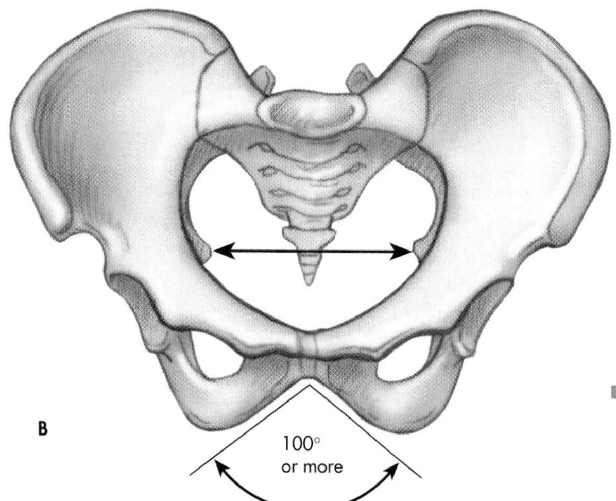

FIGURE 4–9
The male pelvis is shaped like a funnel forming a narrower outlet than the female (A). The female pelvis is shaped like a basin (B).

Answer Column

4.67 **True or False**. The male pelvis is shaped like a funnel forming a narrower outlet than the female.

true

4.68 **True or False**. The female pelvis is shaped like an inverted cone.

false

EXPLANATION FRAME

Drugs that are generally used for skeletal system diseases and disorders include anti-inflammatory agents, antirheumatic drugs, and analgesics.

Anti-inflammatory agents relieve the swelling, tenderness, redness, and pain of inflammation. These agents may be classified as steroidal (corticosteroids) and nonsteroidal (NSAIDs).

Analgesics relieve pain without causing loss of consciousness. They are classified as narcotic and nonnarcotic.

4.69 ___________ are synthetic products that are widely used in the treatment of inflammation, arthritis, and related disorders. The most common adverse reactions associated with NSAIDs are nausea, vomiting, abdominal discomfort, constipation, gastric or duodenal ulcer formation, and gastrointestinal bleeding.

NSAIDs

4.70 Drugs that are generally used for skeletal system disorders/diseases include anti-inflammatory, antirheumatic, and ___________ agents.

analgesic
(an al **JEE** zik)

4.71 ___________ drugs relieve the swelling, redness, and pain of inflammation.

anti-inflammatory
(an tee in **FLAM** ah toh ree)

4.72 ___________ are steroid substances with potent anti-inflammatory effects.

corticosteroids
(kor tih koh **STAIR** oyds)

4.73 ___________ is a low-dose form of methotrexate approved for rheumatoid arthritis.

Rheumatrex
(**ROO** mah treks)

4.74 ___________ are agents that relieve pain without causing loss of consciousness.

analgesics (an al **JEE** ziks)

continued

		Answer Column
4.75	____________ ____________ prevent or relieve rheumatism.	**antirheumatic drugs** (an tih roo **MAT** ik)

4.76 ABBREVIATIONS

Write in the correct abbreviation for the following:

		Answer Column
____________	calcium	**Ca**
____________	degenerative joint disease	**DJD**
____________	fracture	**Fx**
____________	joint	**jt**
____________	long arm cast	**LAC**
____________	long leg cast	**LLC**
____________	nonsteroidal anti-inflammatory drugs	**NSAIDs**
____________	osteoarthritis	**OA**
____________	rheumatoid arthritis	**RA**
____________	short arm cast	**SAC**
____________	traction	**Tx**

EXPLANATION FRAME

Osteoporosis, a condition in which there is a reduction in bone mass, affects more than 25 million Americans. Bone loss may occur during the aging process in the male and female, but proceeds at a faster rate in women.

There are some risk factors involved in developing osteoporosis and these are:

- family history of osteoporosis
- thin, petite build
- early menopause (before 45 years)
- avoided dairy products as a child
- drinking alcoholic beverages
- diet high in salt, caffeine, or fat
- lack of exercise
- never been pregnant
- smoking

		Answer Column
4.77	**True or False.** Bone loss may occur during the aging process in the male and female, but proceeds at a faster rate in women.	**true**
4.78	A condition that results in reduction of bone mass is called ____________.	**osteoporosis** (oss tee oh por **ROH** sis)

Answer Column

4.79 The word elements of the word **oste / o / por / osis** are:

___________	combining form that means bone	**oste / o**
___________	root that means a passage	**por**
___________	suffix that means condition of	**-osis**

IN THE SPOTLIGHT

AGING-CHANGES IN THE BONES, JOINTS, AND MUSCLES

As one ages, certain changes occur in the body. Some of these changes occur in the bones and joints. There is loss of bone mass and bone strength due to the loss of bone mineral content during later life. Calcium salts may be deposited in the matrix and cartilage becomes hard and brittle. Women build bone until about age 35, then begin to lose about 1% of bone mass annually. Men usually start losing bone mass 10 to 20 years later.

Age-related osteoporosis, or loss of bone mass, is often seen in older women and men. Bones in the wrists, hip, and back are most likely to fracture, and if a person has severe osteoporosis, the weight of the body itself can even cause a bone fracture. Low levels of calcium can make an older person more susceptible to osteoporosis and stress fractures. Bone healing in the older adult is slower and impaired due to osteoblasts being less able to use calcium to restructure bone tissue.

Joints begin to wear down as a person ages. They lose some of their function due to arthritis, which is inflammation of a joint. Arthritis can lead to joint pain, along with stiffness and deformity in the joints. The disks between the bones in the spine become less rubbery and more prone to rupture.

Muscles tend to decrease in size as people age. Starting at about age 20, muscle mass begins to decrease. By age 40, most people have lost muscle and increased amounts of fat are deposited into the muscles. These two factors cause the decreased muscle strength that occurs as people age.

All of these changes can affect a person's coordination and posture. Walking may become more difficult, movement is generally slower, and falling becomes more likely. Elderly individuals who are at risk for bone fractures from falling may minimize some of the risk by wearing undergarments that have padded shields at the hips.

The National Academy of Science suggests that people 51 and older consume 1200 mg of calcium daily to help strengthen their bones. It is also recommended that 30 minutes of moderate weight-bearing exercise a day can slow changes in the muscles, joints, and bones. The 30 minutes a day can be done all in one session or can be broken up into smaller increments of time. Individuals can also help protect bones, muscles, and joints by eating a well-balanced diet, not smoking, limiting alcohol intake, and hormone replacement therapy for postmenopausal women.

CASE STUDY

Please read the following case study and then work frames 4.80–4.84. Write in your answer in the answer column. Check your responses with the answers provided at the end of frame 4.84.

A 58-year-old female was seen by a physician and the following is a synopsis of her visit.

PRESENT HISTORY: The patient states that she has noticed that she seems to be shorter and that she has developed a humpback.

SIGNS AND SYMPTOMS: Loss of height, kyphosis, and pain in the lower back.

DIAGNOSIS: Osteoporosis (postmenopausal).

TREATMENT: Estrogen replacement therapy (ESTRADERM—Estradiol Transdermal System); begin a regular exercise program and a diet rich in calcium, phosphorus, magnesium, and vitamins A, C, D, and the B-complex vitamins; and analgesics for bone pain.

PREVENTION: Know the risk factors involved in developing osteoporosis, follow a regular exercise program, and include a diet rich in calcium, phosphorus, magnesium, and vitamins A, C, D, and the B-complex vitamins. Good sources of vitamin A are dairy products, fish, liver oils, animal liver, green and yellow vegetables. Good sources of vitamin D are ultraviolet rays, dairy products, and commercial foods that contain supplemental vitamin D (milk and cereals). Good sources of vitamin C are citrus fruits, tomatoes, melons, fresh berries, raw vegetables, and sweet potatoes. Good sources of the B-complex vitamins are organ meats, dried beans, poultry, eggs, brewer's yeast, fish, whole grains, and dark-green vegetables. Good sources of calcium are dairy products, beans, cauliflower, egg yolk, molasses, leafy green vegetables, tofu, sardines, clams, and oysters. Good sources of phosphorus are dairy products, eggs, fish, poultry, meats, dried peas and beans, whole grain cereals, and nuts. Good sources of magnesium are whole grain cereals, fruits, milk, nuts, vegetables, seafood, and meats.

4.80 Signs and symptoms of osteoporosis include loss of height, ____________, and pain in the lower back.

4.81 To help relieve bone pain in osteoporosis, the physician may prescribe an ____________.

4.82 ____________ is an Estradiol Transdermal System.

4.83 Good sources of vitamin A are dairy products, fish, liver oils, ____________ ____________, green and yellow vegetables.

4.84 Good sources of magnesium are whole grain cereals, fruits, milk, ____________, vegetables, seafood, and meats.

CASE STUDY ANSWERS

4.80 kyphosis
4.81 analgesic
4.82 ESTRADERM
4.83 animal liver
4.84 nuts

REVIEW A: WORD ELEMENTS

This review allows you to check your knowledge of some of the word elements presented in this unit. In the spaces provided, write the meaning of the word elements that are identified as **Prefix (P), Word Root (R), Combining Form (CF), and/or Suffix (S).**

MEDICAL WORD	*WORD ELEMENT*	*MEANING*
1. osteoblast	oste / o (CF)	____________
	-blast (S)	____________
2. chondrocytes	chondr / o (CF)	____________
	-cytes (S)	____________
3. endochondral	endo (P)	____________
	chondr (R)	____________
	-al (S)	____________
4. chondral	chondr (R)	____________
	-al (S)	____________
5. chondralgia	chondr (R)	____________
	-algia (S)	____________
6. chondrectomy	chondr (R)	____________
	-ectomy (S)	____________
7. chondropathology	chondr / o (CF)	____________
	path / o (CF)	____________
	-logy (S)	____________
8. osteoporosis	oste / o (CF)	____________
	por (R)	____________
	-osis (S)	____________
9. osteocarcinoma	oste / o (CF)	____________
	carcin (R)	____________
	-oma (S)	____________
10. osteomyelitis	oste / o (CF)	____________
	myel (R)	____________
	-itis (S)	____________
11. osteomalacia	oste / o (CF)	____________
	-malacia (S)	____________
12. osteotome	oste / o (CF)	____________
	-tome (S)	____________

REVIEW B: MEDICAL TERMS

Please place the correct letter from column II on the appropriate line of column I.

COLUMN I		COLUMN II
________	1. diaphysis	A. narrow space throughout the length of the diaphysis
________	2. epiphyses	B. spongy bone, reticular tissue
________	3. periosteum	C. allows free movement
________	4. compact bone	D. the shaft of a long bone
________	5. medullary canal	E. tough, connective tissue membrane
________	6. endosteum	F. does not permit movement
________	7. cancellous	G. the ends of a developing bone
________	8. synarthrosis	H. the dense, hard layer of bone tissue
________	9. amphiarthrosis	I. permits very slight movement
________	10. diarthrosis	J. the membrane that forms the covering of bones

REVIEW C: TYPES OF BODY MOVEMENTS

Please provide the correct type of body movement for each of the following descriptions.

1. ________ process of turning outward
2. ________ process of lying face downward
3. ________ process of lying face upward
4. ________ process of straightening a flexed limb

REVIEW D: UNSCRAMBLE THE WORDS

Unscramble the following medical terms and place the correct term on the line directly across from the scrambled word.

1. raofenm ________
2. ustaem ________
3. beclertu ________
4. trenahctro ________
5. usnis ________
6. uxallh ________
7. cancaleal ________
8. murfe ________

REVIEW E: DRUGS USED FOR THE SKELETAL SYSTEM

Please provide the correct answer for each of the following descriptions.

1. ____________ steroid substance with potent anti-inflammatory effects
2. ____________ a low-dose form of methrotrexate approved for adult rheumatoid arthritis
3. ____________ agents that relieve pain without causing loss of consciousness
4. ____________ agents that prevent or relieve rheumatism

REVIEW F: ABBREVIATIONS

Please provide the correct abbreviation and/or meaning for the abbreviation.

1. ____________ calcium
2. DJD ____________
3. ____________ fracture
4. jt ____________
5. ____________ long arm cast
6. long leg cast ____________
7. OA ____________
8. rheumatoid arthritis ____________
9. SAC ____________
10. traction ____________

5 THE MUSCULAR SYSTEM: RHEUMATOLOGY AND ORTHOPEDICS

LEARNING CONCEPTS

- the muscular system
- essential terminology
- pronunciation guide
- word elements
- explanation frames
- types of exercise
- RICE: first aid treatment for musculoskeletal injuries
- selected diseases and disorders
- drugs used for the muscular system
- abbreviations
- in the spotlight: achilles tendinitis
- case study: Duchenne's muscular dystrophy
- review exercises

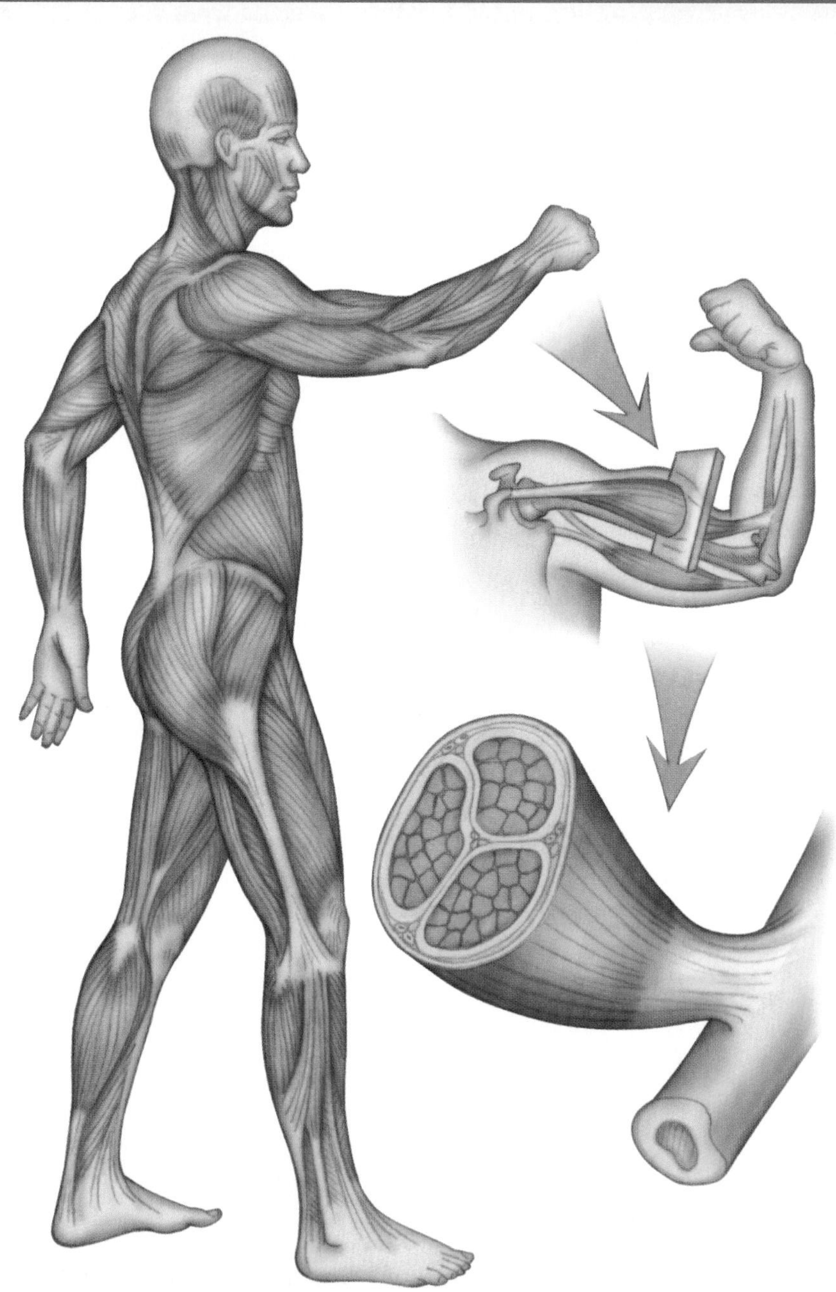

OBJECTIVES

ON COMPLETION OF THIS UNIT, YOU SHOULD BE ABLE TO:

- Briefly describe the muscular system.
- Describe the primary functions of the various organs or structures of the muscular system.
- Identify and give the meaning of the primary word elements for this unit.
- Analyze, build, spell, and pronounce selected medical words.
- Describe the three distinguishable parts of a muscle.
- Describe how muscles perform in groups and define the three basic classifications.
- Define selected types of exercises used for improvement of health or correction of deformity.
- Name and describe some of the most common types of injuries caused by sports and/or exercise.
- Give the first aid treatment for minor musculoskeletal injury.
- Describe selected diseases/disorders of the muscular system.
- Describe selected drugs that are used for muscular system diseases or disorders.
- Define selected abbreviations that pertain to the muscular system.
- Give the types, signs and symptoms, diagnosis, and treatment of Achilles tendinitis.
- Complete the Case Study on Duchenne's muscular dystrophy.
- Successfully complete the review section.

TECH LINK

CD-ROM Use the CD-ROM enclosed with your textbook to gain additional reinforcement through interactive word building exercises, spelling games, labeling activities, and additional quizzes.

www.prenhall.com/rice Use the above address to access the free, interactive Companion Website created specifically for this textbook. Get hints, instant feedback, and textbook references to chapter-related multiple choice and true/false questions, fill-in-the-blank, and labeling exercises. In addition, you will find an audio glossary, and essay questions.

The muscular system is composed of all the muscles in the human body. There are about 600 muscles in the body and they make up approximately 42% of a person's body weight. Muscles are composed of long, slender cells known as fibers. Muscle fibers are of different lengths and shapes and vary in color from white to deep red.

Muscles are classified as skeletal, smooth, and cardiac. Skeletal muscle is also known as voluntary or striated. Smooth muscle is also called involuntary, visceral, or unstriated. Cardiac muscle is involuntary, but striated in appearance. See Figure 5–1.

Skeletal Muscle

Also known as voluntary or striated muscles, skeletal muscles are controlled by the conscious part of the brain and attach to the bones. Skeletal muscles, through contractility, extensibility, and elasticity, are responsible for the movement of the body. These muscles have a cross-striped appearance and thus are known as striated muscles. They vary in size, shape, arrangement of fibers, and means of attachment to bones. Selected skeletal muscles are listed with their functions in Tables 5–1 and 5–2 and shown in Figures 5–2 and 5–3.

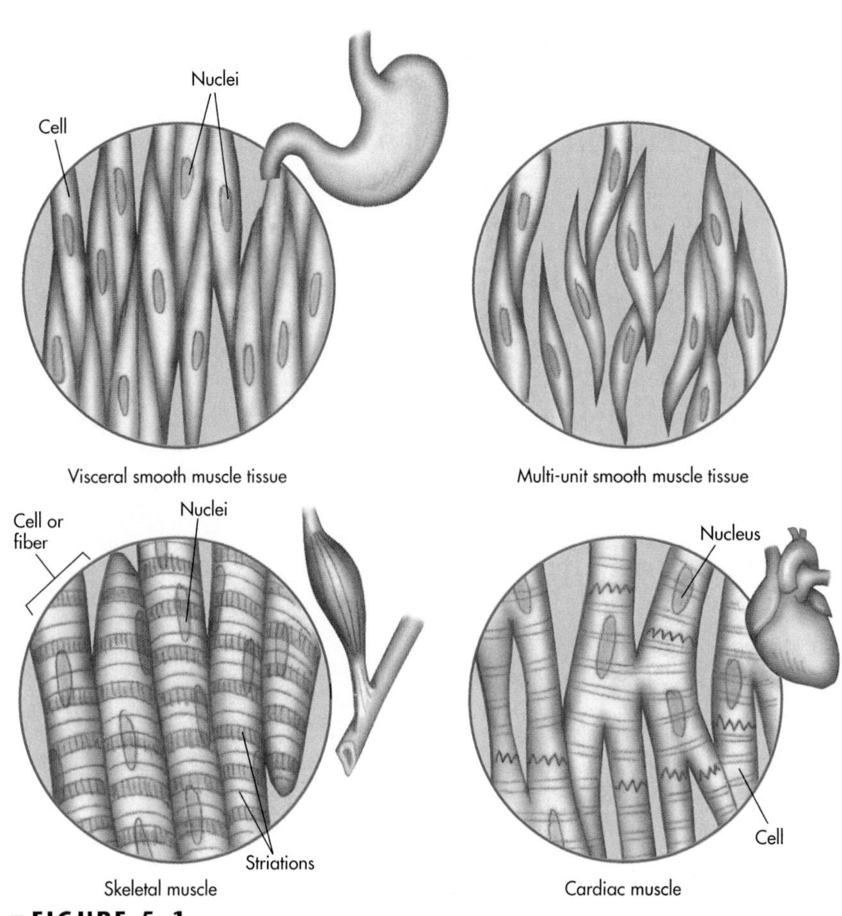

FIGURE 5–1
Types of muscle tissue.

TABLE 5–1 SELECTED SKELETAL MUSCLES (ANTERIOR VIEW)

Muscle	Action
Sternocleidomastoid	Rotates and laterally flexes neck
Trapezius	Draws head back and to the side, rotates scapula
Deltoid	Raises and rotates arm
Rectus Femoris	Extends leg and assists flexion of thigh
Sartorius	Flexes and rotates the thigh and leg
Tibialis Anterior	Dorsiflexes foot and increases the arch in the beginning process of walking
Pectoralis Major	Flexes, adducts, and rotates arm
Biceps Brachii	Flexes arm and forearm and supinates forearm
Rectus Abdominis	Compresses or flattens abdomen
Gastrocnemius	Plantar flexes foot and flexes knee
Soleus	Plantar flexes foot

TABLE 5–2 SELECTED SKELETAL MUSCLES (POSTERIOR VIEW)

Muscle	Action
Trapezius	Draws head back and to the side, rotates scapula
Deltoid	Raises and rotates arm
Triceps	Extends forearm
Latissimus Dorsi	Adducts, extends, and rotates arm; used during swimming
Gluteus Maximus	Extends and rotates thigh
Biceps Femoris	Flexes knee and rotates it outward
Gastrocnemius	Plantar flexes foot and flexes knee
Semitendinosus	Flexes and rotates leg, extends thigh

Smooth Muscle

Also called involuntary, visceral, or unstriated, smooth muscles are not controlled by the conscious part of the brain. They are under the control of the autonomic nervous system and, in most cases, produce relatively slow contraction with greater degree of extensibility. These muscles lack the cross-striped appearance of skeletal muscle and are smooth. Included in this type are the muscles of internal organs of the digestive system, respiratory system, and urinary tract, plus certain muscles of the eye and skin.

Cardiac Muscle

The muscle of the heart (myocardium) is involuntary but striated in appearance. It is controlled by the autonomic nervous system and specialized neuromuscular tissue located within the right atrium.

Muscles are responsible for movement, they help maintain posture through a continual partial contraction of skeletal muscles, and they help produce heat through the chemical changes involved in muscular action. See Table 5–3.

TABLE 5–3 THE MUSCULAR SYSTEM

Organ/Structure	Primary Functions
Muscles	Responsible for movement, help to maintain posture, and produce heat
Skeletal	Through contractility, extensibility, and elasticity, are responsible for the movement of the body
Smooth	Produce relatively slow contraction with greater degree of extensibility in the internal organs, especially organs of the digestive system, respiratory system, and urinary tract, plus certain muscles of the eye and skin, and walls of blood vessels
Caridac	Muscles of the heart, controlled by the autonomic nervous system and specialized neuromuscular tissue located within the right atrium that is capable of causing cardiac muscle to contract rhythmically. The neuromuscular tissue of the heart comprises the sinoatrial node, the atrioventricular node, and the atrioventricular bundle
Tendons	A band of connective tissue serving for the attachment of muscles to bones

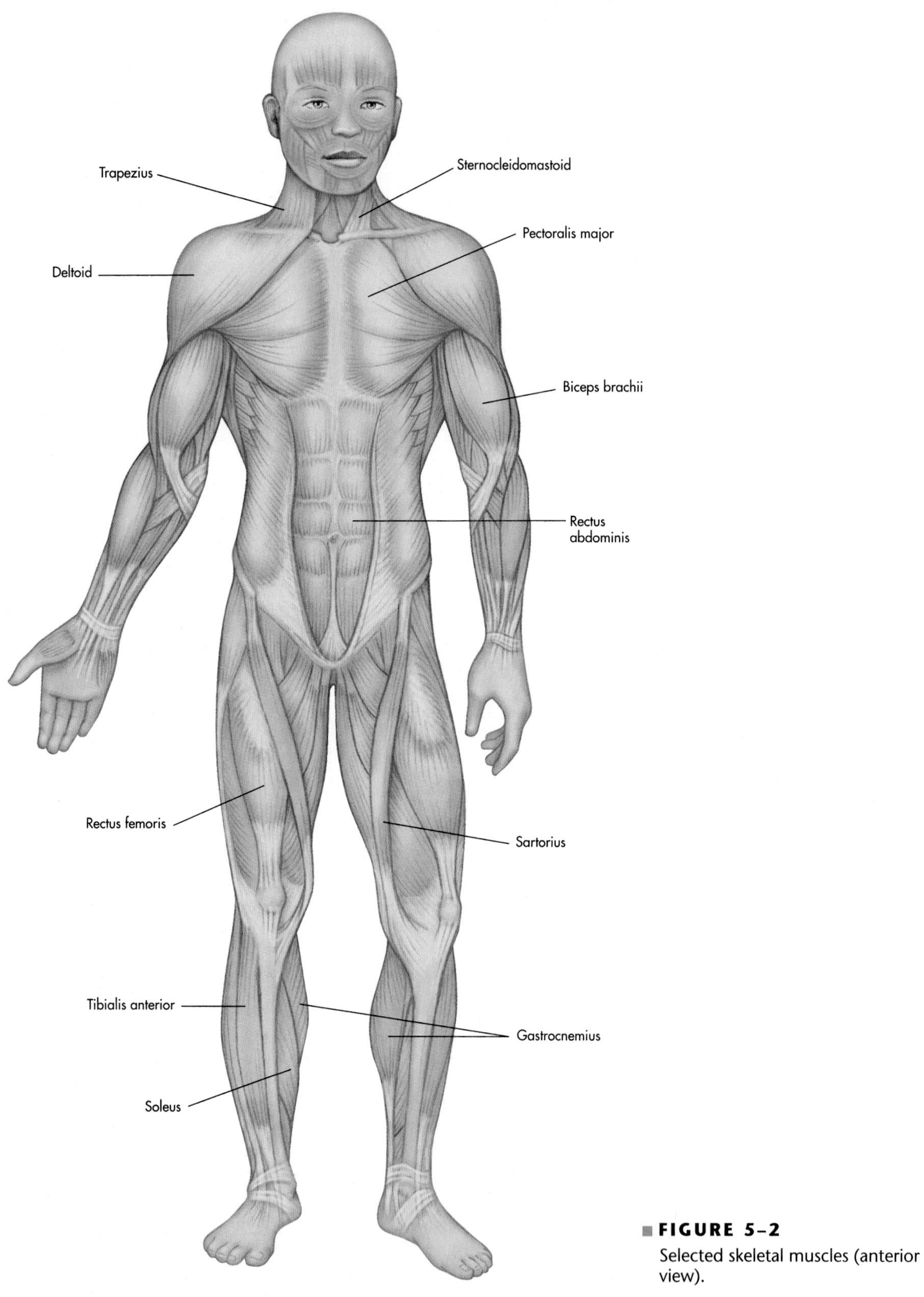

FIGURE 5–2
Selected skeletal muscles (anterior view).

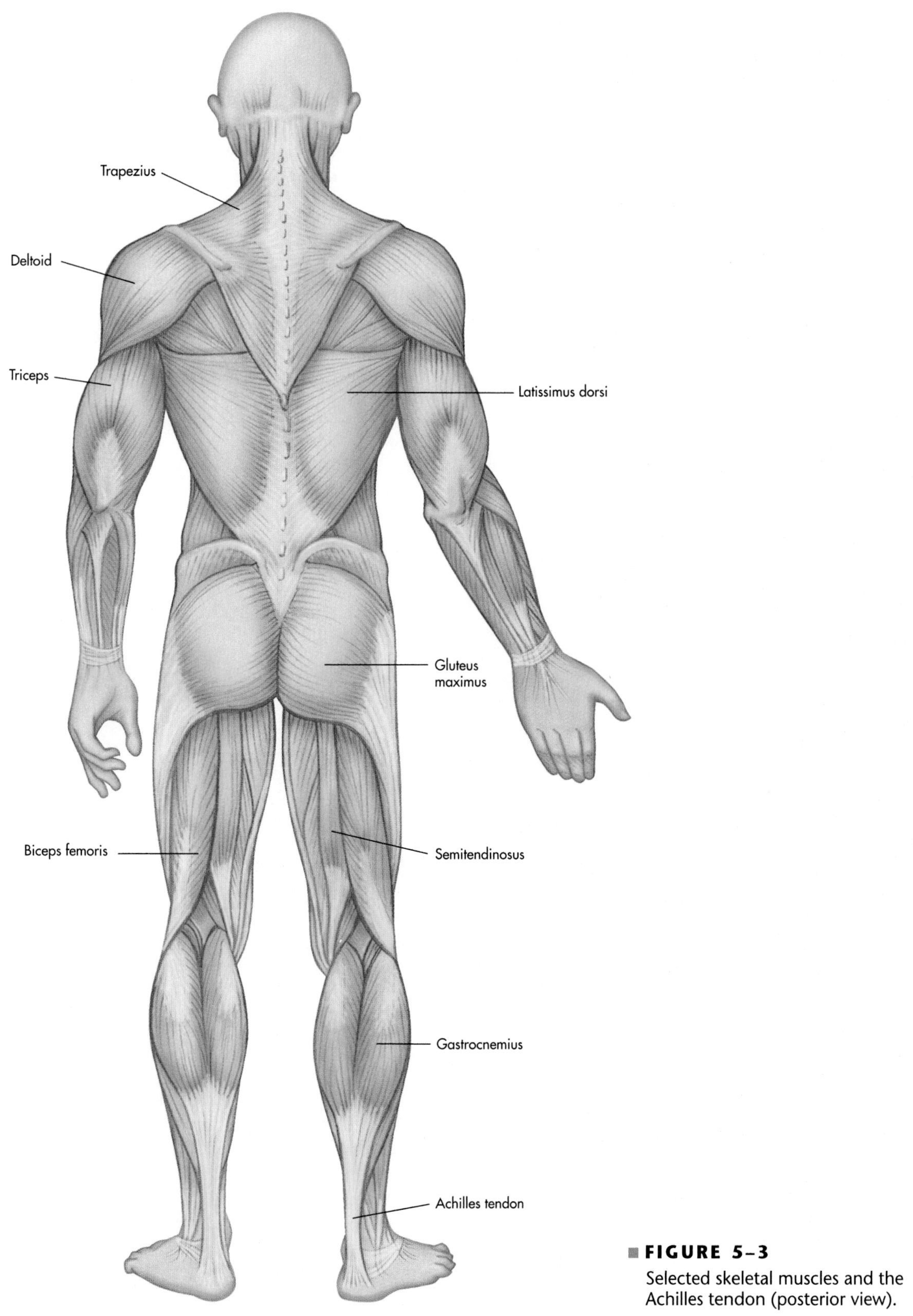

FIGURE 5–3
Selected skeletal muscles and the Achilles tendon (posterior view).

PRIMARY WORD ELEMENTS

The following word elements (prefixes, roots, combining forms, and suffixes) will be used to build medical terms that relate to this unit. Please commit these to memory.

PREFIX

PREFIX	MEANING	PREFIX	MEANING
a	without, lack of	**intra**	within
dys	bad, difficult, painful	**quadri**	four

COMBINING FORM

COMBINING FORM / ROOT	MEANING	COMBINING FORM / ROOT	MEANING
brach / i	arm	**my**	muscle
cry / o	cold	**my / o, my / os**	muscle
fasc / i, fasci / o	band (fascia)	**rhabd / o**	rod
fibr / o	fiber, fibrous tissue	**rheumat / o**	discharge
is / o	equal	**sarc**	flesh
lemma	sheath, rind, husk	**sarc / o**	flesh
log	study	**synov**	joint fluid
melan	black	**ten / o**	tendon
metr	measure	**tendin**	tendon
muscul	muscle	**therm / o**	heat, hot

SUFFIX

SUFFIX	MEANING	SUFFIX	MEANING
-al, -ar, -ic	pertaining to	**-lysis**	destruction
-algia, -dynia	pain	**-malacia**	softening
-asthenia	weakness	**-oma**	tumor
-ceps	head	**-osis**	condition of
-desis	surgical binding	**-plasty**	surgical repair
-ectomy	surgical excision	**-rrhaphy**	suture
-ist	one who specializes	**-therapy**	treatment
-itis	inflammation	**-tomy**	incision
-logy	study of	**-trophy**	nourishment, development

ANSWER COLUMN

5.1 ___________ is the medical specialty that studies rheumatic diseases.

rheumatology
(roo mah **TALL** oh jee)

5.2 The medical term rheumatic means pertaining to ___________.
Rheumatism is a general term that is used to describe acute and chronic conditions characterized by inflammation, soreness and stiffness of muscles, and pain in joints and associated structures.

rheumatism
(**ROO** mah tih zem)

Answer Column

5.3 A __________ is a physician who specializes in rheumatic diseases. The word elements used to build **rheumat / o / log / ist** are:

__________ combining form that means discharge
__________ root that means study
__________ suffix that means one who specializes

Rheumat / o is from the Greek origin of the root rheuma that means discharge. In general use, the word element is used to describe rheumatism.

rheumatologist (roo mah **TALL** oh jist)
rheumat / o
log
-ist

EXPLANATION FRAME

There are several muscular conditions characterized by signs and symptoms of rheumatism: tenderness, soreness, pain, and local spasm. These conditions are fibromyositis, myositis, myalgia, and torticollis.

5.4 __________ is the inflammation of muscle and fibrous tissue. The word elements used to build **fibr / o / my / o / s / itis** are:

__________ combining form that means fiber
__________ combining form that means muscle
__________ suffix that means inflammation

fibromyositis (figh broh mye oh **SIGH** tis)
fibr / o
my / o / s
-itis

5.5 __________ is a medical term that is defined as chronic pain in muscles and soft tissues surrounding joints. *It is often associated with* ***fibromyositis,*** *although it is not an inflammatory process. It is classified by the American College of Rheumatology, and a patient who presents with a history of widespread pain for at least 3 months and pain in 11 of 18 tender point sites on digital palpation may be classified as having* ***fibromyalgia.***

fibromyalgia (figh broh mye **AL** jee ah)

5.6 Other muscular system medical terms associated with rheumatism are:

__________ inflammation of muscle (s)
__________ muscle pain
__________ that literally means "twisted neck"

Torticollis is a deformity of the neck that involves shortening of the neck muscles, which tilts the head to the affected side with the chin pointing to the other side. It may be congenital or acquired.

myositis (mye oh **SIGH** tis)
myalgia (mye **AL** jee ah)
torticollis (tor tih **KOL** iss)

5.7 Muscle __________ are of different lengths and shapes and vary in color from white to deep red.

fibers (**FIGH** bers)

Answer Column

continued

5.8 A plasma membrane surrounding each striated muscle fiber is called __________.

The word elements used to build **sarc / o / lemma** are:

__________ combining form that means flesh

__________ root that means a sheath or rind

Answer: **sarcolemma** (sar koh **LEM** ah); **sarc / o**; **lemma**

5.9 A tumor of striated muscle tissue is called __________.

The word elements used to build **rhabd / o / my / oma** are:

__________ combining form that means rod

__________ root that means muscle

__________ suffix that means tumor

Answer: **rhabdomyoma** (rab doh mye **OH** mah); **rhabd / o**; **my**; **-oma**

5.10 Each muscle consists of a group of fibers held together by connective tissue and enclosed in a fibrous sheath or __________. See Figure 5–4. *A fascia is a thin layer of connective tissue covering, supporting, or connecting the muscles or inner organs of the body.*

Answer: **fascia** (**FASH** ee ah)

5.11 Each fiber within a muscle receives its own nerve impulses and has its own stored supply of __________, which it uses as fuel for energy.

Answer: **glycogen** (**GLIGH** koh jen)

5.12 Muscle has to be supplied with proper nutrition and __________ to perform properly; therefore, blood and lymphatic vessels permeate its tissues.

Answer: **oxygen** (**OK** sih jen)

EXPLANATION FRAME

A muscle has three distinguishable parts: the body or main portion, an origin, and an insertion. Skeletal muscles move body parts by pulling from one bone across its joint to another bone with movement occurring at the diarthrotic joint.

5.13 The point of attachment of a muscle to the part that it moves is called __________.

Answer: **insertion** (in **SIR** shun)

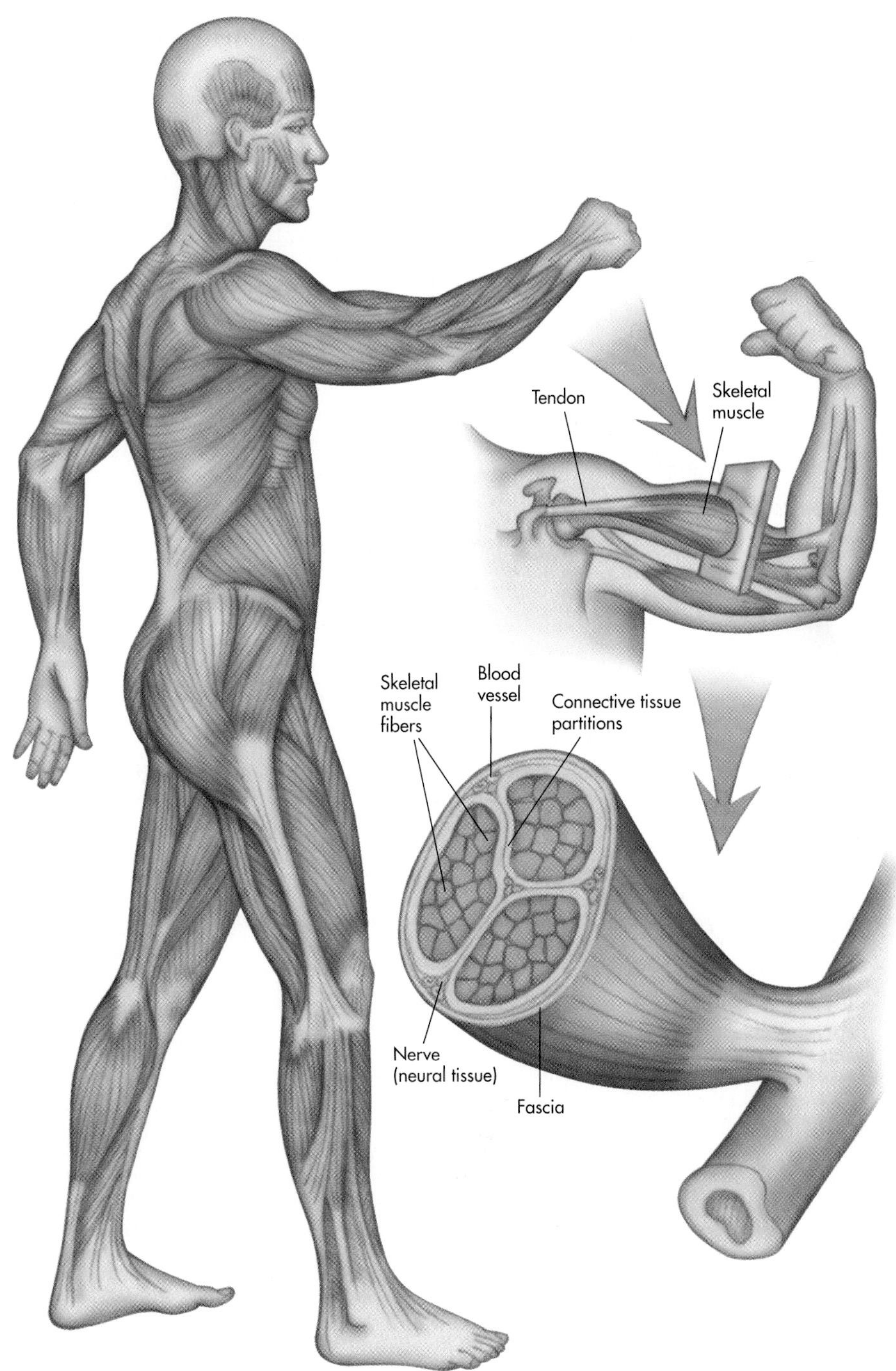

FIGURE 5–4

A skeletal muscle consists of a group of fibers held together by connective tissue. It is enclosed in a fibrous sheath (fascia).

ANSWER COLUMN

continued

5.14 Skeletal muscles have two or more points of attachment. The more fixed attachment is known as the ___________, and the point of attachment of a muscle to the part that it moves is the **insertion.**

origin (OR ih jin)

EXPLANATION FRAME

Muscles and nerves function together as a motor unit. For skeletal muscles to contract, it is necessary to have stimulation by impulses from motor nerves. Muscles perform in groups and are classified as:

Antagonist. A muscle that counteracts the action of another muscle.
Prime mover. A muscle that is primary in a given movement.
Synergist. A muscle that acts with another muscle to produce movement.

5.15 A muscle that acts with another muscle to produce movement is called ___________.

synergist (SIN er jist)

5.16 Muscles are responsible for ___________. The types of movement are locomotion, propulsion of substances through tubes as in circulation and digestion, and changes in the size of openings as in the contraction and relaxation of the iris of the eye.

movement (MOOV ment)

5.17 Muscles help to maintain posture through a continual partial contraction of skeletal muscles. This process is known as ___________.

tonicity (toh **NIS** ih tee)

5.18 Muscles help to produce ___________ through the chemical changes involved in muscular action.

heat (HEET)

5.19 ___________ is the destruction of muscle tissue.

The word elements used to build **my / o / lysis** are:

___________ combining form that means muscle

___________ suffix that means destruction

myolysis (mye **OL** ih sis)

my / o

-lysis

		ANSWER COLUMN
5.20	____________ is a malignant tumor derived from muscle tissue. The word elements that are used to build this term are: ____________ combining form that means muscle ____________ root that means flesh ____________ suffix that means tumor	**myosarcoma** (mye oh sar **KOH** mah) **my / o** **sarc** **-oma**
5.21	A condition in which there is an abnormal darkening of muscle tissue is called ____________. **My / o** (CF) = muscle, **melan** (R) = black, and the suffix **-osis** means condition of.	**myomelanosis** (mye oh mel ah **NOH** sis)
5.22	The suffix **-malacia** means softening. A term that uses this component part is ____________. **My / o** (CF) = muscle, and the suffix **-malacia** = softening. **My / o / malacia** is softening of muscle tissue.	**myomalacia** (mye oh mah **LAY** she ah)
5.23	The medical term for muscle weakness is ____________. The root **my** means muscle and the suffix ____________ means weakness.	**myasthenia** (mye ass **THEE** nee ah) **-asthenia**
5.24	____________ is a diagnostic test to measure electrical activity across muscle membranes by means of electrodes that are attached to a needle that is inserted into the muscle. *Abnormal results may indicate myasthenia gravis and muscular dystrophy.*	**electromyography** (ee lek troh my **OG** rah fee)
5.25	____________ means within a muscle. The word elements used to build this term are: ____________ prefix that means within ____________ root that means muscle ____________ suffix that means pertaining to	**intramuscular** (in trah **MUSS** kyoo lar) **intra** **muscul** **-ar**
5.26	____________ pain involves a muscle and its fascia. The word elements used to build this term are: ____________ combining form that means muscle ____________ combining form that means band (fascia) ____________ suffix that means pertaining to	**myofascial** (mye oh **FASH** ee al) **my / o** **fasc / i** **-al**

Answer Column

continued

5.27 The surgical repair of a fascia is called __________. The word elements used to build this term are:

__________ combining form that means a band

__________ suffix that means surgical repair

fascioplasty (**FASH** ee oh plas tee)

fasci / o

-plasty

5.28 The combining forms **fasci / o** and **fasc / i** and the word root **fasc** mean a band. Now build some medical terms that use these word elements plus the following suffixes: **-ectomy, -desis,** and **-itis.**

__________ surgical excision of a fascia

__________ surgical binding of a fascia

__________ inflammation of a fascia

fasciectomy (fas ee **EK** toh mee)

fasciodesis (fas ee **ODD** eh sis)

fascitis (fah **SIGH** tis)

EXPLANATION FRAME

Tendons bind muscles to bones. See Figure 5–1. Fascia cover, support, or connect muscles or the body's inner organs. Ligaments bind together bones, especially those within joints. A bursa is a saclike cavity; especially one containing a viscid fluid and located at points of friction, such as a joint.

5.29 A band of fibrous connective tissue serving for the attachment of muscles to bones is called a __________. *A tendon can vary in length from less than 1 inch to more than 1 foot. A wide, thin, sheetlike tendon is known as an* ***aponeurosis.***

tendon (**TEN** dun)

5.30 An __________ is a wide, thin, sheetlike tendon that serves to attach muscle to bone or to other tissues.

aponeurosis (ap oh nuh **ROH** sis)

5.31 The word root **tendin** and the combining form **ten / o** mean tendon. Some medical terms that use these word elements are:

__________ inflammation of a tendon

__________ tendon pain

__________ suture of a tendon

__________ incision into a tendon

__________ inflammation of a tendon sheath

Synov *is a word root that means joint fluid.* ***Synovia*** *(also called synovial fluid) is a colorless, viscid, lubricating fluid of joints, bursae, and tendon sheaths secreted within synovial membranes.*

tendinitis (ten dih **NYE** tis)

tenodynia (ten oh **DIN** ee ah)

tenorrhaphy (tah **NOR** ah fee)

tenotomy (teh **NOT** oh mee)

tenosynovitis (ten oh sin oh **VYE** tis)

ANSWER COLUMN

FOR REVIEW

The word elements **tendin** and **ten / o** mean tendon. The root **synov** means joint fluid. The suffixes: **-itis** means inflammation, **-dynia** means pain, **-rrhaphy** means suture, and **-tomy** means incision.

5.32 ___________ is a muscle having three heads with a single insertion. The prefix **tri** means three and the suffix **-ceps** means head. The **triceps brachii** is a muscle located in the upper arm. It extends the forearm and arm.

triceps (TRY seps)

5.33 ___________ is a medical term that means pain in the arm. The word elements used to build **brach / i / algia** are:

___________ combining form that means arm

___________ suffix that means pain

brachialgia (bray kee **AL** jee ah)

brach / i

-algia

5.34 **Quadri** is a prefix that means four. When linked to the suffix **-ceps**, which means ___________, the term **quadriceps** is created. This term describes a muscle that has four heads or points of attachment. The quadriceps femoris is a large muscle that is located in the thigh. It extends the leg.

head (HED)

5.35 Smooth muscle is also called ___________ or unstriated.

visceral (VISS er al)

EXPLANATION FRAME

Dystrophin is a protein found in muscle cells. When the gene that is responsible for this protein is defective and sufficient dystrophin is not produced, muscle wasting occurs.

5.36 ___________ is a protein found in muscle cells.

dystrophin (DIS troh fin)

5.37 ___________ is the faulty muscular development due to lack of nourishment.

The word elements used to build this term are:

___________ prefix that means difficult

___________ suffix that means nourishment, development

dystrophy (DIS troh fee)

dys

-trophy

Answer Column

continued

5.38 __________ __________ is a familial disease characterized by progressive atrophy and wasting of muscles.

muscular dystrophy (**MUSS** kyoo lar **DIS** troh fee)

5.39 __________ muscular dystrophy begins in childhood, is progressive, and affects the shoulder and pelvic girdle muscles.

The disease is seen in males and is transmitted as a sex-linked recessive trait. Death usually occurs at an early age.

Duchenne's (doo **SHENZ**)

5.40 __________ means a lack of nourishment or a wasting of muscular tissue caused by lack of use.

The word elements used to build **a / trophy** are:

__________ prefix that means lack of

__________ suffix that means nourishment, development

atrophy (**AT** roh fee)

a

-trophy

5.41 A __________ is a fibrosis of connective tissue in skin, fascia, muscle, or joint capsule that prevents normal mobility of the related tissue or joint. With a muscular contracture, a muscle shortens and renders the muscle resistant to the normal stretching process.

contracture (kon **TRACK** chur)

5.42 __________ __________ is a slow, progressive contracture of the palmar fascia causing the ring and little fingers to bend into the palm so that they cannot be extended.

Dupuytren's contracture (doo pwee **TRAHNZ**)

5.43 __________ __________ occurs as a result of circulatory impairment due to pressure from a cast, constricting dressing/bandage, or injury of the radial artery. With this type of contracture there is pronation and flexion of the hand, with atrophy of the muscles of the forearm.

Volkmann's contracture (**FOKE** mahnz)

5.44 The surgical excision of a limb, part, or other appendage is called an __________.

amputation (am pew **TAY** shun)

5.45 The medical term for a lack of muscle tone is __________.

flaccid (**FLAK** sid)

ANSWER COLUMN

5.46 The __________ is a partition that separates the chest and abdominal cavities. **Dia** is a prefix that means through and **-phragm** is a suffix that means a fence or partition.

diaphragm (DYE ah fram)

5.47 __________ __________ is a term used to describe the muscles immediately surrounding the shoulder joint. They stabilize the shoulder joint while the entire arm is moved.

rotator cuff
(ROH tay tor **KUFF)**

5.48 __________ is a performed activity of the muscles for the improvement of health or correction of deformity.

exercise (EK ser size)

EXPLANATION FRAME

Types of exercises include:

Active. The patient contracts and relaxes his or her muscles.
Assistive. The patient contracts and relaxes his or her muscles with the assistance of a therapist.
Isometric. Active muscular contraction performed against stable resistance, thereby not shortening the muscle length.
Passive. Exercise is performed by another individual without the assistance of the patient.
Range of motion. Movement of each joint through its full range of motion. Used to prevent loss of motility or to regain usage after an injury or fracture.
Relief of tension. Technique used to promote relaxation of the muscles and provide relief from tension.

5.49 __________ means pertaining to having equal measure.

The word parts used to build this term are:

__________ combining form that means equal
__________ root that means to measure
__________ suffix that means pertaining to

isometric (eye soh **MET** rik)

is / o
metr
-ic

EXPLANATION FRAME

Each year, more and more evidence indicates that regular physical activity can help the human body. Regular aerobic and weight-bearing exercises, such as aerobic dance, brisk walking, weight lifting, and bicycling, improve heart and lung function and muscle tone. To maintain aerobic fit-

(continued)

ANSWER COLUMN

continued

ness, one needs to exercise three times a week for 20 to 30 minutes at his or her target heart rate. Exercise decreases risk factors for heart disease, stroke, and osteoporosis. It improves mood, and researchers have found that people who exercise regularly tend to be less depressed than people who don't exercise at all.

5.50 **True or False.** Regular physical exercise can decrease risk factors for heart disease, stroke, and osteoporosis. — **true**

EXPLANATION FRAME

Exercise carries a number of risks due to the stresses placed on joints, muscles, tendons, and connective tissue. Injuries caused by sports and/or exercise are very common. Some of the most common types of injuries are bone bruise, bursitis, tendonitis, muscle cramps, sprains, stress fractures, strains, bone spurs, and pulled muscles.

The first aid treatment for minor musculoskeletal injury is **RICE.**

R Rest
I Ice
C Compression
E Elevation

5.51 A __________ is the twisting of a joint that causes pain and disability; it is caused by trauma to the joint. The ankle joint is the most often sprained. — **sprain (SPRAYN)**

5.52 A __________ is the excessive, forcible stretching of a muscle or musculotendinous unit. — **strain (STRAYN)**

5.53 **True or False.** Although there are many benefits of exercise, it carries a number of risks due to the stresses placed on joints, muscle, tendons, and connective tissue. — **true**

5.54 **True or False.** The Achilles tendon can become inflamed and/or torn from playing basketball and/or tennis, or during running and brisk walking. — **true**

ANSWER COLUMN

5.55 **True or False.** The best way to prevent injuries due to exercise and/or sports is to build muscle strength gradually.

true

5.56 When there is a minor musculoskeletal injury, the first aid treatment is ___________.

RICE

5.57 ___________ is the treatment of choice for soft tissue injuries and muscle injuries. It causes vasoconstriction of blood vessels and is effective in diminishing bleeding and edema. Ice should not be placed directly onto the skin. **Cry / o** is a combining form that means cold and **-therapy** is a suffix that means treatment.

cryotherapy (krye oh **THER** ah pee)

5.58 **True or False. Thermotherapy** is the treatment using scientific application of heat. **Therm / o** (CF) = heat and the suffix **-therapy** = treatment correctly describes thermotherapy. Heat may be used 48 to 72 hours after an injury. Types: heating pad, hot water bottle, hot packs, infrared light, and immersion of body part in warm water. Extreme care should be followed when using or applying heat.

true

EXPLANATION FRAME

Relaxants are used to treat painful muscle spasms that may result from strains, sprains, and musculoskeletal trauma or disease. Centrally acting muscle relaxants act by depressing the central nervous system and can be administered either orally or by injection. The patient must be informed of the sedative effect produced by these drugs. Drowsiness, dizziness, and blurred vision may diminish the patient's ability to drive a vehicle, operate equipment, or climb stairs.

5.59 ___________ are used to treat painful muscle spasms that may result from strains, sprains, and musculoskeletal trauma or disease.

relaxants (ree **LAK** sants)

5.60 The sedative effect produced by relaxants may cause ___________, dizziness, and blurred vision. The patient must be informed of these effects.

drowsiness (**DROW** zee ness)

ANSWER COLUMN

EXPLANATION FRAME

Other medications that may be used to treat muscular system diseases and disorders include anti-inflammatory agents, antirheumatic drugs, and analgesics.

Anti-inflammatory agents relieve the swelling, tenderness, redness, and pain of inflammation. These agents may be classified as steroidal (corticosteroids) and nonsteroidal (NSAIDs).

Antirheumatic drugs prevent or relieve rheumatism.

Analgesics relieve pain without causing loss of consciousness.

5.61 ____________ drugs prevent or relieve rheumatism.

antirheumatic (an tih roo **MAT** ik)

5.62 ____________ agents relieve the swelling, tenderness, redness, and pain of inflammation.

anti-inflammatory (an tee in **FLAM** ah toh ree)

5.63 ____________ relieve pain without causing loss of consciousness.

analgesics (an al **JEE** ziks)

5.64 ABBREVIATIONS

Write in the correct abbreviation for the following:

		Answer
____________	below elbow	**BE**
____________	below knee	**BK**
____________	deep tendon reflexes	**DTRs**
____________	electromyography	**EMG**
____________	intramuscular	**IM**
____________	muscular dystrophy	**MD**
____________	musculoskeletal	**MS**
____________	physical therapy	**PT**
____________	range of motion	**ROM**
____________	shoulder	**sh**
____________	triceps jerk	**TJ**
____________	weight	**wt**

IN THE SPOTLIGHT

IN THE SPOTLIGHT

ACHILLES TENDINITIS

Achilles tendinitis is an inflammation of the Achilles tendon, a large tendon at the lower end of the gastrocnemius muscle inserted into the os calcis (the heel bone). It is the strongest and thickest tendon in the body and is also referred to as the calcaneal tendon.

Achilles tendinitis is often the result of injury and/or tearing of the tendon fibers. There are two types: insertional, where the tendon attaches to the heel bone, and noninsertional, which occurs slightly higher up the tendon. The signs and symptoms of this disease include local pain, usually slow in onset, and a limp, causing difficulty in walking, running, and jumping. The discomfort varies from being very painful and restrictive, to being only a nuisance. The back of the shoe can cause painful pressure on the attachment of the tendon to the heel bone. Sensitivity at the site of the inflammation is a consistent sign. For noninsertional tendinitis, swelling is frequently seen and felt. Exercise can make the symptoms either better or worse.

The most common cause of this condition is overuse. Frequently, a sudden increase in exercise training, running, mileage, or speed will bring on symptoms. Pressure from the hard back of an athletic shoe can irritate the tendon over the heel. Also, landing hard on the arch of the foot may contribute to the strain on the Achilles tendon.

The best prevention of this condition is proper exercise training and footwear. Stretching the calf muscles attached to the Achilles tendon is important before and after exercise. Using arch supports in footwear can help prevent Achilles tendinitis. Also, one should make sure that the back of the shoe is soft enough not to cause injury to the heel bone.

Diagnosis is based upon the signs and symptoms. X-rays do not often reveal abnormalities, but sometimes hardening of the tendon can be observed, or an abnormal piece of bone or bone spur is seen where the tendon connects to the back of the heel. X-rays may also show an unusual bump of the heel, which can rub and irritate the tendon.

Treatment usually consists of rest or changes in activity, stretching, ice after activity, or nonsteroidal anti-inflammatory drugs (NSAIDs). It is important to note that NSAIDs may cause indigestion, stomach ulcers, or gastrointestinal bleeding. They can also affect the kidneys or liver.

Other forms of treatment may include physical therapy that focuses on stretching and strengthening, massage, alternating hot and cold compresses to the heel bone, and ultrasound. The temporary use of a heel lift, or the insertion of an arch support into the shoe, can also help. Surgery is rarely necessary, but can remove bone spurs or the bony prominence of the heel bone.

CASE STUDY

Please read the following case study and then work frames 5.65–5.68. Write in your answer in the answer column. Check your responses with the answers provided at the end of frame 5.68.

A 3-year-old male child was seen by a physician and the following is a synopsis of the visit.

PRESENT HISTORY: The mother states that she noticed that her son has been falling a lot and seems to be very clumsy. She says that he has a waddling gait, is very slow in running and climbing, and walks on his toes. She is most concerned as she is at risk for carrying the gene that causes muscular dystrophy.

SIGNS AND SYMPTOMS: A waddling gait, very slow in running and climbing, walks on his toes, frequent falling, clumsy.

DIAGNOSIS: Duchenne's muscular dystrophy. The diagnosis was determined by the characteristic symptoms, the family history, a muscle biopsy, an electromyography, and an elevated serum creatine kinase level.

TREATMENT: Physical therapy, deep breathing exercises to help delay muscular weakness, supportive measures such as splints and braces to help minimize deformities and to preserve mobility. Counseling and referral services are essential. For more information you may contact the Muscular Dystrophy Association at: 3300 E. Sunrise Drive, Tucson, AZ 85718. Telephone 1-800-572-1717. E-mail mda@mdausa.org.

5.65 Signs and symptoms of Duchenne's muscular dystrophy include a ____________ gait, frequent falls, clumsiness, slowness in running and climbing, and walking on toes.

5.66 For more information about muscular dystrophy you can call ____________.

5.67 The diagnosis was determined by the characteristic symptoms, the family history, a muscle biopsy, an ____________, and an elevated serum creatine kinase level.

5.68 Treatment for Duchenne's muscular dystrophy includes physical therapy, exercise, and supportive measures such as braces and ____________.

CASE STUDY ANSWERS

5.65 waddling
5.66 1-800-572-1717
5.67 electromyography
5.68 splints

REVIEW A: WORD ELEMENTS

This review allows you to check your knowledge of some of the word elements presented in this unit. In the spaces provided, write the meaning of the word elements that are identified as **Prefix (P), Word Root (R), Combining Form (CF),** and/or **Suffix (S).**

MEDICAL WORD	*WORD ELEMENT*	*MEANING*
1. rheumatologist	rheumat / o (CF)	____________
	log (R)	____________
	-ist (S)	____________
2. fibromyositis	fibr / o (CF)	____________
	my / o / s (CF)	____________
	-itis (S)	____________
3. fibromyalgia	fibr / o (CF)	____________
	my (R)	____________
	-algia (S)	____________
4. tenodynia	ten / o (CF)	____________
	-dynia (S)	____________
5. rhabdomyoma	rhabd / o (CF)	____________
	my (R)	____________
	-oma (S)	____________
6. dystrophy	dys (P)	____________
	-trophy (S)	____________
7. myosarcoma	my / o (CF)	____________
	sarc (R)	____________
	-oma (S)	____________
8. myomelanosis	my / o (CF)	____________
	melan (R)	____________
	-osis (S)	____________
9. myomalacia	my / o (CF)	____________
	-malacia (S)	____________
10. myasthenia	my (R)	____________
	-asthenia (S)	____________
11. fascioplasty	fasci / o (CF)	____________
	-plasty (S)	____________

REVIEW B: MEDICAL TERMS

Please place the correct letter from column II on the appropriate line of column I.

COLUMN I		COLUMN II
______	1. fascia	A. smooth muscle
______	2. tendon	B. surgical excision of a limb
______	3. synovia	C. protein found in muscle cells
______	4. visceral	D. forcible stretching of a muscle
______	5. dystrophin	E. fibrous sheath
______	6. amputation	F. treatment using cold
______	7. sprain	G. means for attachment of muscles to bones
______	8. strain	H. more fixed point of attachment
______	9. cryotherapy	I. twisting of a joint
______	10. origin	J. lubricating fluid of joints

REVIEW C: TYPES OF EXERCISE

Please provide the correct type of exercise for each of the following descriptions.

1. With ______ exercise the patient contracts and relaxes his or her own muscles.
2. With ______ exercise, active muscular contraction is performed against stable resistance.
3. ______ exercise is performed by another individual without the assistance of the patient.
4. ______ ______ ______ is movement of each joint through its full range of motion.
5. ______ ______ ______ is used to promote relaxation of the muscles and provide relief from tension.

REVIEW D: UNSCRAMBLE THE WORDS

Unscramble the following medical terms and place the correct term on the line directly across from the scrambled word.

1. serbif ______
2. negoxy ______
3. nictyiot ______
4. epstric ______
5. phytroa ______
6. accidfl ______
7. actconturer ______
8. magrphiad ______

REVIEW E: DRUGS USED FOR THE MUSCULAR SYSTEM

Please provide the correct answer for each of the following descriptions.

1. ____________ are used to treat painful muscle spasms.
2. ____________ drugs prevent or relieve rheumatism.
3. ____________ agents relieve the swelling, tenderness, redness, and pain of inflammation.
4. ____________ relieve pain without causing loss of consciousness.

REVIEW F: ABBREVIATIONS

Please provide the correct abbreviation and/or meaning for the abbreviation.

1. ____________ below elbow
2. BK ____________
3. ____________ electromyography
4. IM ____________
5. ____________ muscular dystrophy
6. PT ____________

6 THE NERVOUS SYSTEM: NEUROLOGY AND NEUROSURGERY

LEARNING CONCEPTS

- the nervous system
- essential terminology
- pronunciation guide
- word elements
- explanation frames
- stroke's warning signs
- selected diseases and disorders
- drugs used for the nervous system
- abbreviations
- in the spotlight: stroke
- case study: Alzheimer's disease
- review exercises

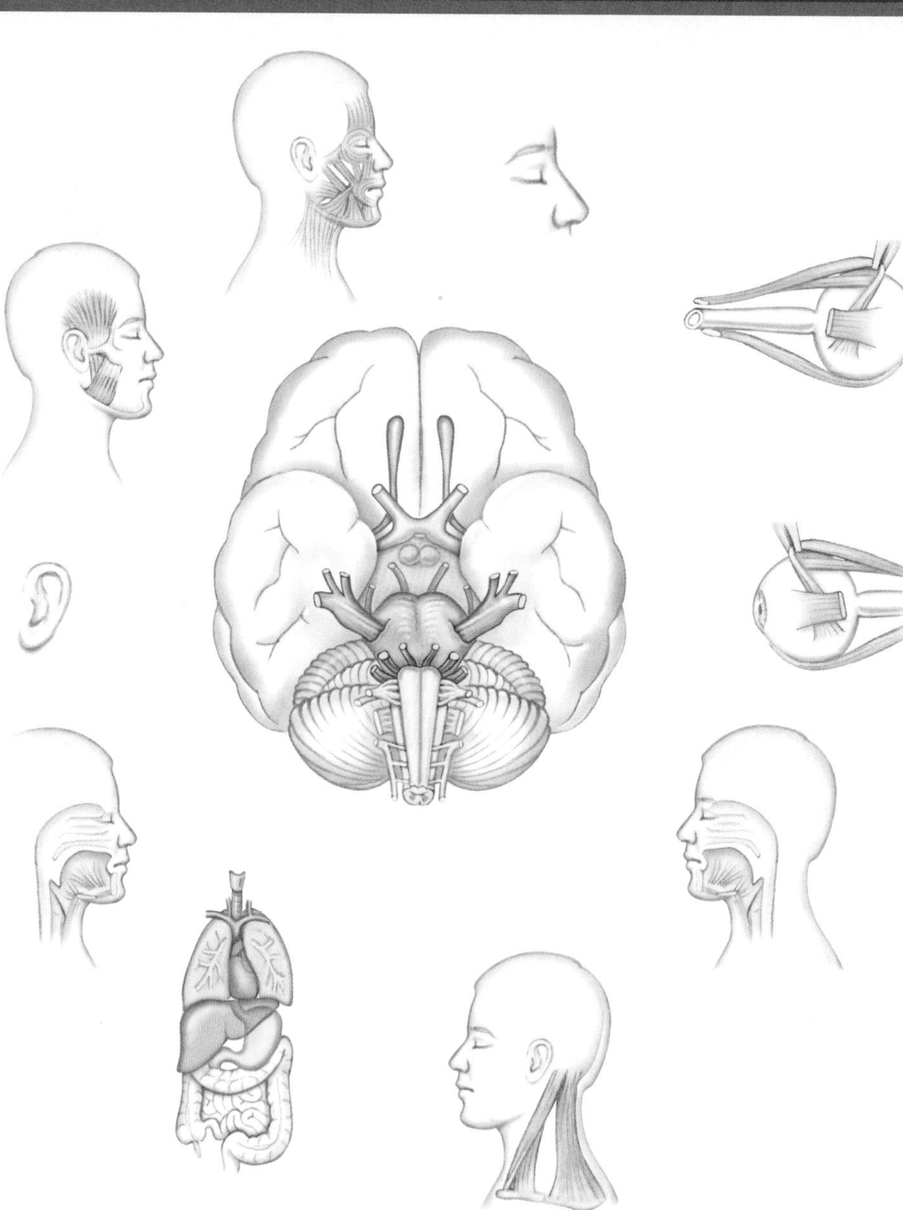

OBJECTIVES

ON COMPLETION OF THIS UNIT, YOU SHOULD BE ABLE TO:

- Briefly describe the nervous system.
- Describe the primary functions of the various organs or structures of the nervous system.
- Identify and give the meaning of the primary word elements for this unit.
- Analyze, build, spell, and pronounce selected medical words.
- List the cranial nerves and functions.
- Describe the major regions of the brain and their functions.
- Describe the spinal cord and its functions.
- List the warning signs of a stroke.
- Describe selected symptoms of a cerebrovascular accident (CVA).
- Describe selected diseases/disorders of the nervous system.
- Describe selected drugs that are used for nervous system diseases or disorders.
- Define selected abbreviations that pertain to the nervous system.
- Describe stroke, giving three names for stroke, how it is classified, and the most important risk factors for a stroke.
- Complete the Case Study on Alzheimer's disease.
- Successfully complete the review section.

The nervous system is usually described as having two interconnected divisions: the CNS, or central nervous system, and the PNS, or peripheral nervous system. The CNS includes the brain and spinal cord. The PNS consists of the network of nerves and neural tissues branching throughout the body from 12 pairs of cranial nerves and 31 pairs of spinal nerves. See Figure 6–1.

There are two principal tissue types in the nervous system. These tissues are made up of neurons or nerve cells and their supporting tissues, collectively called neuroglia. Neurons are the structural and functional units of the nervous system. These cells are specialized conductors of impulses that enable the body to interact with its internal and external environments.

Motor Neurons

Motor neurons cause contractions in muscles and secretions from glands and organs. They also act to inhibit the actions of glands and organs, thereby controlling most of the body's functions. Motor neurons may be described as being efferent processes as they transmit impulses away from the neural cell body to the muscles or organs to be innervated. Motor neurons consist of a nucleated cell body with protoplasmic processes extending away from it in several directions. These processes are known as the axon and dendrites. Most axons are long and are covered with a fatty substance, the myelin sheath, that acts as an insulator and increases the

TECH LINK

CD-ROM Use the CD-ROM enclosed with your textbook to gain additional reinforcement through interactive word building exercises, spelling games, labeling activities, and additional quizzes.

www.prenhall.com/rice Use the above address to access the free, interactive Companion Website created specifically for this textbook. Get hints, instant feedback, and textbook references to chapter-related multiple choice and true/false questions, fill-in-the-blank, and labeling exercises. In addition, you will find an audio glossary, and essay questions.

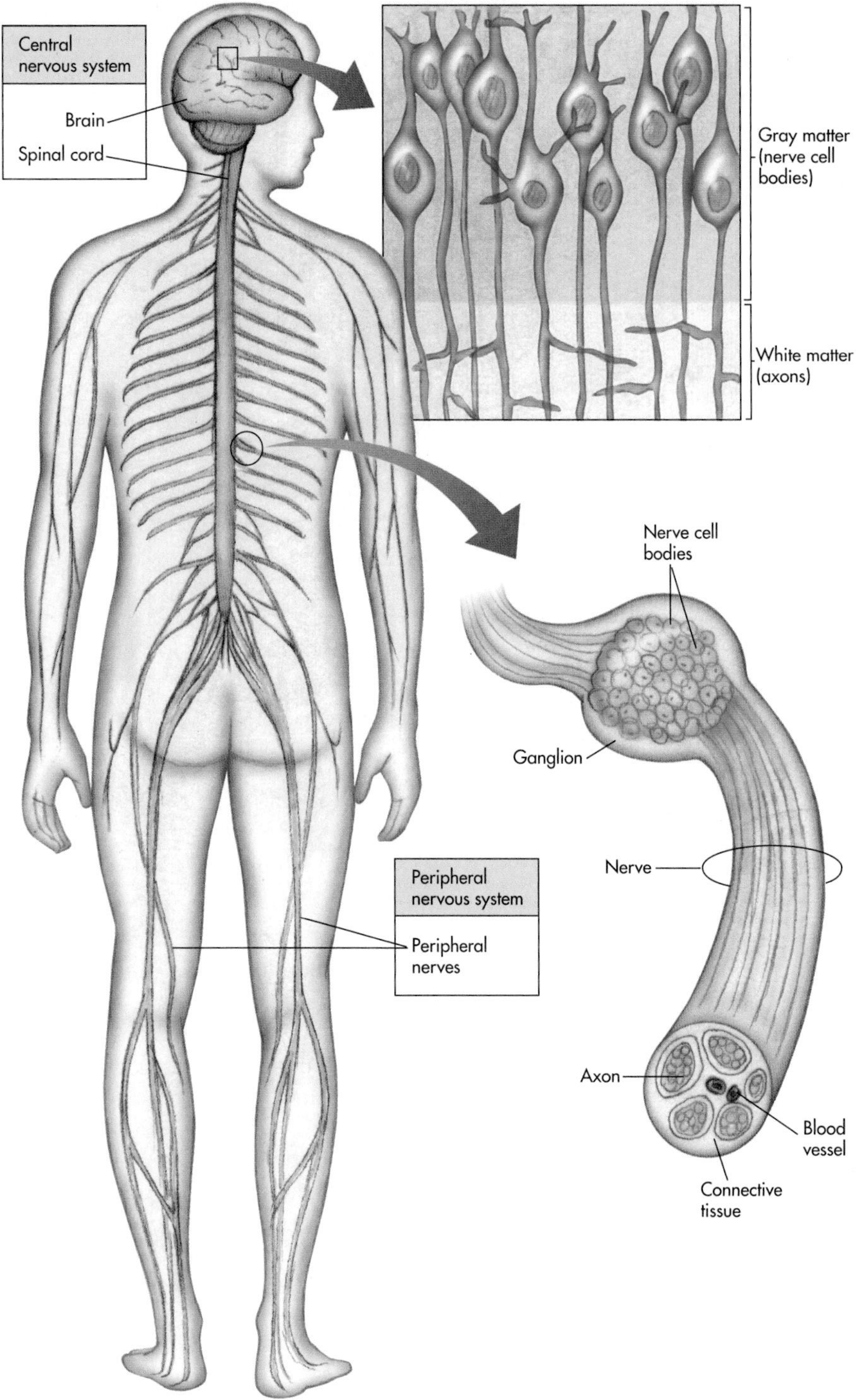

FIGURE 6–1

The nervous system is described as having two interconnected divisions: the central nervous system (CNS) consisting of the brain and spinal cord, and the peripheral nervous system (PNS) consisting of peripheral nerves.

transmission velocity of the nerve fiber it surrounds. Axons may be as long as several feet and reach from the cell body to the area to be activated. Dendrites resemble the branches of a tree, are short, or unsheathed, and transmit impulses to the cell body. Neurons usually have several dendrites and only one axon.

Sensory Neurons

Sensory neurons differ in structure from motor neurons because they do not have true dendrites. The processes transmitting sensory information to the cell bodies of these neurons are called peripheral processes, are sheathed, and resemble axons. They are attached to sensory receptors and transmit impulses to the central nervous system (CNS). In turn, the CNS may stimulate motor neurons in response to this sensory information. Sensory neurons are sometimes referred to as afferent nerves as they carry impulses to the cell body and the central nervous system.

Interneurons

Interneurons are sometimes called central or associative neurons and are located entirely within the central nervous system. They function to mediate impulses between sensory and motor neurons.

The terms nerve fiber, nerve, and tract are used to describe neuronal processes conducting impulses from one location to another.

Nerve Fiber

A nerve fiber is a single elongated process, usually a long axon or a peripheral process from a sensory neuron. Each peripheral nerve fiber is wrapped by a protective membrane called a sheath. There are two types of sheaths, myelinated (thick) and unmyelinated (thin), formed by accessory cells. Some nerve fibers have only the unmyelinated sheath or neurilemma composed of Schwann cells. Myelinated fibers have an inner sheath of myelin, a thick fatty substance, and an outer sheath, the neurilemma. Nerve fibers of the central nervous system (within the brain and spinal cord) do not contain Schwann cells, which are necessary for the regeneration of a damaged nerve fiber. Therefore, damage to fibers of the CNS is permanent, whereas damage to a peripheral nerve may be reversible.

Nerve

A nerve is a bundle of nerve fibers, located outside the brain and spinal cord, that connects to various parts of the body. Nerves are usually described as being afferent (conducting to the CNS) or efferent (conducting to muscles, organs, and glands). Some nerves contain a mixture of afferent and efferent fibers and are called mixed nerves. Nerves are also referred to as sensory (afferent) and motor (efferent).

Tracts

Groups of nerve fibers within the central nervous system are sometimes referred to as tracts when they have the same origin, function, and termination. The spinal cord contains afferent sensory tracts ascending to the brain and efferent motor tracts descending from the brain. The brain itself contains numerous tracts, the largest of which is the corpus callosum joining the left and right hemispheres of the cerebrum.

The central nervous system receives impulses from throughout the body, processes information, and responds with an appropriate action. The network of nerves branching throughout the body from the brain and spinal cord is known as the peripheral nervous system (PNS). A division of the PNS, the autonomic nervous system, controls involuntary bodily functions such as sweating and arterial blood pressure. See Table 6–1.

TABLE 6-1 THE NERVOUS SYSTEM

Organ/Structure	Primary Functions
Neurons (nerve cells)	Structural and functional units of the nervous system. Specialized conductors of impulses that enable the body to interact with its internal and external environments.
Neuroglia	Supporting tissue
Nerve Fibers and Tracts	Conduct impulses from one location to another
Central Nervous System	Receives impulses from throughout the body, processes the information, and responds with an appropriate action
Brain	Governs sensory perception, emotions, consciousness, memory, and voluntary movements
Spinal cord	Conducts sensory impulses to the brain; conducts motor impulses from the brain to body parts; and serves as a reflex center for impulses entering and leaving the spinal cord without involvement of the brain
Peripheral Nervous System	Links the central nervous system with other parts of the body
Cranial nerves (12 pairs)	Provide sensory input and motor control, or a combination of these
Spinal nerves (31 pairs)	Carry impulses to the spinal cord and to muscles, organs, and glands
Autonomic Nervous System	Controls involuntary bodily functions such as sweating and arterial blood pressure

PRIMARY WORD ELEMENTS

The following word elements (prefixes, roots, combining forms, and suffixes) will be used to build medical terms that relate to this unit. Please commit these to memory.

PREFIX

PREFIX	MEANING	PREFIX	MEANING
a, an	without, lack of	**macro**	large
dys	bad, difficult, painful	**micro**	small
hemi	half	**quadri**	four
hydro	water		

COMBINING FORM

COMBINING FORM / ROOT	MEANING	COMBINING FORM / ROOT	MEANING
atel	imperfect	**hem / o**	blood
cephal	head	**log**	study
cephal / o	head	**mening**	membrane (meninges)
cerebell	little brain	**mening / o**	membrane (meninges)
cerebr / o	cerebrum	**myel**	spinal cord
crani / o	skull	**myel / o**	spinal cord
electr / o	electricity	**neur**	nerve
encephal	brain	**neur / o**	nerve
encephal / o	brain		
fibr / o	fiber		

COMBINING FORM / ROOT	MEANING	COMBINING FORM / ROOT	MEANING
pneum / o	lung, air	**psych**	mind
poli / o	gray	**psych / o**	mind
		spin	spine

SUFFIX

SUFFIX	MEANING	SUFFIX	MEANING
-al, -ar, -us	pertaining to	**-oma**	tumor
-algia	pain	**-opsia**	eye, vision
-asthenia	weakness	**-paresis**	weakness
-cele	hernia, tumor, swelling	**-pathy**	disease
-ectomy	surgical excision	**-phagia**	to eat
-graphy	recording	**-phasia**	to speak
-ia, -osis, -y	condition of	**-plasty**	surgical repair
-ist	one who specializes	**-plegia**	stroke, paralysis
-itis	inflammation	**-praxia**	action
-logy	study of	**-taxia**	order
-malacia	softening	**-tome**	instrument to cut
-meter	instrument to measure	**-tomy**	incision

ANSWER COLUMN

6.1 ____________ is the study of the nervous system.
The word elements used to build this term are:
____________ combining form that means nerve
____________ suffix that means study of

neurology (noo **ROL** oh jee)
neur / o
-logy

6.2 A ____________ is a physician who specializes in the study of the nervous system.

neurologist (noo **RAL** oh jist)

6.3 ____________ is a speciality area that is concerned with the surgical approach to treating conditions of the nervous system. The physician who specializes in this area is called a **neurosurgeon.**

neurosurgery (noo roh **SIR** jer ee)

6.4 The brain and spinal cord constitute the ____________ nervous system.

central (**SEN** tral)

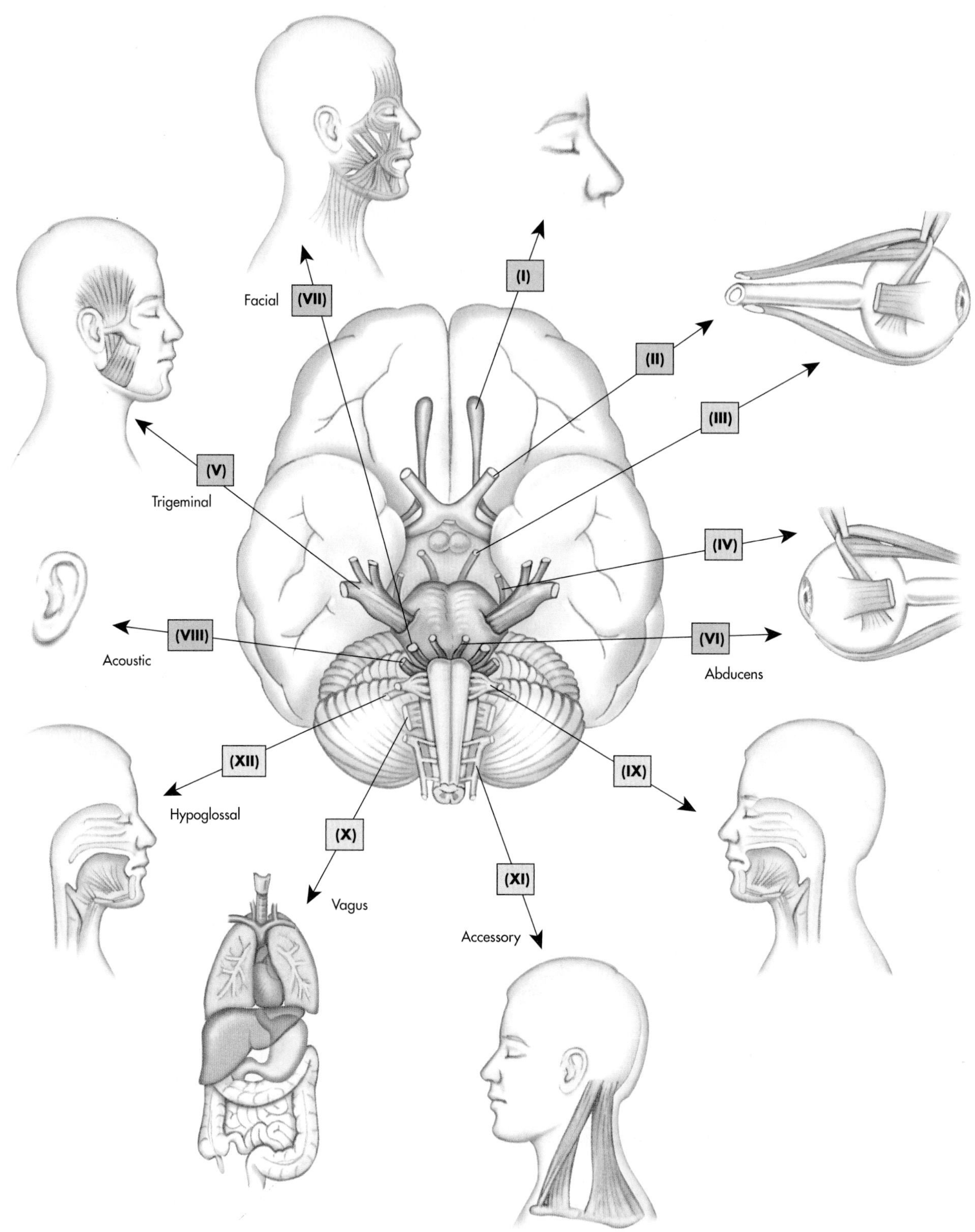

FIGURE 6–2
The relationship of the 12 cranial nerves to specific regions of the brain.

TABLE 6–2 CRANIAL NERVES AND FUNCTIONS

Nerve/Number	Function
Olfactory (I)	Sense of smell
Optic (II)	Vision
Oculomotor (III)	Motor impulses to four of the six external muscles of the eye and to the muscle that raises the eyelid
Trochlear (IV)	Motor impulses to control the superior oblique muscle of the eyeball
Trigeminal (V)	Provide sensory input from the face, nose, mouth, forehead, and top of the head; motor fibers to the muscles of the jaw (chewing)
Abducens (VI)	Conducts motor impulses to the lateral rectus muscle of the eyeball.
Facial (VII)	Controls the muscles of the face and scalp; controls the lacrimal glands of the eye and the submandibular and sublingual salivary glands; input from the tongue for the sense of taste
Acoustic (VIII)	Input for hearing and equilibrium
Glossopharyngeal (IX)	General sense of taste; swallowing; control secretion of saliva
Vagus (X)	Controls muscles of the pharynx and larynx and of the thoracic and abdominal organs; swallowing, voice production, slowing of heartbeat, acceleration of peristalsis
Accessory (XI)	Control of the trapezius and sternocleidomastoid muscles, permitting movement of the head and shoulders
Hypoglossal (XII)	Control of the tongue; tongue movements

ANSWER COLUMN

6.5 The peripheral nervous system (PNS) consists of the network of nerves and neural tissues branching throughout the body from __________ pairs of cranial nerves and 31 pairs of spinal nerves. See Figure 6–2 and Table 6–2.

12

6.6 The combining form **neur / o** and the root **neur** mean nerve. Medical terms that begin with these word elements are:

__________ pain in a nerve or nerves	**neuralgia** (noo **RAL** jee ah)
__________ nervous weakness, exhaustion, prostration	**neurasthenia** (noor ass **THEE** nee ah)
__________ surgical excision of a nerve	**neurectomy** (noo **REK** toh mee)
__________ inflammation of a nerve or nerves	**neuritis** (noo **RYE** tis)
__________ tumor composed of nerve cells	**neuroma** (noo **ROH** mah)
__________ any nerve disease	**neuropathy** (noo **ROP** ah thee)
__________ an emotional condition or disorder	**neurosis** (noo **ROH** sis)
__________ a genetic disorder that affects cell growth of neural tissues	**neurofibromatosis** (noor oh fye broh mah **TOH** sis)

Answer Column

EXPLANATION FRAME

The nervous tissue of the brain consists of millions of nerve cells and fibers. The brain is the largest mass of nervous tissue in the body, weighing about 1380 grams in the male and 1250 grams in the female.

6.7 The combining form **encephal / o** and the root **encephal** mean brain. Medical terms that begin with or contain these word elements are:

		Answer
________	a congenital condition in which there is a lack of development of the brain	**anencephaly** (an en **SEFF** ah lee)
________	a congenital condition of imperfect development of the brain	**atelencephalia** (ah tel en she **FAY** lee ah)
________	the recording of the electrical activity of the brain	**electroencephalography** (ee lek troh en seff ah **LOG** rah fee)
________	inflammation of the brain	**encephalitis** (en seff ah **LYE** tis)
________	herniation of the brain via a congenital or traumatic opening in the skull	**encephalocele** (en **SEFF** ah loh seel)
________	any disease of the brain	**encephalopathy** (en sef ah **LOP** ah thee)
________	inflammation of the brain and its meninges	**meningoencephalitis** (meh ning goh en seff ah **LYE** tis)

EXPLANATION FRAME

When fully developed, the brain fills the cranial cavity and is enclosed by three membranes known collectively as the meninges. From the outside in, these are the dura mater, arachnoid, and pia mater.

6.8 The combining forms **mening / i** and **mening / o** and the root **mening** mean meninges.

Medical terms that begin with these word elements are:

		Answer
________	tumor of the meninges	**meningioma** (meh nin jee **OH** mah)
________	inflammation of the meninges	**meningitis** (men in **JYE** tis)

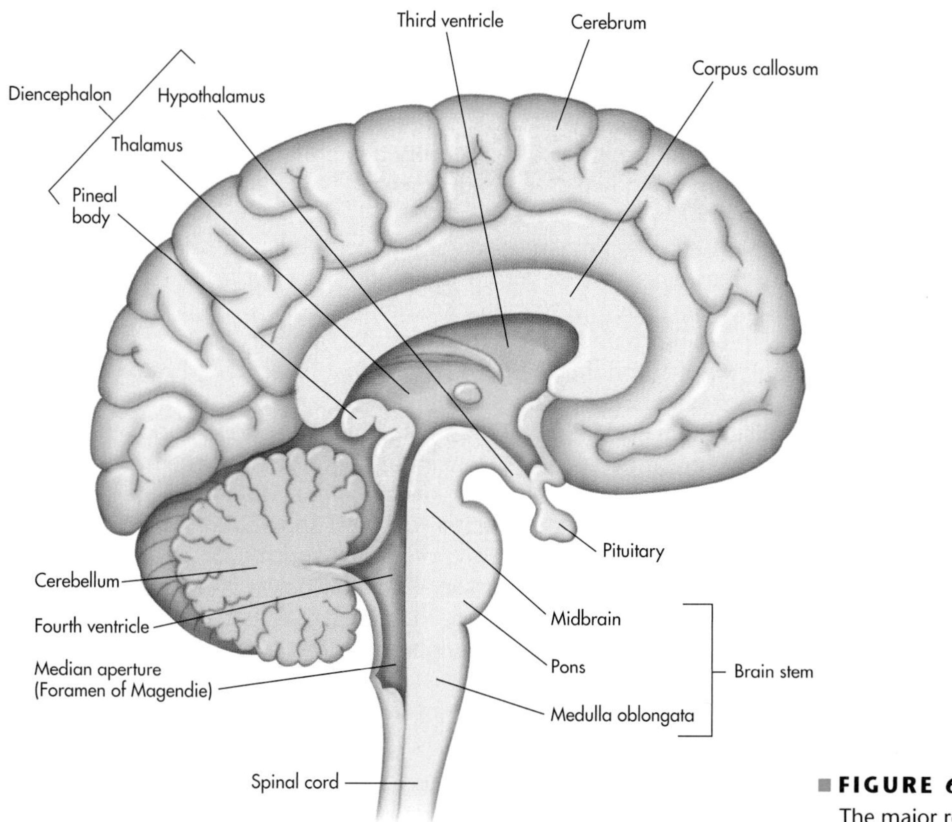

■ **FIGURE 6–3**
The major regions of the brain.

continued

		ANSWER COLUMN
____________	congenital herniation of the skull or spinal column in which the meninges protrude through an opening	**meningocele** (men **IN** goh seel)
____________	congenital herniation of the spinal cord and meninges through a defect in the vertebral column	**meningomyelocele** (men in goh my **ELL** oh seel)
____________	any disease of the meninges	**meningopathy** (men in **GOP** ah thee)
____________	a microorganism of the *Neisseria meningitidis* species, the causative agent of epidemic cerebral meningitis	**meningococcus** (meh ning goh **KOK** us)

EXPLANATION FRAME

The major regions of the adult brain are the cerebrum, diencephalon, midbrain, cerebellum, pons, and the medulla oblongata. The cerebrum represents seven eighths of the brain's total weight. It contains nerve centers governing all sensory and motor activity. See Figure 6–3 and Table 6–3.

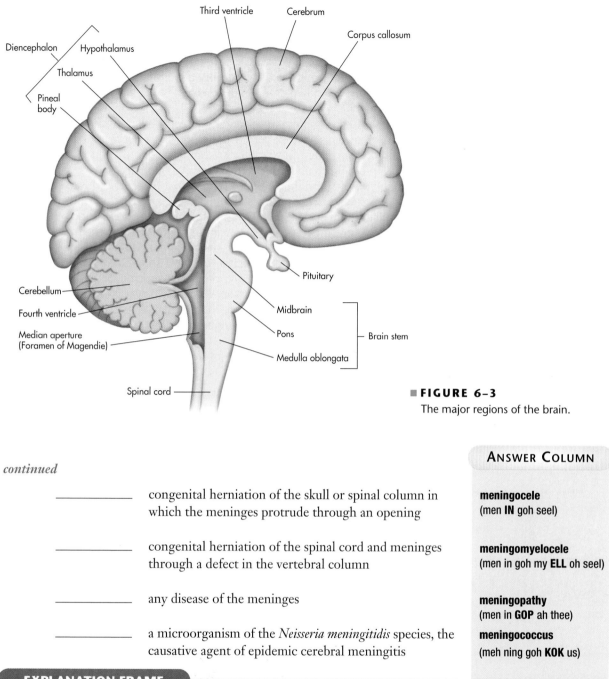

TABLE 6–3 MAJOR REGIONS OF THE BRAIN AND THEIR FUNCTIONS

Brain Area	Functions
Cerebrum	Governs all sensory and motor activity; sensory perception, emotions, consciousness, memory, and voluntary movements
Diencephalon	
Thalamus	Relay center for all sensory impulses (except olfactory) being transmitted to the sensory areas of the cortex. Also relays motor impulses from the cerebellum and the basal ganglia to motor areas of the cortex. Thought to be involved with emotions and arousal mechanisms
Hypothalamus	Principal regulator of autonomic nervous activity that is associated with behavior and expression. It also produces neurosecretions for the control of water balance, sugar and fat metabolism, regulation of body temperature, sleep-cycle control, appetite, and sexual arousal. Additionally, the hypothalamus produces hormones for the posterior pituitary gland
Midbrain	Two-way conduction pathway; relay center for visual and auditory impulses. Contains afferent and efferent pathways connecting major motor areas of the forebrain and hindbrain, thereby serving as a two-way conduction pathway. Also found in the midbrain are four small masses of gray cells known collectively as the corpora quadrigemina. The upper two, called the superior colliculi, are associated with visual reflexes. The lower two, or inferior colliculi, are involved with the sense of hearing
The Hindbrain	
Cerebellum	Coordination of voluntary movement
Pons	Links the cerebellum and medulla to higher cortical areas; two-way conduction pathway between areas of the brain and other areas of the body; influences respiration
Medulla oblongata	Cardiac, respiratory, and vasomotor control center. Regulation and control of breathing, swallowing, coughing, sneezing, and vomiting. Also regulates arterial blood pressure, thereby exerting control over the circulation of blood

ANSWER COLUMN

6.9 The ___________ ___________ regulates and controls breathing, swallowing, coughing, sneezing, and vomiting. It also controls arterial blood pressure and circulation of the blood.

medulla oblongata (meh **DULL** ah ob long **GAH** tah)

6.10 The combining form **cerebell / o** and the root **cerebell** mean little brain. *The cerebellum is part of the hindbrain and plays an important role in coordination of voluntary muscular movement.*

Medical terms that begin with these word elements are:

___________ pertaining to the cerebellum

cerebellar (ser eh **BELL** ar)

___________ inflammation of the cerebellum

cerebellitis (ser eh bell **EYE** tis)

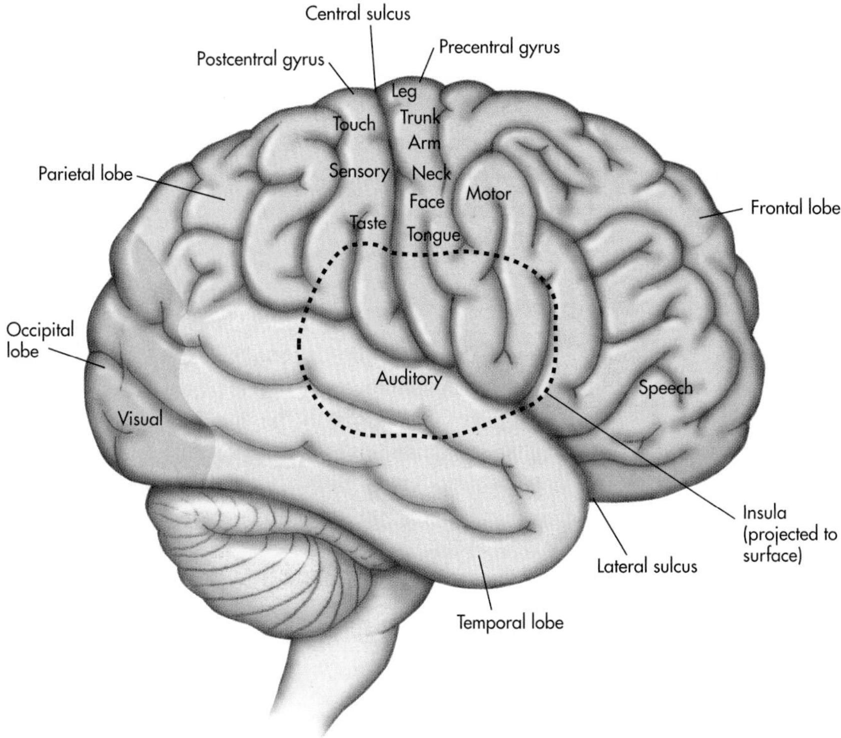

FIGURE 6–4
The brain, its lobes, and principal sulci. The location of certain sensory and motor areas are shown.

ANSWER COLUMN

EXPLANATION FRAME

The cerebral cortex is divided into lobes as a means of identifying certain locations. These lobes correspond to the overlying bones of the skull and are the frontal, parietal, temporal, and occipital lobes. See Figure 6–4.

6.11 The brain's major motor area is located in the __________ lobe.

frontal (FRUN tal)

6.12 The __________ lobe contains centers for sensory input from all parts of the body.

parietal (pah **RYE** eh tal)

6.13 The __________ lobe contains the centers for auditory and language input.

temporal (TEM por al)

Answer Column

6.14 The __________ lobe is considered to be the primary sensory area for vision.

occipital (ock **SIP** ih tal)

6.15 The combining form **cerebr / o** means cerebrum.
Medical terms that begin with **cerebr / o** are:

__________ softening of the cerebrum

cerebromalacia (ser ee broh mah **LAY** she ah)

__________ pertaining to the cerebrum and spinal cord

cerebrospinal (ser eh broh **SPY** nal)

EXPLANATION FRAME

The head is the superior part of the body that contains the brain and the organs of special senses. The skull is the bony framework of the head, composed of 8 cranial bones, the 14 bones of the face, and the teeth. It is also known as the cranium.

6.16 The combining form **cephal / o** and the root **cephal** mean head.
Medical terms that begin with or contain these word elements are:

__________ head pain; headache

cephalalgia (seff ah **LAL** jee ah)

__________ instrument used to measure intracranial blood pressure

cephalohemometer (sef ah loh hee **MOM** eh ter)

__________ pertaining to an increased amount of cerebrospinal fluid within the brain

hydrocephalus (high droh **SEFF** ah lus)

__________ an abnormal condition in which the head is large

macrocephalia (mak roh seh **FAY** lee ah)

__________ pertaining to a very small head

microcephalia (mye kroh seh **FAY** lee ah)

6.17 The combining forms **crani / o** and **cran / i** mean cranium (skull). Now, build some medical terms that use these combining forms plus the following suffixes: **-ectomy, -cele, -plasty,** and **-tomy.**

__________ surgical excision of a portion of the skull

craniectomy (kray nee **EK** toh mee)

__________ herniation of the brain substances through the skull

craniocele (**KRAY** nee oh seel)

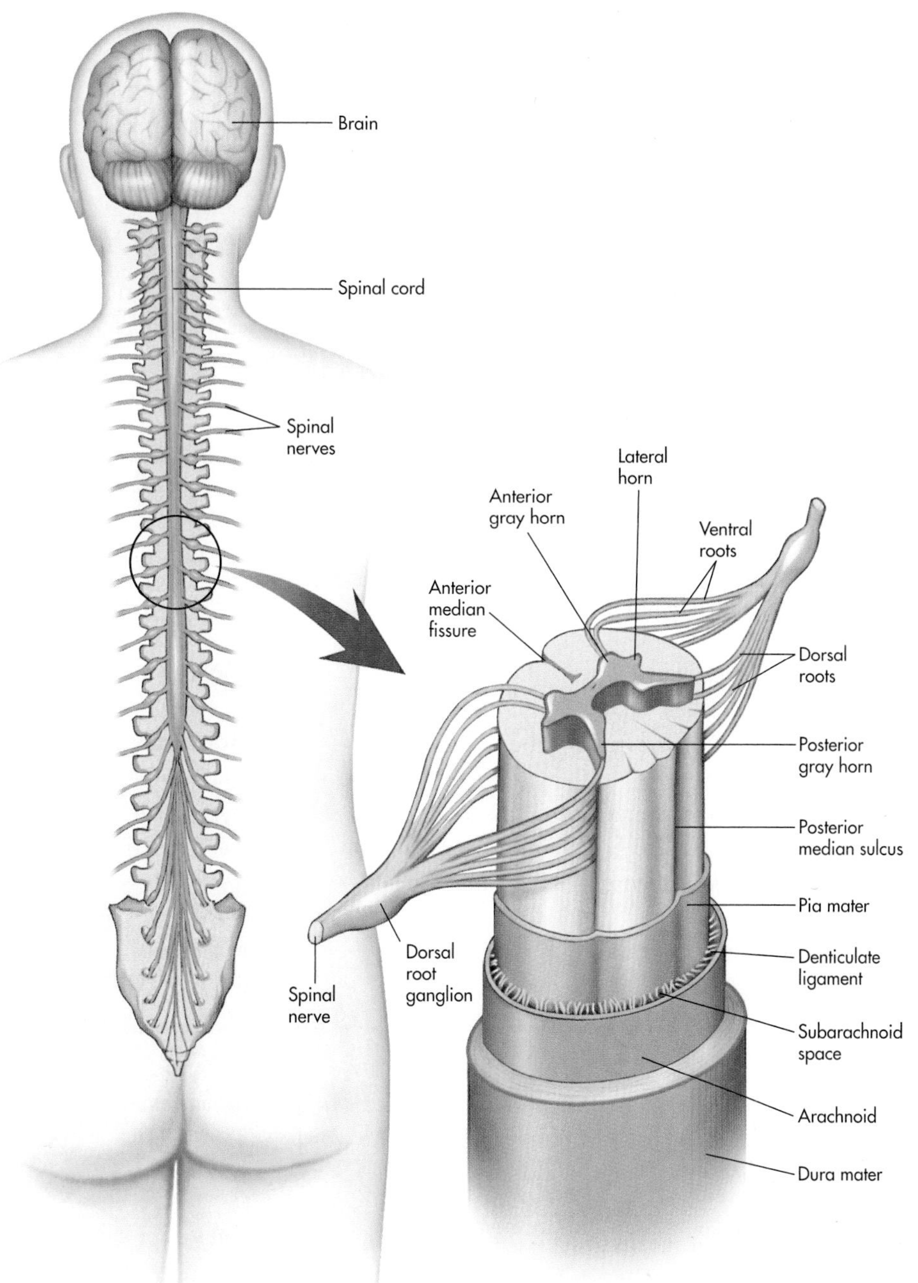

■ **FIGURE 6–5**
The brain, spinal cord, and spinal nerves. An expanded view of a spinal nerve is shown.

continued

		ANSWER COLUMN
__________	surgical repair of the skull	**cranioplasty** (**KRAY** nee oh plas tee)
__________	surgical incision of the skull	**craniotomy** (kray nee **OTT** oh mee)

ANSWER COLUMN

EXPLANATION FRAME

The spinal cord is an ovoid column of nervous tissue and is about 44 cm in length. It extends from the medulla to the 2nd lumbar vertebra in the spinal canal. All nerves to the trunk and limbs are issued from the spinal cord. The functions of the spinal cord are to conduct sensory impulses to the brain, to conduct motor impulses from the brain, and to serve as a reflex center for impulses entering and leaving the spinal cord without involvement of the brain. See Figure 6–5.

6.18 The combining form **myel / o** and the root **myel** mean spinal cord. Now, build some medical terms that use these word elements plus the following suffixes: **-itis, -plasia, -graphy, -pathy,** and **-tome**.

		Answer
________	inflammation of the spinal cord	**myelitis** (my eh **LYE** tis)
________	difficult or defective formation of the spinal cord	**myelodysplasia** (my eh loh dis **PLAY** zee ah)
________	X-ray recording of the spinal cord	**myelography** (my eh **LOG** rah fee)
________	any disease of the spinal cord	**myelopathy** (my eh **LOP** ah thee)
________	instrument used to cut or dissect the spinal cord	**myelotome** (**MY** eh loh tohm)

6.19 ________ is inflammation of the gray matter of the spinal cord. It is an acute viral infection that can be prevented by immunization. The word elements used to build this term are:

poliomyelitis (poh lee oh my ell **EYE** tis)

		Answer
________	combining form that means gray	**poli / o**
________	root that means spinal cord	**myel**
________	suffix that means inflammation	**-itis**

EXPLANATION FRAME

With a spinal cord injury, a part or parts of the body inferior to the point of injury may be affected. The damage to the cord usually leads to some degree of permanent disability. Types of disabilities may include **hemiplegia, paraplegia,** and **quadriplegia.**

Answer Column

6.20 __________ is paralysis that affects one half of the body. The word elements used to build this term are:

__________ prefix that means half

__________ suffix that means paralysis, stroke

hemiplegia (hem ee **PLEE** jee ah)

hemi

-plegia

6.21 __________ is paralysis of both legs and, in some cases, the lower portion of the body. The prefix **para** means beside.

paraplegia (pair ah **PLEE** jee ah)

6.22 __________ is paralysis of all four extremities. The prefix **quadri** means four.

quadriplegia (kwod rih **PLEE** jee ah)

EXPLANATION FRAME

A cerebrovascular accident (CVA), apoplexy, and stroke are terms that identify a condition in which there is a sudden loss of consciousness caused by an embolus, a thrombus, or a rupture of an artery in the brain.

STROKE'S WARNING SIGNS

- Sudden numbness or weakness of face, arm, or leg, especially on one side of the body
- Sudden confusion; trouble speaking or understanding
- Sudden trouble seeing in one or both eyes
- Sudden trouble walking, dizziness, loss of balance or coordination
- Sudden, severe headache with no known cause

6.23 The classic symptoms of a CVA are: hemiparesis, hemiplegia, impaired consciousness, severe headache, aphasia, dysphasia, and hemianopsia. Other symptoms may include dysphagia, dyskinesia, ataxia, and apraxia.

__________ slight paralysis that affects one side of the body

__________ paralysis that affects one half of the body

__________ lack of the ability to speak

__________ difficulty in speaking

hemiparesis (hem ee par **EE** sis)

hemiplegia (hem ee **PLEE** jee ah)

aphasia (ah **FAY** zee ah)

dysphasia (dis **FAY** zee ah)

ANSWER COLUMN

6.24 __________ is the lack of vision in half the field of vision in one or both eyes. The word elements used to build this term are:
__________ prefix that means half
__________ prefix that means lack of
__________ suffix that means eye, vision

hemianopsia (hem ee ah **NOP** see ah)
hemi
an
-opsia

6.25 __________ is a loss or lack of the ability to use objects properly. The word elements used to build this term are:
__________ prefix that means lack of
__________ suffix that means action

apraxia (ah **PRAK** see ah)
a
-praxia

6.26 __________ is a loss or lack of the ability to eat or swallow. The suffix **-phagia** means to eat.

aphagia (ah **FAY** jee ah)

6.27 __________ is a loss or lack of muscular coordination. The suffix **-taxia** means order.

ataxia (ah **TAK** see ah)

FOR REVIEW: PREFIXES AND SUFFIXES

a lack of
dys difficult
hemi half
-phagia to eat
-phasia to speak
-plegia stroke, paralysis
-praxia action
-opsia eye, vision
-taxia order

6.28 __________ is an eating disorder characterized by episodic binge eating with or without self-induced vomiting.

bulimia (boo **LIM** ee ah)

6.29 __________ __________ is a complex psychological disorder in which the individual refuses to eat or has an aberrant eating pattern.

anorexia nervosa (an oh **REK** see ah ner **VOH** suh)

Answer Column

6.30 The medical term for fainting is __________.
Fainting is a temporary loss of consciousness caused by a lack of blood supply to the brain.

syncope (SIN koh pee)

6.31 __________ is an unconscious state or stupor from which the patient cannot be aroused.

coma (COH mah)

6.32 __________ is a loss of consciousness, temporary or prolonged, caused by a blow to the head.

concussion (kon KUSH un)

EXPLANATION FRAME

Herpes zoster is an acute viral disease characterized by painful vesicular eruptions along the segment of the spinal or cranial nerves; also called shingles.

6.33 **True or False**. Another term for herpes zoster is shingles.

true

EXPLANATION FRAME

Amyotrophic lateral sclerosis (ALS) is a condition in which there is muscle weakness, atrophy, and spasticity caused by degeneration of motor neurons of the spinal cord, medulla, and cortex. It is also called Lou Gehrig's disease.

6.34 **True or False.** Amyotrophic lateral sclerosis is also called Lou Gehrig's disease.

true

6.35 __________ disease is a severe form of senile dementia that may be due to some defect in the neurotransmitter system. *There is cortical destruction that causes variable degrees of confusion, memory loss, and other cognitive defects.*

Alzheimer's (ALTZ high merz)

Answer Column

6.36 __________ is a disorder of cerebral function resulting from abnormal electrical activity or malfunctioning of the chemical substances of the brain.

epilepsy (**EP** ih lep see)

6.37 __________ __________ is a chronic disease of the CNS. *Plaques occur in the brain and spinal cord causing tremor, weakness, incoordination, paresthesia, and disturbances in vision and speech.*

multiple sclerosis (**MULL** tih pl skleh **ROH** sis)

6.38 __________ __________ is a chronic disease caused by a defect in the myoneural conduction system. *It is characterized by progressive muscular weakness, primarily of the face and neck. Secondarily, it may involve the muscles of the trunk and extremities.*

myasthenia gravis (my ass **THEE** nee ah **GRAV** iss)

6.39 __________ is a loss of sensation or an impairment of motor function; also called paralysis. *Bell's palsy is a facial paralysis due to a lesion of the facial nerve.*

palsy (**PAWL** zee)

6.40 __________ is a chronic disease of the nervous system. *It is characterized by a loss of equilibrium and by salivation, frustration, nausea, dryness of the mouth, and muscular tremors; also called paralysis agitans, shaking palsy.*

Parkinson's (**PARK** in sons)

6.41 __________ syndrome is an acute disease that causes edema of the brain and increased intracranial pressure, hypoglycemia, and fatty infiltration of the liver and other vital organs. *It occurs in children and has a relationship to aspirin administration. Children should not be given aspirin for acute febrile illnesses.*

Reye's (**RISE**)

6.42 __________ is severe pain along the course of the sciatic nerve.

sciatica (sigh **AT** ih kah)

6.43 __________ a chronic condition consisting of recurrent attacks of drowsiness and sleep during the daytime.

narcolepsy (**NAR** koh lep see)

ANSWER COLUMN

EXPLANATION FRAME

Psychiatry is the branch of medicine that deals with the diagnosis, treatment, and prevention of mental disorders.

6.44 The combining form **psych / o** and the root **psych** mean mind. Medical terms that begin with these word elements are:

		Answer
___________	a physician who specializes in the study, treatment, and prevention of mental disorders	**psychiatrist** (sigh **KIGH** ah trist)
___________	a method of obtaining a detailed account of past and present mental and emotional experiences and repressions	**psychoanalysis** (sigh koh an **NAL** ih sis)
___________	the science dealing with mental processes, both normal and abnormal, and their effects upon behavior	**psychology** (sigh **KALL** oh jee)
___________	an individual with a psychopathic personality	**psychopath** (**SIGH** koh path)
___________	a condition that refers to a mental disorder of such magnitude in which there is a personality disintegration and loss of contact with reality	**psychosis** (sigh **KOH** sis)
___________	pertaining to the relationship of the mind and body	**psychosomatic** (sigh koh soh **MAT** ik)
___________	a drug that affects psychic function, behavior, or experience	**psychotropic** (sigh koh **TROP** ik)

EXPLANATION FRAME

Drugs that are generally used for nervous system diseases and disorders include analgesics, analgesics-antipyretics, sedatives and hypnotics, antiparkinsonism drugs, anticonvulsants, and anesthetics.

6.45 ___________ relieve pain without causing loss of consciousness.

analgesics (an al **JEE** ziks)

6.46 Analgesics- ___________ act to relieve pain and reduce fever.

antipyretics (an tih pye **RET** iks)

6.47 ___________ are used to produce a calming effect without causing sleep.

sedatives (**SED** ah tivs)

6.48 ___________ are used to produce sleep.

hypnotics (hip **NOT** iks)

Answer Column

6.49 ___________ drugs exert an inhibitory effect upon the parasympathetic nervous system.

antiparkinsonian
(an tih par kin **SOH** nee an)

6.50 ___________ inhibit the spread of seizure activity in the motor cortex.

anticonvulsants
(an tih kon **VULL** sants)

6.51 ___________ are used to produce loss of sensation, muscle relaxation, and/or complete loss of consciousness.

anesthetics
(an ess **THET** iks)

6.52 ABBREVIATIONS

Write in the correct abbreviation for the following:

___________	Alzheimer's disease	**AD**
___________	amyotrophic lateral sclerosis	**ALS**
___________	central nervous system	**CNS**
___________	cerebral palsy	**CP**
___________	computerized tomography	**CT**
___________	cerebrovascular accident (stroke)	**CVA**
___________	electroencephalogram	**EEG**
___________	multiple sclerosis	**MS**
___________	positron emission tomography	**PET**
___________	peripheral nervous system	**PNS**
___________	transient ischemic attacks	**TIAs**

EXPLANATION FRAME

TIAs are temporary episodes of impaired neurologic functioning due to a lack of blood flow to a portion of the brain. They are called "little strokes" and are often important signals of an impending CVA (stroke).

IN THE SPOTLIGHT

STROKE

A stroke may be referred to as a cerebrovascular accident (CVA), apoplexy, or a "brain attack."

A stroke occurs when the blood supply to a part of the brain is suddenly interrupted (ischemic) or when a blood vessel in the brain bursts, spilling blood into the spaces surrounding the brain cells (hemorrhagic). Thus, strokes are classified as ischemic or hemorrhagic. With an ischemic stroke the brain cells die from lack of oxygen. Ischemic strokes may occur because of atherosclerosis, carotid stenosis, carotid dissection, polycythemia vera, cardiogenic embolism, atrial fibrillation, congestive heart failure, heart attack, and severe migraine headaches.

Hemorrhagic strokes occur when blood vessels in the brain burst and release blood into the area around the brain cells. The blood then damages the brain cells. The products released when cells die cause swelling in the brain. Since the skull does not allow much room for expansion, this swelling can damage the brain tissue even further. Hemorrhagic strokes may occur because of hypertension, anticoagulants, hemophilia A or hemophilia B, thrombocytopenia, rupture of a cerebral aneurysm, sickle cell disease, arteriovenous malformation, head injuries, and eclampsia.

Stroke is the third leading cause of death in the United States, right after heart disease and cancer. A person's risk of stroke doubles each year after the age of 55. Strokes occur approximately twice as often in blacks and Hispanics as they do in whites and men have a 50% higher chance of stroke than women. Stroke seems to run in some families. Family members may have a genetic tendency for stroke or share a lifestyle that contributes to stroke. The most important risk factors for stroke are hypertension, heart disease, diabetes, and cigarette smoking. Other risks include heavy alcohol consumption, high blood cholesterol levels, illicit drug use, and genetic or congenital conditions. Some risk factors for stroke apply only to women. Primary among these are pregnancy, childbirth, and menopause.

CASE STUDY

Please read the following case study and then work frames 6.53–6.56. Write in your answer in the answer column. Check your responses with the answers provided at the end of frame 6.56.

A 68-year-old female was seen by a physician and the following is a synopsis of the visit.

PRESENT HISTORY: The husband states that he is very concerned about his wife. He has noticed that she has become confused and forgets where she puts things, and even puts things in the wrong place. Last Monday she put the iron in the freezer. The patient had very little to say about herself.

SIGNS AND SYMPTOMS: Chief Complaint: Confusion, memory loss, and inappropriate placing of iron in the freezer.

DIAGNOSIS: Alzheimer's disease. The diagnosis was determined by a complete physical examination, a medical history, neuropsychological testing, an electroencephalogram (EEG), and a computerized tomography (CT) scan.

TREATMENT: The patient was placed on EXELON 1.5 mg bid. The physician advised that if this dose is well tolerated after a minimum of 2 weeks of treatment, the dose may be increased to 3.0 mg bid. Subsequent increases may be 4.5 mg and then to 6.0 mg bid. The maximum dose is 6.0 mg bid (12 mg/day). EXELON is a cholinesterase inhibitor indicated for the treatment of mild to moderate dementia of the Alzheimer's type. While the precise mechanism of action is unknown, it is postulated that EXELON facilitates cholinergic neurotransmission by blocking the breakdown of acetylcholine. This may explain the beneficial effect of EXELON. In clinical studies, patients treated with EXELON showed significant benefit in global functioning (based on evaluation of activities of daily living, behavior, and cognition) when compared with placebo-treated patients. Although there is no cure for Alzheimer's, this medication may help slow the progression of symptoms of the disease and/or may help patients maintain function longer than they would without therapy. Management of a patient with Alzheimer's involves support and assistance to the patient and her family. For more information you may call the Alzheimer's Association at 1-800-272-3900.

PREVENTION: There is no known prevention.

6.53 Signs and symptoms of Alzheimer's disease include confusion, ____________ loss, and the inappropriate placing of an object.

6.54 For more information about Alzheimer's disease you can call 1-800- ____________.

6.55 The diagnosis was determined by a complete physical examination, a medical history, neuropsychological testing, an ____________, and a computerized tomography scan.

6.56 Management of Alzheimer's involves support and ____________.

CASE STUDY ANSWERS

6.53 memory

6.54 272-3900

6.55 electroencephalogram (EEG)

6.56 assistance

REVIEW A: WORD ELEMENTS

This review allows you to check your knowledge of some of the word elements presented in this unit. In the spaces provided, write the meaning of the word elements that are identified as **Prefix (P), Word Root (R), Combining Form (CF),** and/or **Suffix (S).**

MEDICAL WORD	*WORD ELEMENT*	*MEANING*
1. neurology	neur / o (CF)	__________
	-logy (S)	__________
2. craniectomy	cran / i (CF)	__________
	-ectomy (S)	__________
3. craniocele	crani / o (CF)	__________
	-cele (S)	__________
4. cranioplasty	crani / o (CF)	__________
	-plasty (S)	__________
5. myelitis	myel (R)	__________
	-itis (S)	__________
6. myelopathy	myel / o (CF)	__________
	-pathy (S)	__________
7. poliomyelitis	poli / o (CF)	__________
	myel (R)	__________
	-itis (S)	__________
8. hemiplegia	hemi (P)	__________
	-plegia (S)	__________
9. paraplegia	para (P)	__________
	-plegia (S)	__________
10. quadriplegia	quadri (P)	__________
	-plegia (S)	__________
11. hemianopsia	-hemi (P)	__________
	an (P)	__________
	-opsia (S)	__________
12. apraxia	a (P)	__________
	-praxia (S)	__________

REVIEW B: MEDICAL TERMS

Please place the correct letter from column II on the appropriate line of column I.

COLUMN I		COLUMN II
________	1. neuralgia	A. loss of muscular coordination
________	2. encephalitis	B. centers for auditory and language input
________	3. syncope	C. headache
________	4. frontal lobe	D. lack of the ability to eat or swallow
________	5. parietal lobe	E. inflammation of the brain
________	6. temporal lobe	F. fainting
________	7. occipital lobe	G. centers for sensory input
________	8. cephalalgia	H. pain in a nerve or nerves
________	9. aphagia	I. brain's major motor area
________	10. ataxia	J. area for vision

REVIEW C: DISEASES AND DISORDERS

Please provide the correct disease or disorder for each of the following descriptions.

1. ________ is an unconscious state or stupor from which the patient cannot be aroused.
2. ________ is loss of consciousness caused by a blow to the head.
3. ________ is a severe form of senile dementia.
4. ________ is an acute disease that causes edema of the brain. It occurs in children.
5. ________ is severe pain along the course of the sciatic nerve.

REVIEW D: UNSCRAMBLE THE WORDS

Unscramble the following medical terms and place the correct term on the line directly across from the scrambled word.

1. alentrc ________
2. bellcerera ________
3. poraltem ________
4. hasiapa ________
5. epsypile ________
6. yslap ________
7. kinparson's ________
8. catiaisc ________

REVIEW E: DRUGS USED FOR THE NERVOUS SYSTEM

Please provide the correct answer for each of the following descriptions.

1. ____________ are used to produce a calming effect without causing sleep.
2. ____________ are used to produce sleep.
3. ____________ inhibit the spread of seizure activity in the motor cortex.
4. ____________ are used to produce loss of sensation and complete loss of consciousness.

REVIEW F: ABBREVIATIONS

Please provide the correct abbreviation and/or meaning for the abbreviation.

1. ____________ Alzheimer's disease
2. ALS ____________
3. ____________ central nervous system
4. CVA ____________
5. ____________ electroencephalogram
6. MS ____________

7 SPECIAL SENSES: OTORHINOLARYNGOLOGY AND OPHTHALMOLOGY

LEARNING CONCEPTS

- the ears and the eyes
- essential terminology
- pronunciation guide
- word elements
- explanation frames
- hearing loss
- selected diseases and disorders
- drugs used for the special senses
- abbreviations
- in the spotlight: glaucoma
- case study: otitis media
- review exercises

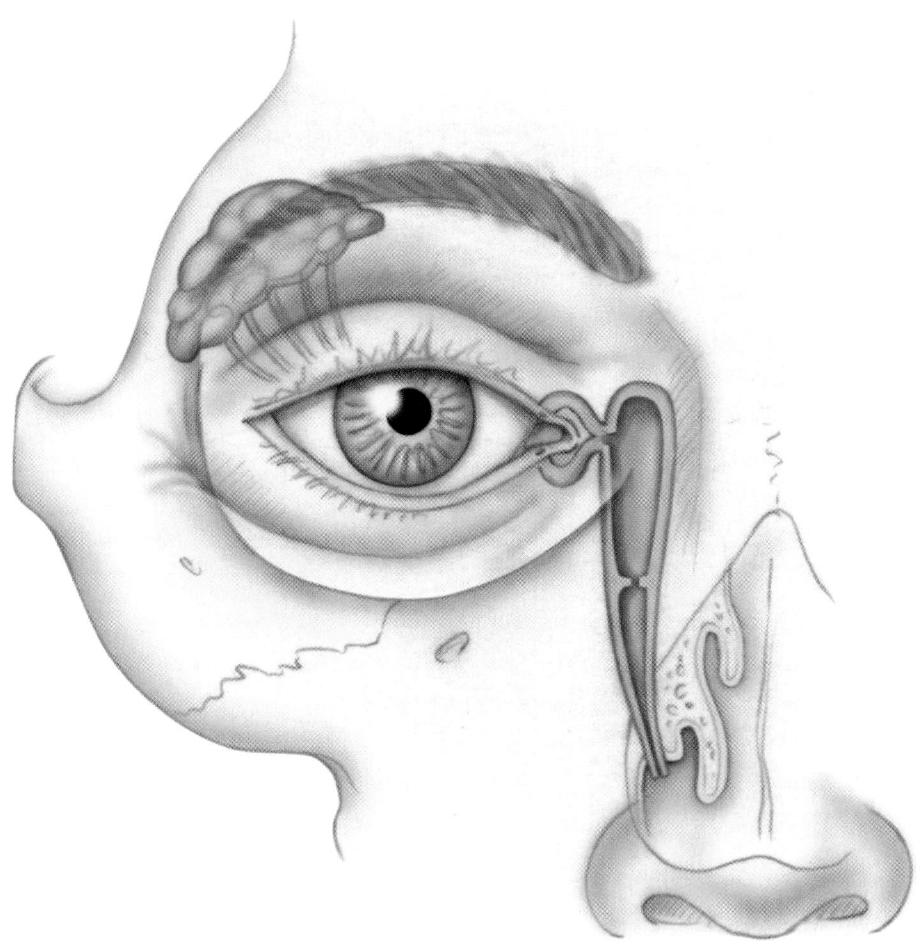

OBJECTIVES

ON COMPLETION OF THIS UNIT, YOU SHOULD BE ABLE TO:

- Briefly describe the ears and the eyes.
- Identify and give the meaning of the primary word elements for this unit.
- Analyze, build, spell, and pronounce selected medical words.
- Describe the primary functions of the various organs or structures of the ear.
- State when one should have his or her hearing checked.
- Describe selected drugs that are used for ear diseases or disorders.
- Define selected abbreviations that pertain to the ear.
- Describe the primary functions of the various organs or structures of the eye
- Describe glaucoma and list the risk factors associated with developing glaucoma.
- Describe selected drugs that are used for eye diseases or disorders.
- Define selected abbreviations that pertain to the eye.
- Describe selected diseases/disorders of the ears and the eyes.
- Complete the Case Study on Otitis Media Acute.
- Successfully complete the review section.

TECH LINK

CD-ROM Use the CD-ROM enclosed with your textbook to gain additional reinforcement through interactive word building exercises, spelling games, labeling activities, and additional quizzes.

www.prenhall.com/rice Use the above address to access the free, interactive Companion Website created specifically for this textbook. Get hints, instant feedback, and textbook references to chapter-related multiple choice and true/false questions, fill-in-the-blank, and labeling exercises. In addition, you will find an audio glossary, and essay questions.

THE EARS AND THE EYES

The ears are the site of hearing and equilibrium. They contain specially designed anatomic structures that receive sound vibrations, are sensitive to the force of gravity, and react to the movement of the head. These anatomic structures are connected to sensory areas of the brain by specialized fibers from the eighth cranial nerve. The ears are generally described as having three distinct divisions: the external ear, the middle ear, and the inner ear.

The eyes are composed of special anatomic structures that work together to facilitate sight. Light passes through the cornea, the pupil, the lens, and the vitreous body to stimulate sensory receptors (rods and cones) on the retina or innermost layer of the eye. Vision is made possible through the coordinated actions of nerves that control the movement of the eyeball, the amount of light admitted by the pupil, the focusing of that light on the retina by the lens, and the transmission of the resulting sensory impulses to the brain by the optic nerve.

PRIMARY WORD ELEMENTS

The following word elements (prefixes, roots, combining forms, and suffixes) will be used to build medical terms that relate to this unit. Please commit these to memory.

PREFIX

PREFIX	MEANING	PREFIX	MEANING
a	without, lack of	**endo**	within
dipl	double	**hyper**	above, excessive
em	in	**peri**	around

COMBINING FORM

COMBINING FORM / ROOT	MEANING	COMBINING FORM / ROOT	MEANING
acoust	hearing	**myring**	drum membrane
ambly	dull	**myring / o**	drum membrane
aud / i	to hear	**neur / o**	nerve
audi / o	to hear	**nyctal**	blind
auditor	hearing	**ocul, opt**	eye
aur	ear	**ophthalm / o, opt / o**	eye
blephar	eyelid	**ot**	ear
blephar / o	eyelid	**ot / o**	ear
cycl / o	ciliary body	**phac**	lens
dacry, dacry / o	tear	**phac / o**	lens
kerat	cornea	**presby**	old
kerat / o	cornea	**py / o**	pus
labyrinth	maze	**rhin / o, nas / o**	nose
labyrinth / o	maze	**scler**	hardening
lacrim	tear	**tinnit**	a jingling
laryng / o	larynx	**ton / o**	tone, tension
mast	breast	**tympan**	eardrum
myc	fungus		

SUFFIX

SUFFIX	MEANING	SUFFIX	MEANING
-al, -ic, -us	pertaining to	**-metry**	measurement
-algia, -dynia	pain	**-oid**	resemble, form
-cusis	hearing	**-opia, -opsia**	eye, vision
-ectomy	surgical excision	**-osis**	condition of
-gram	record	**-plasty**	surgical repair
-ist	one who specializes	**-ptosis**	drooping
-itis	inflammation	**-rrhea**	flow, discharge
-lith	stone	**-scope**	instrument
-logy	study of	**-tic**	pertaining to
-lymph	clear fluid	**-tome**	instrument to cut
-meter	instrument to measure	**-tomy**	incision

Answer Column

7.1 ____________ is the study of the ear, nose, and larynx. The word elements used to build this term are:

____________	combining form that means ear	**ot / o**
____________	combining form that means nose	**rhin / o**
____________	combining form that means larynx	**laryng / o**
____________	suffix that means study of	**-logy**

otorhinolaryngology (oh toh rye noh lair in **GOL** oh jee)

7.2 An ____________ is a physician who specializes in the study of the ear, nose, and larynx.

otorhinolaryngologist (oh toh rye noh lair in **GOL** oh jist)

EXPLANATION FRAME

The ear is generally described as having three distinct divisions: the external ear, the middle ear, and the inner ear. See Figure 7–1 and Table 7–1.

The **external ear** is the appendage on the side of the head consisting of the auricle, the external acoustic meatus or auditory canal, and the tympanic membrane or eardrum. The auricle collects sound waves that then pass through the auditory canal to vibrate the tympanic membrane that separates the external ear from the middle ear. The auditory canal is an S-shaped tubular structure about 2.5 cm long. Numerous glands line the canal and secrete cerumen or earwax to lubricate and protect the ear.

7.3 ____________ and ____________ are two medical terms that mean pertaining to the sense of hearing.

auditory acoustic (**AW** dih tor ee) (ah **KOOS** tik)

The word elements used to build these terms are:

____________	root that means hearing	**auditor**
____________	suffix that means pertaining to	**-y**
____________	root that means hearing	**acoust**
____________	suffix that means pertaining to	**-ic**

7.4 The combining forms **aud / i** and **audi / o** mean to hear.
Medical terms that begin with these word elements are:

____________	a record of hearing by audiometry	**audiogram** (**AW** dee oh gram)
____________	one who specializes in disorders of hearing	**audiologist** (aw dee **OL** oh jist)
____________	study of hearing disorders	**audiology** (aw dee **OL** oh jee)
____________	an instrument used to measure hearing	**audiometer** (aw dee **OM** eh ter)

TABLE 7-1 SPECIAL SENSES: THE EAR

Organ/Structure	Primary Functions
The External Ear	
Auricle (pinna)	Collects and directs sound waves into the auditory canal and then into the tympanic membrane
Auditory canal (external acoustic meatus)	Numerous glands line the canal and secrete earwax to lubricate and protect the ear
Tympanic membrane (eardrum)	Separates the external ear from the middle ear
The Middle Ear	
Contains the ossicles: malleus, incus, and stapes; has five openings; and is lined with mucous membrane	Transmits sound vibrations Equalizes external/internal air pressure on the tympanic membrane Exerts control over potentially damaging or disruptive loud sounds
The Inner Ear	
Cochlea	Contains the organ of Corti, the organ of hearing
Vestibule	Contains the utricle and saccule, membranous pouches containing perilymph. The utricle communicates with the semicircular canals and contains hair cell sensory receptors connected to fibers from the eighth cranial nerve. These hair cells react to the force of gravity and movement and are a part of the sense of equilibrium
The semicircular canals	Contain nerve endings in the form of hair cells that note changes in the position of the head and report such movement to the brain through fibers leading to the eighth cranial nerve

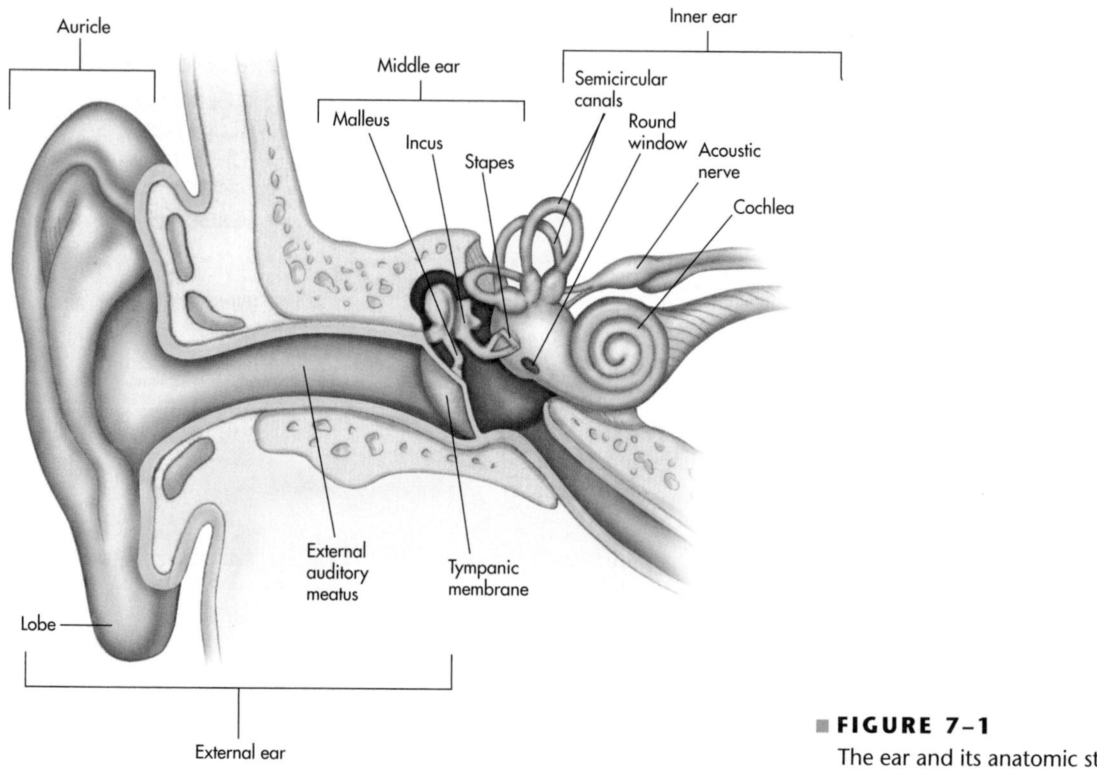

FIGURE 7–1
The ear and its anatomic structures.

continued

		Answer Column
___________	measurement of the hearing sense	**audiometry** (aw dee **OM** eh tree)
___________	capable of being heard	**audible** (**AW** dih bil)

FOR REVIEW: SUFFIXES

-gram record
-ist one who specializes
-logy study of
-meter instrument to measure
-metry measurement

7.5 The combining form **ot /o** and the roots **ot** and **aur** mean ear. Medical terms that begin with these word elements are:

___________	pertaining to the ear	**aural** (**AW** ral)
___________	pertaining to the ear	**otic** (**OH** tik)
___________	inflammation of the ear	**otitis** (oh **TYE** tis)
___________	pain in the ear, earache; also called **ot / algia**	**otodynia** (oh toh **DIN** ee ah)
___________	ear stone	**otolith** (**OH** toh lith)
___________	a fungus condition of the ear	**otomycosis** (oh toh my **KOH** sis)
___________	study of ear conditions with nerve complications	**otoneurology** (oh toh noo **ROL** oh jee)
___________	pertaining to the ear and pharynx	**otopharyngeal** (oh toh fair **IN** jee al)
___________	surgical repair of the ear	**otoplasty** (**OH** toh plass tee)
___________	flow of pus from the ear	**otopyorrhea** (oh toh pye oh **REE** ah)
___________	a hardening condition of the ear characterized by progressive deafness	**otosclerosis** (oh toh sklair **OH** sis)
___________	an instrument used to examine the ear	**otoscope** (**OH** toh scope)

FOR REVIEW: SUFFIXES

-al and **-ic** pertaining to
-itis inflammation
-dynia pain
-lith stone
-logy study of
-osis condition of
-plasty surgical repair
-rrhea flow
-scope instrument

ANSWER COLUMN

EXPLANATION FRAME

Beyond the tympanic membrane, is the **middle ear;** a tiny cavity in the temporal bone of the skull. This cavity contains three small bones or ossicles instrumental to the hearing process. These ossicles are the malleus, incus, and stapes. Sometimes referred to as the hammer, anvil, and stirrup because of their shapes, these bones mechanically transmit sound vibrations from the tympanic membrane, to which the malleus is attached, through the incus to the stapes, which attaches to a thin membrane covering a small opening, the oval window, that marks the beginning of the inner ear. During transmission, tympanic vibrations may be amplified as much as 22 times their original force.

7.6 The combining form **myring / o** and the root **myring** mean drum membrane.

Medical terms that begin with these word elements are:

		Answer
____________	surgical excision of the tympanic membrane	**myringectomy** (mir in **JEK** toh mee)
____________	surgical repair of the tympanic membrane	**myringoplasty** (mir **IN** goh plass tee)
____________	an instrument used to examine the eardrum	**myringoscope** (mih **RING** goh scope)
____________	an instrument used for cutting the eardrum	**myringotome** (mih **RING** goh tohm)
____________	incision of the tympanic membrane	**myringotomy** (mir in **GOT** oh mee)

7.7 The root **tympan** means eardrum.

Medical terms that begin with this word element are:

		Answer
____________	surgical excision of the tympanic membrane	**tympanectomy** (tim pah **NEK** toh mee)
____________	pertaining to the eardrum	**tympanic** (tim **PAN** ik)
____________	inflammation of the eardrum	**tympanitis** (tim pan **EYE** tis)
____________	surgical repair of the eardrum	**tympanoplasty** (tim pan oh **PLASS** tee)

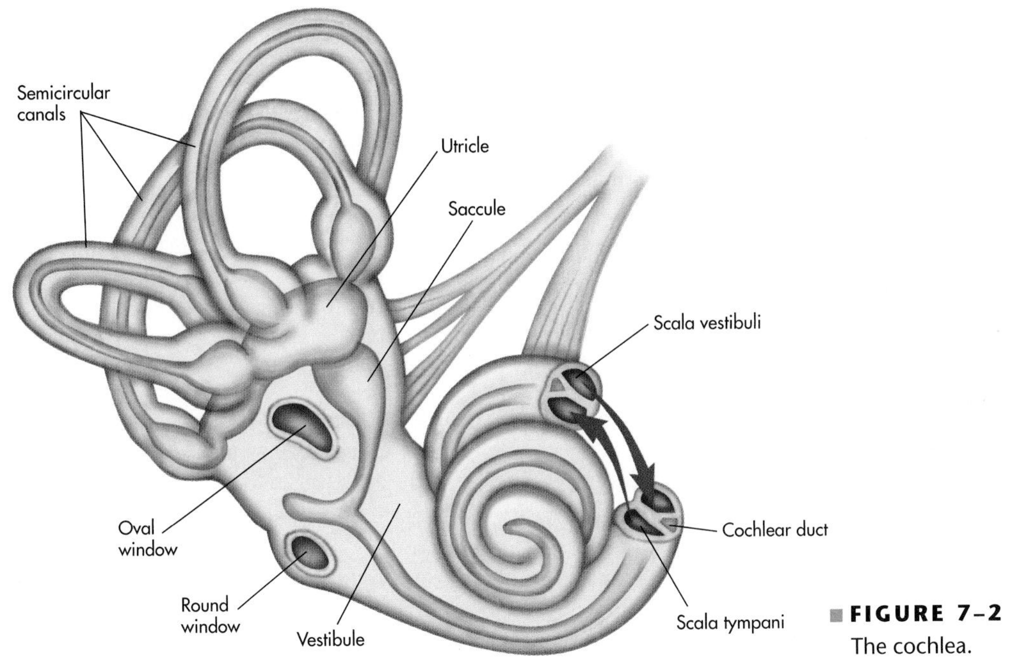

FIGURE 7–2
The cochlea.

ANSWER COLUMN

EXPLANATION FRAME

The **inner ear** consists of a membranous labyrinth or maze located within a bony labyrinth. These structures are called labyrinths because of their complicated shapes. The bony labyrinth, located in the temporal bone, consists of the cochlea, vestibule, and three semicircular canals. See Figure 7–2. Nerve endings in the form of hair cells located in various parts of the inner ear serve as receptors for the senses of hearing and equilibrium.

7.8 ____________ means a state of balance. In the inner ear, the semicircular canals are the site of the organs of balance.

equilibrium
(ee kwih **LIB** ree um)

7.9 The combining form **labyrinth / o** and the root **labyrinth** mean maze. Medical terms that begin with these word elements are:

____________ surgical excision of the labyrinth

____________ inflammation of the labyrinth

____________ incision of the labyrinth

labyrinthectomy
(lab ih rin **THEK** toh mee)
labyrinthitis
(lab ih rin **THIGH** tis)
labyrinthotomy
(lab ih rin **THOT** oh mee)

Answer Column

7.10 ____________ is a clear fluid contained within the labyrinth of the ear. The prefix **endo** means within and the suffix **-lymph** means clear fluid, serum.

endolymph (EN doh limf)

7.11 ____________ is the serum fluid of the inner ear. The prefix **peri** means around and the suffix **-lymph** means clear fluid, serum.

perilymph (PER ih limf)

7.12 The medical term for earwax is ____________.

Cerumen (earwax) is the yellowish substance secreted by the glands in the canal of the external ear. Cerumen lubricates and protects the ear.

cerumen (she **ROO** men)

EXPLANATION FRAME

Hearing declines naturally with age. Three fifths of all people over the age of 65 and 90% of those over age 80 have some degree of hearing impairment.

Hearing loss usually occurs gradually and one may not realize when the problem has progressed far enough to warrant wearing a hearing aid. A simple test to determine if you have a hearing loss is to rub your thumb and forefinger together about 6 to 8 inches from your ear. If you don't hear the characteristic scratching noise, you may have a problem.

The National Hearing Aid Society suggests you have your hearing checked if you:

- Turn up the volume of the television or radio to the point that others complain.
- Strain to hear conversation.
- Misunderstand words or ask people to repeat what they have said.
- Watch other people's face intently when you listen to them.
- Realize the effort to hear leaves you irritated and tired.
- Feel that people just don't speak as clearly as they used to.
- Experience ear infections, ringing in the ears, or dizziness.

7.13 ____________ is the medical term that means impairment of hearing in old age. The word elements used to build this term are:

____________ root that means old

____________ suffix that means hearing

presbycusis
(pres bih **KYOO** sis)

presby

-cusis

ANSWER COLUMN

7.14 ________ is the complete or partial loss of the ability to hear.

deafness (DEF ness)

7.15 A ringing or jingling sound in the ear is called ____________.
The word elements used to build this term are:

____________ root that means a jingling

____________ suffix that means pertaining to

tinnitus (tin **EYE** tus)

tinnit

-us

7.16 ____________ is a feeling of dizziness, an illusion of movement. *Vertigo may be caused by a lesion or other process affecting the brain, the eighth cranial nerve, or the labyrinthine system of the ear.*

vertigo (VER tih goh)

7.17 ____________ is a tumor-like mass filled with epithelial cells and cholesterol. *It can occur in the meninges, central nervous system, but it is most common in the middle ear and mastoid area.*

cholesteatoma
(koh lee stee ah **TOH** mah)

7.18 ____________ means formed like a breast. The mastoid process is located on the temporal bone. The root **mast** means breast and the suffix **-oid** means resemble, form. Other medical terms that begin with **mast** are:

____________ pain in the mastoid

____________ inflammation of the mastoid

____________ surgical excision of the mastoid

mastoid (MASS toyd)

mastoidalgia
(mass toyd **AL** jee ah)

mastoiditis
(mass toyd **EYE** tis)

mastoidectomy
(mass toyd **ECK** toh mee)

7.19 ____________ disease is a recurrent and progressive condition that affects the inner ear (labyrinth) and presents a group of symptoms. *Vertigo and dizziness are the classic symptoms, and the patient experiences nausea, tinnitus, and a sensation of fullness or pressure in the ears.*

Ménière's (may nee **ARZ**)

EXPLANATION FRAME

Drugs that are generally used for ear diseases and disorders include analgesics, analgesics-antipyretics, antibiotics, anticholinergics, and antihistamines.

ANSWER COLUMN

7.20 __________ relieve pain without causing loss of consciousness.

analgesics (an al **JEE** ziks)

7.21 Analgesics- __________ act to relieve pain and reduce fever.

antipyretics (an tih pye **RET** iks)

7.22 __________ are used to treat infectious diseases that are caused by bacteria.

antibiotics (an tih bye **OT** iks)

7.23 __________ are used to block the passages of impulses through the parasympathetic nerves.

anticholinergics (an tih koh lin **ER** jiks)

7.24 __________ are used to counteract the effects of histamine.

antihistamines (an tih **HISS** tah meens)

7.25 ABBREVIATIONS

Write in the correct abbreviation for the following:

		Answer
__________	auris dexter (right ear)	**AD**
__________	auris sinistra (left ear)	**AS**
__________	auris unitas (both ears)	**AU**
__________	bone conduction	**BC**
__________	ear, nose, and throat	**ENT**
__________	eye, ear, nose, and throat	**EENT**
__________	hearing distance	**HD**
__________	otitis media	**OM**
__________	otology	**oto**
__________	serous otitis media	**SOM**

7.26 __________ is the study of the eye.

The word elements used to build this term are:

__________ combining form that means eye

__________ suffix that means study of

ophthalmology (off thal **MALL** oh jee)

ophthalm / o

-logy

ANSWER COLUMN

7.27 An ___________ is a physician who specializes in the study of the eye. The word elements used to build this term are:

___________ combining form that means eye

___________ root that means study of

___________ suffix that means one who specializes

ophthalmologist (off thal **MALL** oh jist)

ophthalm / o

log

-ist

EXPLANATION FRAME

The eye is composed of special anatomic structures that work together to facilitate sight. The **external structures** of the eye are the orbit, the muscles of the eye, the eyelids, the conjunctiva, and the lacrimal apparatus. See Figure 7–3 and Table 7–2 The orbit is a cone-shaped cavity in the front of the skull that contains the eyeball. Connecting the eyeball to the orbital cavity are six short muscles that provide it with support and rotary movement. Each eye has a pair of eyelids that protect the eyeball from intense light, foreign particles, and impact. Lining the underside of each eyelid and reflected onto the anterior portion of the eyeball is a mucous membrane known as the conjunctiva. Included in the lacrimal apparatus are those structures that produce, store, and remove the tears that cleanse and lubricate the eye.

7.28 The combining forms **ophthalm / o** and **opt / o** and the roots **opt** and **ocul** mean eye. Medical terms that contain these word elements are:

___________ pertaining to the eye

___________ any eye disease

___________ an instrument used to examine the interior of the eye

___________ pertaining to the eye

___________ an instrument used to measure the strength of the muscles of the eye

ocular (**OK** you lar)

ophthalmopathy (off thal **MOP** ah thee)

ophthalmoscope (off **THAL** moh scope)

optic (**OP** tik)

optomyometer (op toh my **OM** eh ter)

7.29 The suffix **-opia** means eye, vision. Medical terms that end with this suffix are:

___________ dullness of vision

___________ a defect in the refractive powers of the eye in which images fail to come to focus on the retina

amblyopia (am blee **OH** pee ah)

ametropia (am eh **TROH** pee ah)

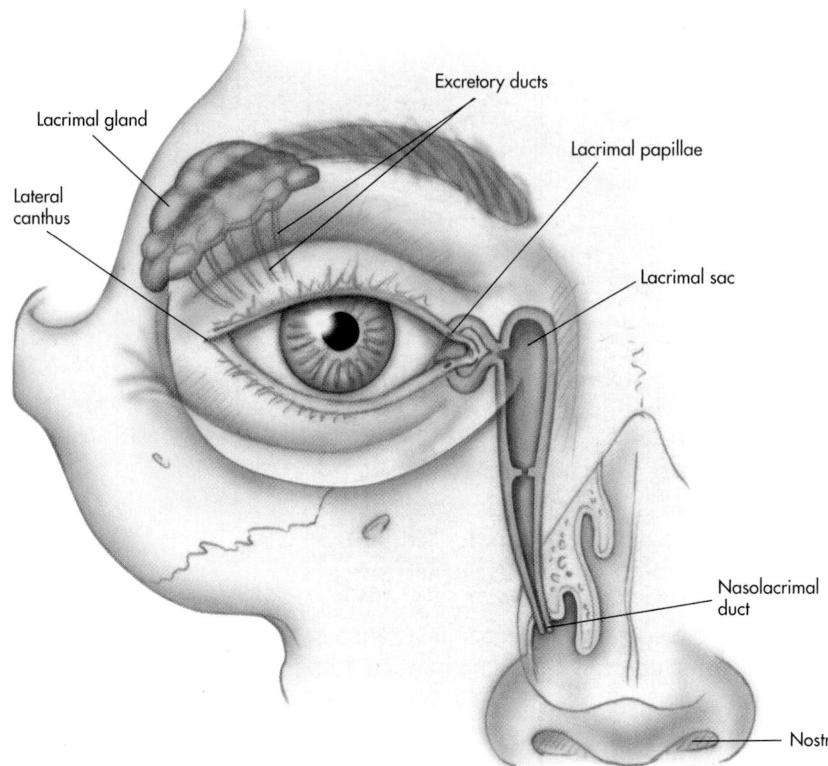

FIGURE 7–3
The lacrimal apparatus and its anatomic structures.

TABLE 7–2 SPECIAL SENSES: THE EYE

Organ/Structure	Primary Functions
The Orbit	Contains the eyeball. Cavity is lined with fatty tissue that cushions the eyeball and has several openings through which blood vessels and nerves pass
The Muscles of the Eye	Six short muscles provide support and rotary movement of the eyeball
The Eyelids	Protect the eyeballs from intense light, foreign particles, and impact
The Conjunctiva	Acts as a protective covering for the exposed surface of the eyeball
The Lacrimal Apparatus	Produces, stores, and removes tears that cleanse and lubricate the eye
The Eyeball	Organ of vision
Sclera	The outer layer known as the "white" of the eye consists of the cornea, which bends light rays and helps to focus them on the surface of the retina
Choroid	Pigmented vascular membrane that prevents internal reflection of light
Ciliary body	Smooth muscle forming a part of the ciliary body that governs the convexity of the lens. The ciliary body secretes nutrient fluids that nourish the cornea, the lens, and surrounding tissues
Iris	Colored membrane attached to the ciliary body. It has a circular opening in its center, the pupil, and two muscles that contract to regulate the amount of light admitted by the pupil
Retina	Innermost layer. Contains photoreceptive cells that translate light waves focused on its surface into nerve impulses
The lens	Sharpens the focus of light on the retina (accommodation)

continued

Answer Column

___________	double vision	**diplopia** (dip **LOH** pee ah)
___________	normal vision	**emmetropia** (em eh **TROH** pee ah)
___________	a defect known as farsightedness	**hyperopia** (high per **OH** pee ah)
___________	a defect known as nearsightedness	**myopia** (my **OH** pee ah)
___________	a defect known as night blindness	**nyctalopia** (nik tah **LOH** pee ah)
___________	farsightedness that occurs normally with aging	**presbyopia** (prez bee **OH** pee ah)

EXPLANATION FRAME

A surgical procedure that may be performed to correct nearsightedness (myopia) is called a radial keratotomy. Delicate spoke-like incisions are made in the cornea to flatten it, thereby shortening the eyeball so that light reaches the retina. Not all patients have their vision improved, and complications could lead to blindness.

7.30 The combining form **kerat / o** and the root **kerat** mean cornea. Medical terms that begin with these word elements are:

___________	inflammation of the cornea	**keratitis** (kair ah **TYE** tis)
___________	an instrument used to measure the curve of the cornea	**keratometer** (kair ah **TOM** eh ter)
___________	surgical repair of the cornea	**keratoplasty** (**KAIR** ah toh plas tee)
___________	incision of the cornea	**keratotomy** (kair ah **TOT** oh mee)

7.31 The combining form **blephar / o** and the root **blephar** mean eyelid. Medical terms that begin with these word elements are:

___________	inflammation of the edges of the eyelids	**blepharitis** (blef ah **RYE** tis)
___________	a drooping of the upper eyelids	**blepharoptosis** (blef ah rop **TOH** sis)
___________	a spasmodic contraction or twitching of the orbicularis oculi muscle due to eyestrain, nervous irritability, or habit spasm	**blepharospasm** (**BLEF** ah roh spazm)

ANSWER COLUMN

7.32	A __________ is a small, hard, painless cyst of a meibomian gland (one of the sebaceous follicles of the eyelids).	**chalazion** (kah **LAY** zee on)
7.33	A __________ is an inflammation of one or more of the sebaceous glands of the eyelid; also called hordeolum.	**sty, stye** (**STY**)
7.34	__________ means pertaining to tears. The word elements used to build this term are: __________ root that means tear __________ suffix that means pertaining to	**lacrimal** (**LAK** rim al) **lacrim** **-al**
7.35	The combining form **dacry / o** and the root **dacry** also mean tear. Medical terms that begin with these word elements are: __________ inflammation of the tear sac(s) __________ a tumor-like swelling caused by obstruction of the tear duct(s)	 **dacryocystitis** (dak ree oh sis **TYE** tis) **dacryoma** (dak ree **OH** mah)
7.36	__________ is a paralysis of the ciliary muscle. The word elements used to build this term are: __________ combining form that means ciliary body __________ suffix that means stroke, paralysis	**cycloplegia** (sigh kloh **PLEE** jee ah) **cycl / o** **-plegia**
7.37	__________ is inflammation of the conjunctiva caused by allergy, trauma, chemical injury, bacterial, viral, or rickettsial infection. The type called "pinkeye" is infectious and contagious.	**conjunctivitis** (kon junk tih **VYE** tis)

EXPLANATION FRAME

The eyeball, its various structures, and the nerve fibers connecting it to the brain make up the **internal eye**. The eyeball is the organ of vision. The three layers of the eyeball are the **sclera**, the **uvea**, and the **retina**.

The eyeball's outer layer is composed of the **sclera** or white of the eye and the cornea or anterior transparent portion of the eye's fibrous outer surface. The curved surface of the cornea is important in that it bends light rays and helps to focus them on the surface of the retina. The **uvea** is the middle layer, lying just below the sclera, and it consists of the iris, the ciliary body, and the choroid. The innermost layer or **retina** contains photoreceptive cells that translate light waves focused on its surface into nerve impulses. See Figure 7–4 and Table 7–2.

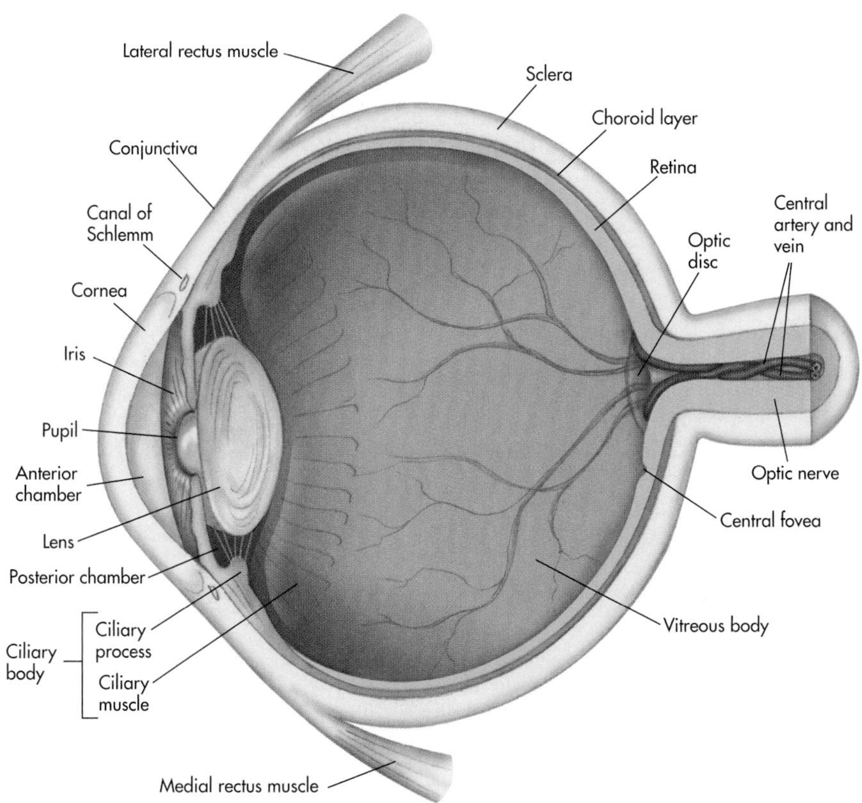

FIGURE 7–4
The eyeball and its anatomic structures.

Answer Column

7.38 The ____________ is a colored membrane attached to the ciliary body and suspended between the lens and the cornea in the aqueous humor. *It has a circular opening in its center, the pupil, and two muscles that contract or dilate to regulate the amount of light admitted by the pupil.*

iris (EYE ris)

7.39 The ____________ is the opening in the center of the iris.

pupil (PYOO pil)

7.40 The photoreceptive cells of the retina are the rods and ____________. *There are approximately 6 million cone cells grouped into a small area called the macula lutea. The cones are light-sensitive and receive color stimuli. There are approximately 120 million rods that are sensitive to dim light. They contain rhodopsin, a pigment necessary for night vision.*

cones (KOHNS)

7.41 The process of sharpening the focus of light on the retina is known as ____________.

accommodation (ah kom oh **DAY** shun)

EXPLANATION FRAME

The function of the lens is to sharpen the focus of light on the retina. This process, called accommodation, is reflexive in nature and combines changes in the size of the pupil, the curvature of the lens, and the convergence of the optic axes to keep the image in the same place on both retinae.

Accommodation occurs for both near and distant vision.

Visual acuity is the measurement of the acuteness or sharpness of vision. A Snellen eye chart may be used, and the patient reads letters of various sizes from a distance of 20 feet. Normal vision is 20/20. See Figure 7–5.

7.42 An opacity of the crystalline lens is called a ____________.

cataract (KAT ah rakt)

EXPLANATION FRAME

Opacity is the state of being opaque. Opaque means not transparent. With cataract(s), the lens become cloudy; therefore, light image cannot get through as easily and vision becomes faint and hazy. This condition usually develops over several years and most often occurs in adults past middle age.

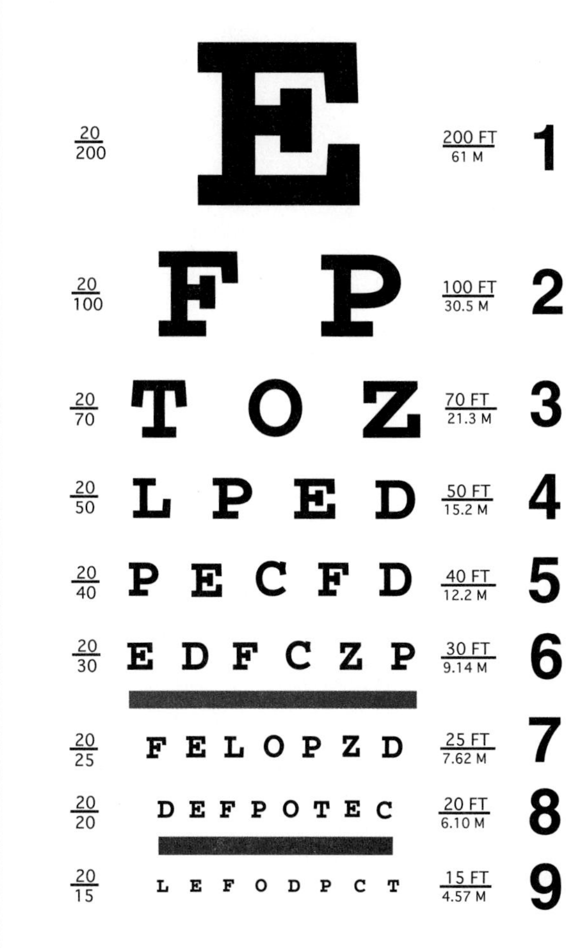

FIGURE 7–5
The Snellen eye chart. Individuals with normal vision can read line 8 of a full-sized chart at 20 feet (6.10 meters).

ANSWER COLUMN

7.43 The combining form **phac / o** means lens.
Medical terms that begin with this word element are:

__________ surgical destruction and removal of the lens in the treatment of a cataract or cataracts

__________ a condition of hardening of the lens

Answer: **phacolysis** (fah **KOL** ih sis); **phacosclerosis** (fak oh skleh **ROH** sis)

7.44 __________ is a disease characterized by increased intraocular pressure, which results in atrophy of the optic nerve and can cause blindness.

Answer: **glaucoma** (glau **KOH** mah)

Answer Column

7.45 A ____________ is an instrument that is used to measure intraocular pressure.

The word elements used to build this term are:

____________ combining form that means tone

____________ suffix that means instrument to measure

tonometer (toh **NOM** eh ter)

ton / o

-meter

7.46 An eye disorder in which optic axes cannot be directed to the same object is called ____________. Different forms of strabismus are: **esotropia** (eye turns inward; *crossed eye*), **exotropia** (eye turns outward; *walleye*), and **hypertropia** (upward deviation of the visual axis of one eye).

strabismus (strah **BIZ** mus)

EXPLANATION FRAME

Drugs that are generally used for diseases and disorders of the eye include those that are used for glaucoma, during diagnostic examination of the eye, and in intraocular surgery. Antibiotic, antifungal, and antiviral drugs are used in the treatment of eye infections.

7.47 ____________, cholinergics, and cholinesterase inhibitors are drugs that are used to treat glaucoma.

diuretics (dye yoor **RET** iks)

7.48 ____________ are agents that cause the pupil to dilate.

mydriatics (mid ree **AT** iks)

7.49 ____________ are used to treat infectious diseases. Those that are used for the eye may be in the form of an ointment, cream, or solution.

antibiotics (an tih bye **OT** iks)

7.50 ____________ agents are used in treating fungal infections of the eye, such as blepharitis, conjunctivitis, and keratitis.

antifungal (an tih **FUNG** gal)

7.51 ____________ agents are used to treat viral infections of the eye. *Stoxil, or Herplex (idoxuridine), is a potent antiviral agent used in the treatment of keratitis caused by the herpes simplex virus.*

antiviral (an tih **VYE** ral)

ANSWER COLUMN

7.52 ABBREVIATIONS

Write in the correct abbreviation for the following:

		Answer
____________	accommodation	**Acc**
____________	emmetropia	**EM**
____________	hypermetropia (hyperopia)	**HT**
____________	intraocular pressure	**IOP**
____________	left eye	**LE**
____________	myopia	**MY**
____________	near visual acuity	**NVA**
____________	oculus dexter (right eye)	**OD**
____________	oculus sinister (left eye)	**OS**
____________	oculi unitas (both eyes)	**OU**
____________	right eye	**RE**
____________	esotropia	**ST**
____________	visual acuity	**VA**
____________	visual field	**VF**
____________	exotropia	**XT**
____________	plus or convex	**+**
____________	minus or concave	**–**

IN THE SPOTLIGHT

GLAUCOMA

Glaucoma is an eye disease in which the normal fluid pressure inside the eyes slowly rises, leading to vision loss—or even blindness. There are several types of glaucoma. The most common is called primary open-angle glaucoma (POAG). This type of glaucoma accounts for 90% of all cases. Other types include closed-angle glaucoma, congenital glaucoma, and normal-tension glaucoma.

At the front of the eye, there is a small space called the anterior chamber. Clear fluid flows in and out of the chamber to bathe and nourish nearby tissues. In glaucoma, for still unknown reasons, the fluid drains too slowly out of the eyes. As the fluid builds up, the pressure inside the eye rises. Unless this pressure is controlled, it may cause damage to the optic nerve and other parts of the eye and loss of vision occurs.

It is estimated that 3 million Americans have glaucoma. At least half do not know they have it, because at first glaucoma usually has no symptoms. Untreated, glaucoma is a leading cause of irreversible blindness in the United States. In the later stages of the disease some symptoms may occur and these are:

- Loss of side vision (peripheral vision)
- Difficulty focusing on close work
- Seeing colored rings or halos around light
- Headaches and eye pain
- Frequent changes of prescription glasses
- Difficulty adjusting eyes to the dark

Although anyone can develop glaucoma, some people are at higher risk. Risk factors of glaucoma are:

- Everyone over 60 years of age
- Blacks over age 40
- People with a family history of glaucoma
- Diabetes

Regular and complete eye exams are very important. It is recommended that a check for glaucoma be done:

- At age 35 and at age 40
- After age 40, every 2 to 3 years
- After age 60, every 1 to 2 years
- If there are any of the risk factors of glaucoma, every 1 to 2 years after age 30

Although open-angle glaucoma cannot be cured, it can usually be controlled. Individual treatments will vary from person to person. Treatments may include medications (eyedrops or pills), laser surgery, eye surgery, and drainage implant devices.

CASE STUDY

Please read the following case study and then work frames 7.53–7.56. Write in your answer in the answer column. Check your responses with the answers provided at the end of frame 7.56.

A 4-year-old female was seen by a physician and the following is a synopsis of the visit.

PRESENT HISTORY: The mother states that her daughter has been complaining of an earache, ringing in the ears, and has been running a fever. She is irritable and doesn't want to eat.

SIGNS AND SYMPTOMS: Chief Complaints: otodynia (otalgia), tinnitus, fever, irritability, and anorexia.

DIAGNOSIS: Otitis Media Acute. The diagnosis was determined by a physical examination of the ear (otoscopy). A culture of the fluid taken from the ear showed the presence of bacteria—*Streptococcus pneumoniae.*

TREATMENT: The physician ordered an analgesic for pain (Tylenol) and an antibiotic (amoxicillin) for the infection.

PREVENTION: Since most middle ear infections are caused by an upper respiratory infection that has spread through the eustachian tube, URIs should be treated promptly.

7.53 Signs and symptoms of otitis media include otodynia, ____________ (ringing in the ears), fever, irritability, and anorexia.

7.54 Otodynia (otalgia) is the medical term for ____________.

7.55 The diagnosis was determined by a physical examination of the ear called an ____________ and a culture of the fluid taken from the ear.

7.56 Treatment included an analgesic (Tylenol) and an ____________ (amoxicillin).

CASE STUDY ANSWERS

7.53 tinnitus 7.55 otoscopy

7.54 earache 7.56 antibiotic

REVIEW A: WORD ELEMENTS

This review allows you to check your knowledge of some of the word elements presented in this unit. In the spaces provided, write the meaning of the word elements that are identified as **Prefix (P), Word Root (R), Combining Form (CF),** and/or **Suffix (S).**

MEDICAL WORD	*WORD ELEMENT*	*MEANING*
1. otorhinolaryngology	ot / o (CF)	__________
	rhin / o (CF)	__________
	laryng / o (CF)	__________
	-logy (S)	__________
2. auditory	auditor (R)	__________
	-y (S)	__________
3. acoustic	acoust (R)	__________
	-ic (S)	__________
4. audiometer	audi / o (CF)	__________
	-meter (S)	__________
5. otitis	ot (R)	__________
	-itis (S)	__________
6. tinnitus	tinnit (R)	__________
	-us (S)	__________
7. ophthalmology	ophthalm / o (CF)	__________
	-logy (S)	__________
8. lacrimal	lacrim (R)	__________
	-al (S)	__________
9. cycloplegia	cycl / o (CF)	__________
	-plegia (S)	__________
10. keratitis	kerat (R)	__________
	-itis (S)	__________
11. tonometer	ton / o (CF)	__________
	-meter (S)	__________
12. ophthalmopathy	ophthalm / o (CF)	__________
	-pathy (S)	__________

REVIEW B: MEDICAL TERMS

Please place the correct letter from column II on the appropriate line of column I.

COLUMN I		COLUMN II
________	1. aural	A. a state of balance
________	2. otoscope	B. impairment of hearing in old age
________	3. myringotomy	C. dullness of vision
________	4. equilibrium	D. an instrument used to examine the ear
________	5. presbycusis	E. opening in the center of the iris
________	6. ocular	F. incision of the tympanic membrane
________	7. ambylopia	G. pertaining to the ear
________	8. emmetropia	H. colored membrane attached to the ciliary body
________	9. iris	I. normal vision
________	10. pupil	J. pertaining to the eye

REVIEW C: DISEASES AND DISORDERS

Please provide the correct disease or disorder for each of the following descriptions.

1. ________ is a recurrent and progressive condition that affects the inner ear and presents a group of symptoms.
2. ________ is complete or partial loss of the ability to hear.
3. ________ is a tumor-like mass filled with epithelial cells and cholesterol.
4. ________ is a disease characterized by increased intraocular pressure.
5. ________ is an opacity of the crystalline lens.

REVIEW D: UNSCRAMBLE THE WORDS

Unscramble the following medical terms and place the correct term on the line directly across from the scrambled word.

1. yniadoto ________
2. mphyloden ________
3. umencer ________
4. tigorev ________
5. iapoym ________
6. niozalcha ________
7. modataccoionm ________
8. musbisarts ________

REVIEW E: DRUGS USED FOR THE SPECIAL SENSES

Please provide the correct answer for each of the following descriptions.

1. ____________ are used to treat infectious diseases that are caused by bacteria.
2. ____________ are used to counteract the effects of histamine.
3. ____________ are agents that cause the pupil to dilate.
4. ____________ agents are used to treat fungal infections of the eye.

REVIEW F: ABBREVIATIONS

Please provide the correct abbreviation and/or meaning for the abbreviation.

1. ____________ eye, ear, nose, and throat
2. both ears ____________
3. ____________ right ear
4. MY ____________
5. ____________ near visual acuity
6. OD ____________

8 THE ENDOCRINE SYSTEM: ENDOCRINOLOGY

LEARNING CONCEPTS

- the endocrine system
- essential terminology
- pronunciation guide
- word elements
- explanation frames
- diabetes mellitus: warning signs and symptoms
- selected diseases and disorders
- drugs used for the endocrine system
- abbreviations
- in the spotlight: Addison's disease
- case study: diabetes mellitus
- review exercises

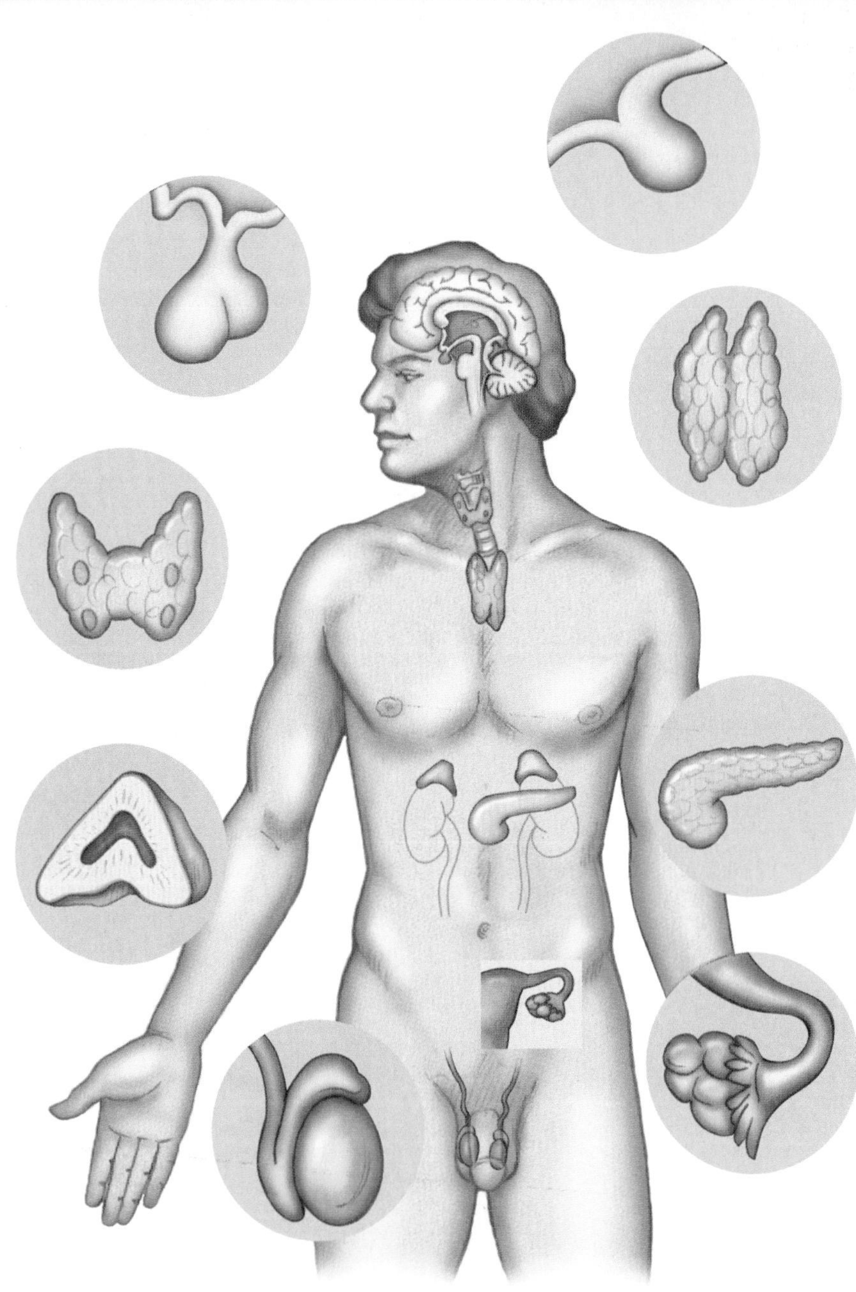

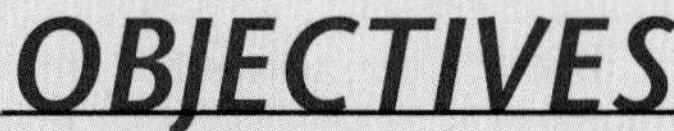

OBJECTIVES

ON COMPLETION OF THIS UNIT, YOU SHOULD BE ABLE TO:

- Briefly describe the endocrine system.
- Describe the primary functions of the various glands of the endocrine system.
- Give the hormones and hormonal functions of the various endocrine glands.
- Identify and give the meaning of the primary word elements for this unit.
- Analyze, build, spell, and pronounce selected medical words.
- Describe selected diseases/disorders of the endocrine system.
- List the warning signs and symptoms of diabetes mellitus.
- List six functions of epinephrine (Adrenalin, adrenaline).
- Describe selected drugs that are used for endocrine system diseases or disorders.
- Define selected abbreviations that pertain to the endocrine system.
- Give the cause, signs and symptoms, diagnosis, and treatment of Addison's disease.
- Complete the Case Study on Diabetes Mellitus Type I IDDM.
- Successfully complete the review section.

TECH LINK

CD-ROM Use the CD-ROM enclosed with your textbook to gain additional reinforcement through interactive word building exercises, spelling games, labeling activities, and additional quizzes.

www.prenhall.com/rice Use the above address to access the free, interactive Companion Website created specifically for this textbook. Get hints, instant feedback, and textbook references to chapter-related multiple choice and true/false questions, fill-in-the-blank, and labeling exercises. In addition, you will find an audio glossary, and essay questions.

The endocrine system is made up of glands and the hormones they secrete. Although the endocrine glands are the body's main hormone producers, some other organs such as the brain, heart, lungs, liver, skin, thymus, the placenta during pregnancy, and the gastrointestinal mucosa produce and release hormones.

The primary glands of the endocrine system are the pituitary, pineal, thyroid, parathyroid, islets of Langerhans, adrenals, ovaries in the female, and testes in the male. See Table 8–1.

The vital function of the endocrine system involves the production and regulation of chemical substances called hormones. A hormone is a chemical transmitter that is released in small amounts and transported via the bloodstream to a target organ or other cells. The word hormone is derived from the Greek language and means "to excite" or "to urge on." As the body's chemical messengers, hormones transfer information and instructions from one set of cells to another. They regulate growth, development, mood, tissue function, metabolism, and sexual function in the male and female. See Table 8–2.

Many pathological conditions are caused by or associated with hyposecretion or hypersecretion of specific hormones of the endocrine system. Too much or too little of any hormone can be harmful to the body. Controlling the production of or replacing specific hormones can treat many hormonal disorders and/or conditions.

The endocrine system and the nervous system work closely together to help maintain homeostasis. The hypothalamus, a collection of specialized cells that are located in the lower central part of the brain, is the primary link between the endocrine and the nervous systems. Nerve cells in the hypothalamus control the pituitary gland by producing chemicals that either stimulate or suppress hormone secretions from the pituitary.

TABLE 8–1 THE ENDOCRINE SYSTEM

Gland	Primary Functions
Pituitary (Hypophysis)	Master gland; regulatory effects on other endocrine glands
Anterior lobe	Influences growth and sexual development; thyroid function, adrenocortical function; regulates skin pigmentation
Posterior lobe	Stimulates the reabsorption of water and elevates blood pressure; stimulates the release of milk and the uterus to contract during labor, delivery, and parturition
Pineal	Helps regulate the release of gonadotropin and controls body pigmentation
Thyroid	Vital role in metabolism and regulates the body's metabolic processes, influences bone and calcium metabolism, helps maintain plasma calcium homeostasis
Parathyroid	Maintenance of a normal serum calcium level, plays a role in the metabolism of phosphorus
Pancreas (Islets of Langerhans)	Regulates blood glucose levels and plays a vital role in metabolism of carbohydrates, proteins, and fats
Adrenals (Suprarenals)	
Adrenal cortex	Regulates carbohydrate metabolism, anti-inflammatory effect; helps body cope during stress; regulates electrolyte and water balance; promotes development of male characteristics
Adrenal medulla	Synthesizes, secretes, and stores catecholamines (dopamine, epinephrine, norepinephrine)
Ovaries	Promote growth, development, and maintenance of female sex organs
Testes	Promote growth, development, and maintenance of male sex organs

TABLE 8–2 SUMMARY OF THE ENDOCRINE GLANDS, HORMONES, AND HORMONAL FUNCTIONS

Endocrine Glands	Hormones	Hormonal Functions
Pituitary Gland		
Anterior lobe	Growth hormone (GH)	Growth and development of bones, muscles, and other organs
	Adrenocorticotropin hormone (ACTH)	Growth and development of the adrenal cortex
	Thyroid-stimulating hormone (TSH)	Growth and development of the thyroid gland
	Follicle-stimulating hormone (FSH)	Stimulates the growth of ovarian follicles in the female and sperm in the male
	Luteinizing hormone (LH)	Stimulates the development of the corpus luteum in the female and the production of testosterone in the male
	Prolactin hormone (PRL)	Stimulates the mammary glands to produce milk after childbirth
	Melanocyte-stimulating hormone (MSH)	Regulates skin pigmentation and promotes the deposit of melanin in the skin after exposure to sunlight
Posterior lobe	Antidiuretic hormone (ADH)	Stimulates the reabsorption of water by the renal tubules and has a pressor effect that elevates the blood pressure
	Oxytocin	Acts on the mammary glands to stimulate the release of milk and stimulates the uterus to contract during labor, delivery, and parturition
Pineal Gland	Melatonin	Helps regulate the release of gonadotropin and influences the body's internal clock
	Serotonin	Neurotransmitter, vasoconstrictor, and smooth muscle stimulant; acts to inhibit gastric secretion
Thyroid Gland	Thyroxine	Maintenance and regulation of the basal metabolic rate (BMR)
	Triiodothyronine	Influences the basal metabolic rate
	Calcitonin	Influences calcium metabolism
Parathyroid Glands	Parathormone hormone (PTH)	Plays a role in maintenance of a normal serum calcium level and in the metabolism of phosphorus
Islets of Langerhans	Glucagon	Facilitates the breakdown of glycogen to glucose
	Insulin	Plays a role in maintenance of normal blood sugar
	Somatostatin	Suppresses the release of glucagon and insulin
Adrenal Glands		
Cortex	Cortisol	Principal steroid hormone. Regulates carbohydrate, protein, and fat metabolism; gluconeogenesis; increases blood sugar level; anti-inflammatory effect; helps body cope during times of stress
	Corticosterone	Steroid hormone. Essential for normal use of carbohydrates, the absorption of glucose, and gluconeogenesis. Also influences potassium and sodium metabolism

(*continues*)

TABLE 8-2 *(Continued)*

Endocrine Glands	Hormones	Hormonal Functions
	Aldosterone	Principal mineralocorticoid. Essential in regulating electrolyte and water balance
	Testosterone	Development of male secondary sex characteristics
	Androsterone	Development of male secondary sex characteristics
Medulla	Dopamine	Dilates systemic arteries, elevates systolic blood pressure, increases cardiac output, increases urinary output
	Epinephrine (adrenaline)	Vasoconstrictor, vasopressor, cardiac stimulant, antispasmodic, and sympathomimetic
	Norepinephrine	Vasoconstrictor, vasopressor, and neurotransmitter
Ovaries	Estrogens (estradiol, estrone, and estriol)	Female sex hormones. Essential for the growth, development, and maintenance of female sex organs and secondary sex characteristics. Promotes the development of the mammary glands, and plays a vital role in a woman's emotional well-being and sexual drive
	Progesterone	Prepares the uterus for pregnancy
Testes	Testosterone	Essential for normal growth and development of the male accessory sex organs. Plays a vital role in the erection process of the penis and, thus, is necessary for the reproductive act, copulation
Thymus Gland	Thymosin	Promotes the maturation process of T lymphocytes
	Thymopoietin	Influences the production of lymphocyte precursors and aids in their process of becoming T lymphocytes
Gastrointestinal Mucosa	Gastrin	Stimulates gastric acid secretion
	Secretin	Stimulates pancreatic juice, bile, and intestinal secretion
	Pancreozymin	Stimulates the pancreas to produce pancreatic juice
	Cholecystokinin	Contraction and emptying of the gallbladder
	Enterogastrone	Regulates gastric secretions

PRIMARY WORD ELEMENTS

The following word elements (prefixes, roots, combining forms, and suffixes) will be used to build medical terms that relate to this unit. Please commit these to memory.

PREFIX

PREFIX	MEANING	PREFIX	MEANING
ad	toward	**hyper**	above, excessive
dia	through	**hypo**	below, deficient
endo	within	**poly**	excessive, many, much
ex	out, away from	**pro**	before

COMBINING FORM

COMBINING FORM / ROOT	MEANING	COMBINING FORM / ROOT	MEANING
acr / o	extremity, point	**neur / o**	nerve
aden	gland	**ophthalm**	eye
aden / o	gland	**pituitar**	phlegm
calc	calcium	**ren**	kidney
crin / o	to secrete	**scler**	hardening
ger	old age	**thym, thym / o**	thymus
glyc	glucose	**thyr**	thyroid, shield
insul, insulin	insulin	**thyr / o**	thyroid, shield
letharg	drowsiness	**trop**	turning
myx	mucus		

SUFFIX

SUFFIX	MEANING	SUFFIX	MEANING
-al, -ic	pertaining to	**-logy**	study of
-algia	pain	**-malacia**	softening
-betes	to go	**-megaly**	enlargement, large
-dipsia	thirst	**-oid**	resemble
-ectomy	surgical excision	**-oma**	tumor
-edema	swelling	**-pathy**	disease
-emia	blood condition	**-pexy**	surgical fixation
-ia, -ism, -osis	condition of	**-phagia**	to eat
-ist	one who specializes	**-physis**	growth
-itis	inflammation	**-ptosis**	drooping

8.1 ____________ is the study of the endocrine system.
The word elements used to build this term are:
____________ prefix that means within
____________ combining form that means to secrete
____________ suffix that means study of

ANSWER COLUMN

endocrinology
(en doh krin **ALL** oh jee)
endo
crin / o
-logy

ANSWER COLUMN

8.2 An ____________ is a physician who specializes in the study of the endocrine system.

endocrinologist
(en doh krin **ALL** oh jist)

EXPLANATION FRAME

The organs of the endocrine system are called glands. These glands are called endocrine because they produce internal secretions—hormones. They are ductless and they secrete their hormones into the bloodstream. The medical term **endocrine** means to secrete within. **Endo** is a prefix that means within and **crine** is a root that means to secrete.

Diseases and disorders of the endocrine system generally involve excessive (**hyper**) or deficient (**hypo**) production or utilization of hormones.

8.3 The combining form **aden / o** and the root **aden** mean gland. Medical terms that begin with these word elements are:

____________ pain in a gland; SYN: adenodynia

____________ surgical excision of a gland

____________ a tumor of a gland

____________ a softening of a gland

____________ a condition of hardening of a gland

____________ any disease condition of a gland

adenalgia
(ad eh **NAL** jee ah)
adenectomy
(ad eh **NEK** toh mee)
adenoma
(ad eh **NOH** mah)
adenomalacia
(ad eh noh mah **LAY** shee ah)
adenosclerosis
(ad eh noh skleh **ROH** sis)
adenosis
(ad eh **NOH** sis)

FOR REVIEW: SUFFIXES/ROOT

-algia pain
-ectomy surgical excision
-malacia softening
-oma tumor
-osis condition of
scler (R) hardening

EXPLANATION FRAME

The pituitary gland is a small gray gland located at the base of the brain. See Figure 8–1. It is approximately 1 cm in diameter and weighs about 0.6 gram. The pituitary gland is called the master gland of the body because of its regulatory effects on many of the other endocrine glands. The pituitary gland is also known as the hypophysis. It is divided into the anterior lobe or adenohypophysis and the posterior lobe or neurohypophysis.

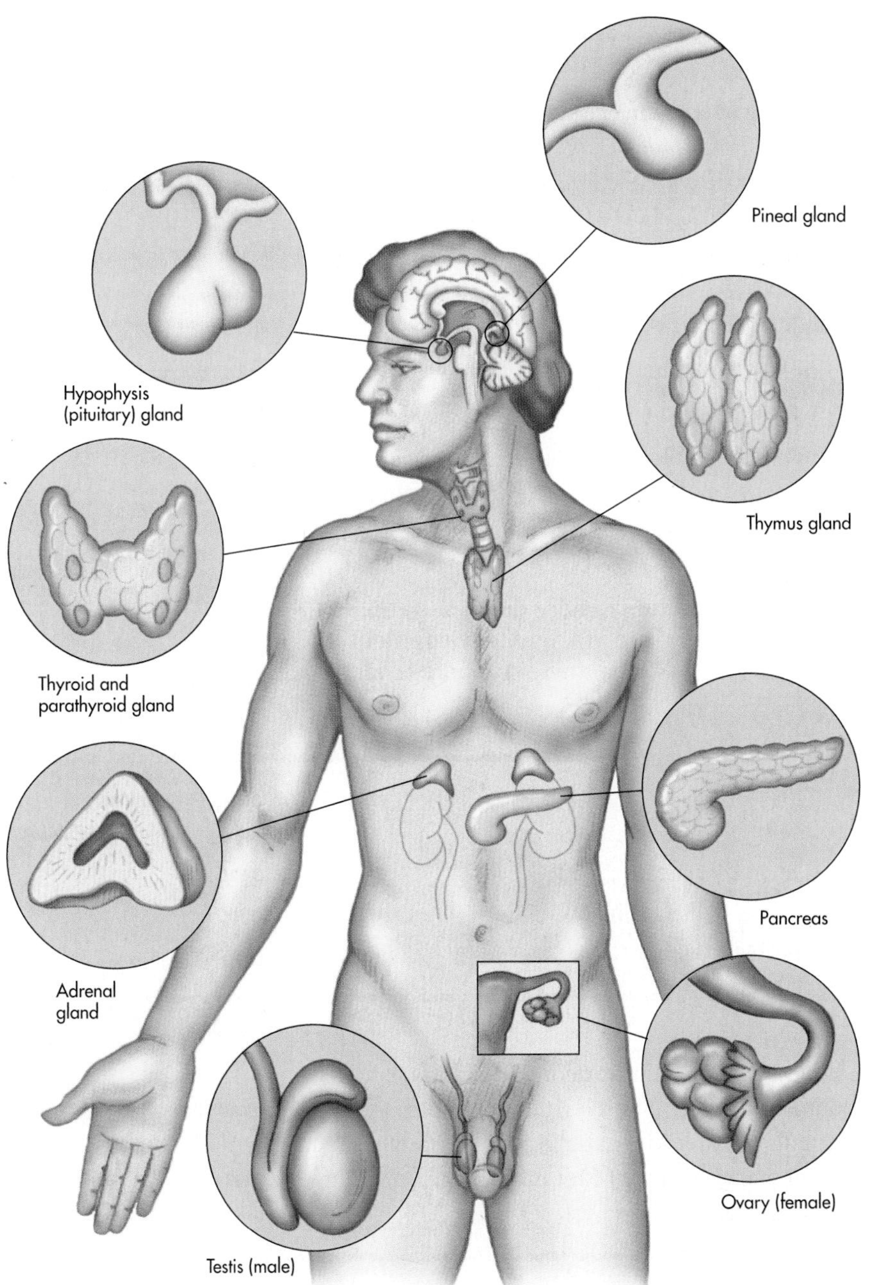

FIGURE 8–1
The primary glands of the endocrine system.

Answer Column

8.4 The ________ gland is known as the master gland of the body. *Pituitary means pertaining to phlegm (thick mucus). Phlegm was one of the four "humors" of early physiology. In ancient medicine a humor was any of the four juices or fluids (blood, phlegm, black bile, yellow bile) of which the body was thought to be composed.*

pituitary
(pih **TOO** ih tair ee)

8.5 ________ is any condition of the pituitary gland.
The word elements used to build this term are:
________ root that means phlegm
________ suffix that means condition of

pituitarism
(pih **TOO** ih tah rizm)
pituitar
-ism

EXPLANATION FRAME

The adenohypophysis or anterior lobe of the pituitary gland secretes several hormones that are essential for the growth and development of bones, muscles, other organs, sex glands, the thyroid gland, and the adrenal cortex.

8.6 The word elements used to build ________ are:
________ combining form that means gland
________ prefix that means deficient, below, under
________ suffix that means growth

adenohypophysis
(ad eh noh high **POFF** ih sis)
aden / o
hypo
-physis

8.7 Growth hormone, also called somatotropin hormone (STH), is essential for the growth and development of bones, muscles, and other organs. Hyposecretion of this hormone may result in ________ and Simmond's disease. Hypersecretion of the hormone may result in ________ during early life and acromegaly in adults.

dwarfism
(**DWARF** izm)
gigantism
(**JYE** gan tizm)

8.8 ________ is enlargement of the extremities.
The word elements used to build this term are:
________ combining form that means extremity
________ suffix that means enlargement, large

acromegaly
(ak roh **MEG** ah lee)
acr / o
-megaly

ANSWER COLUMN

EXPLANATION FRAME

The neurohypophysis or posterior lobe of the pituitary gland secretes two known hormones: antidiuretic hormone and oxytocin. Antidiuretic hormone (ADH) is also known as vasopressin (VP). It stimulates the reabsorption of water by the renal tubules. Hyposecretion of this hormone may result in **diabetes insipidus**. Oxytocin acts on the mammary glands to stimulate the release of milk and stimulates the uterus to contract during labor, delivery, and parturition.

8.9 The word elements used to build __________ are:
__________ combining form that means nerve
__________ prefix that means deficient, below, under
__________ suffix that means growth

neurohypophysis
(noo roh high **POFF** ih sis)
neur / o
hypo
-physis

8.10 With __________ __________ the patient excretes copious amounts of colorless and dilute urine. *Urine output of 5 to 10 liters/24 hours is common. The disease is treated by the use of vasopressin replacement therapy by injection or nasal spray.*

diabetes insipidus
(dye ah **BEE** teez in **SIP** ih dus)

EXPLANATION FRAME

The pineal gland (body) is a small, pine cone–shaped gland located near the posterior end of the corpus callosum. See Figure 8–1. The pineal gland secretes melatonin and serotonin. Melatonin is a hormone that may be released at night to help regulate the release of gonadotropin and aids in promoting sleep. Serotonin is a hormone that is a neurotransmitter, vasoconstrictor, and smooth muscle stimulant and acts to inhibit gastric secretion.

8.11 __________ is a tumor of the pineal body.

pinealoma
(pin ee ah **LOH** mah)

8.12 __________ is surgical excision of the pineal body.

pinealectomy
(pin ee-al **EK** toh mee)

ANSWER COLUMN

EXPLANATION FRAME

The thyroid gland is a large, bilobed gland located in the neck. See Figure 8–1. The thyroid gland is approximately 5 cm long and 3 cm wide and weighs approximately 30 grams. It plays a vital role in metabolism and regulates the body's metabolic processes. It secretes thyroxine (T4), triiodothyronine (T3), and calcitonin.

8.13 The combining form **thyr / o** and the root **thyr** mean thyroid, shield. Medical terms that begin with these word elements are:

		Answer
____________	resembling a shield	**thyroid** (**THIGH** royd)
____________	surgical excision of the thyroid gland	**thyroidectomy** (thigh royd **EK** toh mee)
____________	inflammation of the thyroid gland	**thyroiditis** (thigh royd **EYE** tis)
____________	downward drooping of the thyroid gland	**thyroptosis** (thigh rop **TOH** sis)
____________	any condition of abnormal functioning of the thyroid gland	**thyrosis** (thigh **ROH** sis)
____________	a poisonous condition of the thyroid gland	**thyrotoxicosis** (thigh roh toks ih **KOH** sis)

8.14 Hyposecretion of the thyroid hormones T_3 and T_4 results in cretinism during infancy, myxedema during adulthood, and Hashimoto's disease, which is a chronic thyroid disease.

____________ is a congenital deficiency in secretion of the thyroid hormones.

cretinism (**KREE** tin izm)

____________ is a condition of mucus swelling resulting from hypofunction of the thyroid gland. The root **myx** means mucus and the suffix **-edema** means swelling.

myxedema (miks eh **DEE** mah)

8.15 Hypersecretion of the thyroid hormones T_3 and T_4 results in hyperthyroidism, which is also called thyrotoxicosis, and Graves' disease; exophthalmic goiter, toxic goiter, or Basedow's disease.

____________ means pertaining to an abnormal protrusion of the eye. The word elements used to build this term are:

exophthalmic (eks off **THAL** mik)

ANSWER COLUMN

continued

___________	prefix that means out, away from	**ex**
___________	root that means eye	**ophthalm**
___________	suffix that means pertaining to	**-ic**

8.16 ___________ is also known as thyrocalcitonin and is a thyroid hormone that influences bone and calcium metabolism. It helps maintain plasma calcium homeostasis.

calcitonin (kal sih **TOH** nin)

EXPLANATION FRAME

The parathyroid glands are small, yellowish-brown bodies occurring as two pairs and located on the dorsal surface and lower aspects of the thyroid gland. See Figure 8–1. The hormone secreted by the parathyroids is parathormone (PTH), which is essential for the maintenance of a normal serum calcium level. It also plays a role in the metabolism of phosphorus.

8.17 Hyposecretion of PTH may result in hypoparathyroidism, which may result in tetany. ___________ is defined as a nervous syndrome, characterized by intermittent tonic spasms that usually involve the extremities.

tetany (**TET** ah nee)

8.18 Hypersecretion of PTH may result in hyperparathyroidism, which may result in osteoporosis, kidney stones, and hypercalcemia. ___________ means excessive buildup of calcium in the blood. The word elements used to build this term are:

hypercalcemia (high per kal **SEE** mee ah)

___________	prefix that means excessive, above	**hyper**
___________	root that means calcium	**calc**
___________	suffix that means blood condition	**-emia**

EXPLANATION FRAME

The islets of Langerhans are small clusters of cells located within the pancreas. See Figure 8–1. They are composed of three major types of cells: alpha, beta, and delta. The alpha cells secrete the hormone glucagon. The beta cells secrete the hormone insulin. The delta cells secrete the hormone somatostatin.

8.19 ___________ facilitates the breakdown of glycogen to glucose, thereby elevating the blood sugar.

glucagon (**GLOO** koh gon)

ANSWER COLUMN

8.20 ___________ is essential for maintenance of a normal level of blood sugar, which is 70–110 mg/100 mL of blood. *Insulin can be synthetically produced in various types and was first discovered and used successfully by Sir F. G. Banting.*

insulin
(IN soo lin)

EXPLANATION FRAME

Diabetes mellitus is a complex disorder of metabolism. It affects 14 million Americans, with care and treatment costing $20 billion annually. **Hyposecretion** or inadequate use of insulin may result in diabetes mellitus. The National Diabetes Data Group of the National Institutes of Health has categorized the various forms of diabetes mellitus as Type I—insulin-dependent diabetes mellitus (IDDM); Type II—noninsulin-dependent diabetes mellitus (NIDDM); Type III—women who have developed glucose intolerance in association with pregnancy; and Type IV—diabetes associated with pancreatic disease, hormonal changes, the adverse effects of drugs, and other anomalies.

WARNING SIGNS AND SYMPTOMS OF DIABETES MELLITUS

Type I insulin-dependent diabetes mellitus (IDDM)

- Frequent urination **(polyuria)**
- Excessive thirst **(polydipsia)**
- Extreme hunger **(polyphagia)**
- Unexplained weight loss
- Blurred vision

Type II noninsulin-dependent diabetes mellitus (NIDDM)

- Any type I symptom
- Tingling or numbing in feet
- Frequent vaginal or skin infection

8.21 The classic symptoms of diabetes mellitus are designated as the "**polys**": polyuria, polydipsia, and polyphagia. The prefix **poly** means excessive, many, much and the suffixes:

___________ means urine — **-uria**
___________ means thirst — **-dipsia**
___________ means to eat — **-phagia**

Answer Column

8.22 ____________ mellitus is a disease characterized by excessive discharge of urine (polyuria), polydipsia, and polyphagia.

The word elements used to build **dia / betes** are:

____________ prefix that means through

____________ suffix that means to go

diabetes
(dye ah **BEE** teez)

dia

-betes

8.23 ____________ is a condition in which the glucose in the blood is abnormally low. ____________ is a prefix that means deficient; ____________ is a root that means glucose and ____________ is a suffix that means blood condition. *Symptoms of hypoglycemia include acute fatigue, restlessness, malaise, irritability, weakness, sweating, hunger, dizziness, trembling, headache, and CNS manifestations—confusion, visual disturbances, stupor, coma, seizures, and behavior that may be mistaken for drunkenness.*

hypoglycemia
(high poh glye **SEE** mee ah)
hypo **glyc**
-emia

8.24 ____________ is a condition where there is an excessive amount of insulin in the blood. It may be caused by a tumor on the islets of Langerhans or an overdose of insulin. It is also known as insulin shock.

The word elements used to build this term are:

____________ prefix that means excessive, above, beyond

____________ root that means insulin

____________ suffix that means condition of

hyperinsulinism
(high per **IN** soo lin izm)

hyper

insulin

-ism

EXPLANATION FRAME

The adrenal glands (suprarenals) are two small, triangular-shaped glands located on top of each kidney. See Figure 8–1. Each gland weighs about 5 grams and consists of an outer portion or cortex and an inner portion called the medulla. The adrenal cortex secretes a group of hormones: the glucocorticoids, the mineralocorticoids, and the androgens.

8.25 ____________ literally means toward the kidney.

The word elements used to build this term are:

____________ prefix that means toward

____________ root that means kidney

____________ suffix that means pertaining to

adrenal
(ad **REE** nal)

ad

ren

-al

Answer Column

8.26 Medical terms that pertain to the adrenal gland are:

___________	surgical excision of the adrenal gland	**adrenalectomy** (ad ree nal **EK** toh mee)
___________	any disease of the adrenal gland	**adrenopathy** (ad ren **OP** ah thee)
___________	pertaining to nourishing or stimulating to the adrenal glands	**adrenotropic** (ah dree noh **TROP** ik)

8.27 ___________ is a glucocorticoid hormone and it is the principal steroid hormone secreted by the cortex. It is also called hydrocortisone.

cortisol
(**KOR** tih sol)

8.28 Hyposecretion of cortisol may result in ___________ disease or hypoadrenocorticism.

Addison's
(**AD** ih sons)

8.29 Hypersecretion of cortisol may result in ___________ syndrome. The patient with this condition experiences fatigue, muscular weakness, and changes in body appearance. *Prolonged administration of large doses of ACTH can cause Cushing's syndrome. A "buffalo hump" and a "moon face" are characteristic signs of Cushing's syndrome.*

Cushing's
(**CUSH** ingz)

8.30 ___________ is the principal mineralocorticoid secreted by the adrenal cortex. *It is essential in regulating electrolyte and water balance by promoting sodium and chloride retention and potassium excretion. Hyposecretion of this hormone may result in a reduced plasma volume.*

aldosterone
(al **DOSS** ter ohn)

8.31 Hypersecretion of aldosterone may result in a condition known as primary ___________.

aldosteronism
(al **DOSS** teh roh nizm)

8.32 Androgen refers to a substance or hormone that promotes the development of male characteristics. The two main androgen hormones are ___________ and androsterone. These hormones are essential for the development of the male secondary sex characteristics.

testosterone
(tess **TOSS** ter ohn)

ANSWER COLUMN

8.33 The __________ medulla synthesizes, secretes, and stores catecholamines, specifically dopamine, epinephrine, and norepinephrine.

adrenal
(ad **REE** nal)

8.34 __________ acts to dilate systemic arteries, elevates systolic blood pressure, increases cardiac output, and increases urinary output. It is a neurotransmitter and when produced as a drug, it may be used in the treatment of shock.

dopamine
(**DOH** pah meen)

EXPLANATION FRAME

Epinephrine (Adrenalin, adrenaline) acts as a vasoconstrictor, vasopressor, cardiac stimulant, antispasmodic, and sympathomimetic. Its main function is to assist in the regulation of the sympathetic branch of the autonomic nervous system. It can be synthetically produced and may be administered parenterally (by injection), topically (on a local area of the skin), or by inhalation (by nose or mouth). Other functions are:

- It elevates the systolic blood pressure.
- It increases the heart rate and cardiac output.
- It dilates the bronchial tubes.
- It dilates the pupils.
- It increases glycogenolysis, thereby hastening the release of glucose from the liver. This action elevates the blood sugar level and provides the body with a spurt of energy.

The thymus is a bilobed body located in the mediastinal cavity in front of and above the heart. See Figure 8–2. It is composed of lymphoid tissue and is a part of the lymphoid system. It is a ductless gland-like body and secretes the hormones thymosin and thymopoietin.

8.35 __________ promotes the maturation process of T lymphocytes (thymus-dependent).

thymosin
(thigh **MOH** sin)

8.36 __________ is a hormone that influences the production of lymphocyte precursors and aids in their process of becoming T lymphocytes.

thymopoietin
(thigh moh **POY** eh tin)

8.37 The combining form **thym / o** and the root **thym** mean thymus. Medical terms that begin with these word elements are:

continued

Answer Column

		Answer
____________	surgical excision of the thymus gland	**thymectomy** (thigh **MEK** toh mee)
____________	inflammation of the thymus gland	**thymitis** (thigh **MY** tis)
____________	a tumor of the thymus gland	**thymoma** (thigh **MOH** mah)
____________	surgical fixation of an enlarged thymus in a new position	**thymopexy** (thigh moh **PEKS** ee)

8.38 ____________ is a medical term that means pertaining to drowsiness. The word elements used to build this term are:

		Answer
		lethargic (leth **AR** jik)
____________	root that means drowsiness	**letharg**
____________	suffix that means pertaining to	**-ic**

8.39 ____________ is a condition of premature old age occurring in children. The word elements used to build this term are:

		Answer
		progeria (proh **JEE** ree ah)
____________	prefix that means before	**pro**
____________	root that means old age	**ger**
____________	suffix that means condition of	**-ia`**

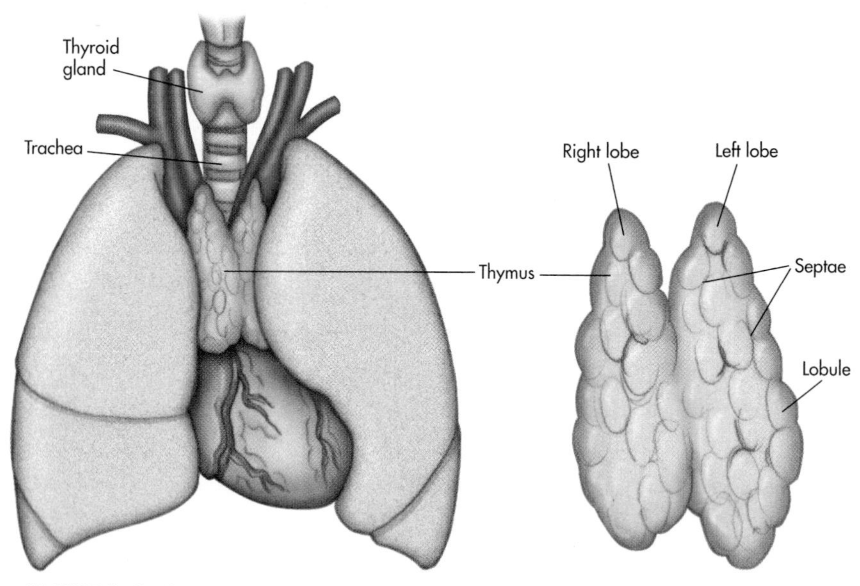

FIGURE 8–2
The thymus gland. Appearance and position (A), with anatomic structures (B).

ANSWER COLUMN

EXPLANATION FRAME

Drugs that are generally used for endocrine system diseases and disorders include thyroid hormones, antithyroid hormones, insulin, and oral hypoglycemic agents.

8.40 ____________ hormones are used as supplements or replacement therapy in hypothyroidism, myxedema, and cretinism.

thyroid (**THIGH** royd)

8.41 ____________ hormones are used in the treatment of hyperthyroidism.

antithyroid (an tih **THIGH** royd)

8.42 ____________ is used in the treatment of insulin-dependent diabetes mellitus, noninsulin-dependent diabetes mellitus when other regimens are not effective, and ketoacidosis.

insulin (**IN** soo lin)

8.43 Oral ____________ agents are used to stimulate insulin secretion from pancreatic cells in noninsulin-dependent diabetics with some pancreatic function.

hypoglycemic (high poh glye **SEE** mik)

8.44 ABBREVIATIONS

Write in the correct abbreviation for the following:

		Answer
____________	adrenocorticotropic hormone	**ACTH**
____________	antidiuretic hormone (vasopression)	**ADH**
____________	blood glucose	**BG, bG**
____________	basal metabolic rate	**BMR**
____________	diabetes insipidus	**DI**
____________	diabetes mellitus	**DM**
____________	insulin-dependent diabetes mellitus	**IDDM**
____________	noninsulin-dependent diabetes mellitus	**NIDDM**
____________	parathormone	**PTH**
____________	somatotropin hormone	**STH**
____________	triiodothyronine	T_3
____________	thyroxine	T_4
____________	vasopressin	**VP**

IN THE SPOTLIGHT

ADDISON'S DISEASE

Addison's disease occurs when the cortex of the adrenal gland is damaged and there is a deficiency in the production of the adrenocortical hormones. The most common cause of this condition is the result of the body attacking itself (autoimmune disease). For unknown reasons, the immune system views the adrenal cortex as a foreign body, something to attack and destroy. Other causes of Addison's disease include infections of the adrenal glands, spread of cancer to the glands, or hemorrhage into the glands.

Addison's disease is named for the nineteenth-century English physician, Thomas Addison, who identified and described the condition. It can occur at any age, including infancy, and is equally prevalent among males and females. It is a rare disease, occurring about 1 in 100,000 Americans.

The signs and symptoms of Addison's disease may include:

- Weight loss
- Anorexia
- Weakness and lethargy
- Increased pigmentation of the skin and mucous membranes
- Low blood sugar
- Joint and muscle aches
- Persistent fever
- Nausea, vomiting, diarrhea, abdominal discomfort

The signs and symptoms usually develop slowly over several months, but they may appear suddenly. In acute adrenal failure (addisonian crisis), the signs and symptoms include dehydration, shock, and loss of consciousness. This condition is life-threatening and requires immediate medical care. Prescribed adrenocortical steroids along with intravenous fluids and sodium are administered to the patient.

The diagnosis of Addison's disease is determined by blood and urine tests that measure the amount of corticosteroid hormones present. With Addison's the level of the hormones is very low. When Addison's disease is diagnosed early, treatment generally consists of replacement of the adrenocortical hormones and supplemental sodium. Both the patient and family are taught the importance of lifelong replacement therapy and the proper technique of how to give an intramuscular injection of hydrocortisone. The patient is advised to wear or carry medical identification at all times.

CASE STUDY

Please read the following case study and then work frames 8.45–8.48. Write in your answer in the answer column. Check your responses with the answers provided at the end of frame 8.48.

A 20-year-old female was seen by a physician and the following is a synopsis of the visit.

PRESENT HISTORY: The patient states that she has been very thirsty, hungry, and urinating a lot. She says that diabetes runs in her family, and she is concerned that she may be developing the disease.

SIGNS AND SYMPTOMS: Chief Complaints: polydipsia, polyphagia, polyuria.

DIAGNOSIS: Diabetes Mellitus Type I IDDM. The diagnosis was determined by the characteristic symptoms, family history, a blood glucose test, and a glucose tolerance test.

TREATMENT: The management of diabetes mellitus Type I is based on trying to normalize insulin activity and blood glucose levels to reduce the development of complications of the disease. The patient was instructed in insulin therapy, diet therapy, an exercise program, and lifestyle modifications. The patient was taught how to properly administer insulin, with dosage based on her blood glucose test performed before breakfast, lunch, and dinner. A follow-up visit was scheduled for 2 weeks with instructions to call if there were any questions or problems.

8.45 Signs and symptoms of diabetes mellitus Type I include ____________, polyphagia, and polyuria.

8.46 Polyphagia is the medical term for excessive ____________.

8.47 The diagnosis was determined by the characteristic symptoms, family history, a blood glucose test, and a ____________ tolerance test.

8.48 Treatment for diabetes mellitus Type I includes insulin therapy, ____________ therapy, an exercise program, and lifestyle changes.

CASE STUDY ANSWERS

8.45 polydipsia

8.46 eating

8.47 glucose

8.48 diet

REVIEW A: WORD ELEMENTS

This review allows you to check your knowledge of some of the word elements presented in this unit. In the spaces provided, write the meaning of the word elements that are identified as **Prefix (P), Word Root (R), Combining Form (CF),** and/or **Suffix (S)**.

MEDICAL WORD	*WORD ELEMENT*	*MEANING*
1. endocrinology	endo (P)	________
	crin / o (CF)	________
	-logy (S)	________
2. adenalgia	aden (R)	________
	-algia (S)	________
3. adenomalacia	aden / o (CF)	________
	-malacia (S)	________
4. pituitarism	pituitar (R)	________
	-ism (S)	________
5. adenohypophysis	aden / o (CF)	________
	hypo (P)	________
	-physis (S)	________
6. acromegaly	acr / o (CF)	________
	-megaly (S)	________
7. neurohypophysis	neur / o (CF)	________
	hypo (P)	________
	-physis (S)	________
8. exophthalmic	ex (P)	________
	ophthalm (R)	________
	-ic (S)	________
9. hypercalcemia	hyper (P)	________
	calc (R)	________
	-emia (S)	________
10. polyuria	poly (P)	________
	-uria (S)	________
11. polyphagia	poly (P)	________
	-phagia (S)	________

REVIEW B: MEDICAL TERMS

Please place the correct letter from column II on the appropriate line of column I.

COLUMN I		COLUMN II
________	1. adenoma	A. resembling a shield
________	2. pituitary	B. toward the kidney
________	3. pinealectomy	C. surgical fixation of the thymus gland
________	4. thyroid	D. premature old age occurring in children
________	5. adrenal	E. a tumor of a gland
________	6. thymopexy	F. surgical excision of the pineal body
________	7. lethargic	G. excessive amount of insulin in the blood
________	8. progeria	H. abnormally low blood glucose level
________	9. hypoglycemia	I. pertaining to drowsiness
________	10. hyperinsulinism	J. master gland of the body

REVIEW C: DISEASES AND DISORDERS

Please provide the correct disease or disorder for each of the following descriptions.

1. ________ is enlargement of the extremities.
2. ________ ________ is a condition in which the patient excretes copious amounts of urine.
3. ________ disease is due to hyposecretion of cortisol.
4. ________ disease is due to hypersecretion of cortisol.
5. ________ ________ is a disease characterized by polyuria, polydipsia, and polyphagia.

REVIEW D: UNSCRAMBLE THE WORDS

Unscramble the following medical terms and place the correct term on the line directly across from the scrambled word.

1. sisoneda ________
2. dismwarf ________
3. tismangig ________
4. sisoryth ________
5. anytet ________
6. sulinin ________
7. solicort ________
8. onealdoster ________

REVIEW E: DRUGS USED FOR THE ENDOCRINE SYSTEM

Please provide the correct answer for each of the following descriptions.

1. ___________ hormones are used as replacement therapy in hypothyroidism and/or myxedema.
2. ___________ hormones are used in the treatment of hyperthyroidism.
3. ___________ is used in the treatment of insulin-dependent diabetes mellitus.
4. ___________ agents are used to stimulate insulin secretion from pancreatic cells.

REVIEW F: ABBREVIATIONS

Please provide the correct abbreviation and/or meaning for the abbreviation.

1. ___________ adrenocorticotropic hormone
2. ADH ___________
3. ___________ diabetes insipidus
4. DM ___________
5. ___________ parathormone
6. VP ___________

9 THE CARDIOVASCULAR SYSTEM: CARDIOLOGY

LEARNING CONCEPTS

- the cardiovascular system
- essential terminology
- pronunciation guide
- word elements
- explanation frames
- the heart
- the heartbeat
- primary pulse points
- heart disease
- predisposing factors
- blood pressure
- arrhythmias
- blood vessels: arteries, veins, and capillaries
- selected diseases and disorders
- drugs used for the cardiovascular system
- abbreviations
- in the spotlight: heart attack
- case study: angina pectoris
- review exercises

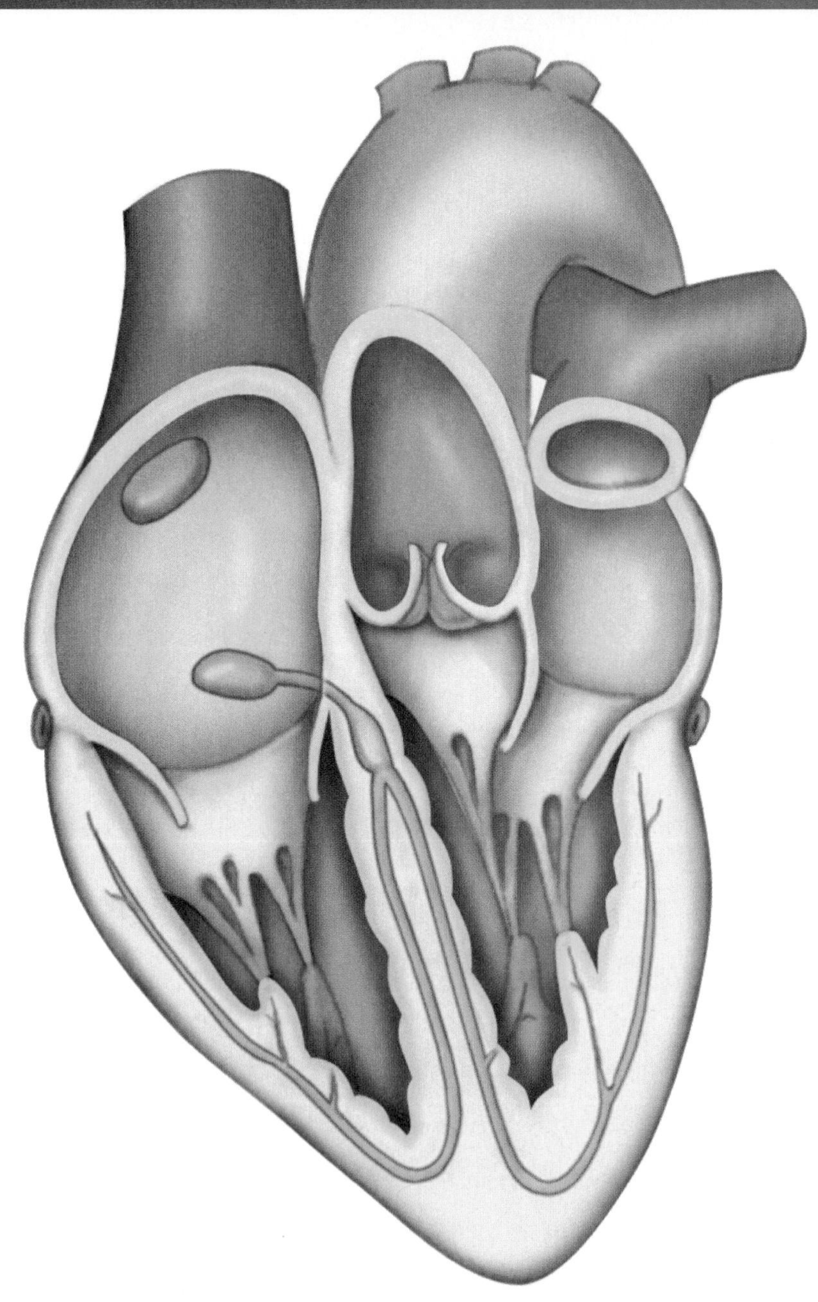

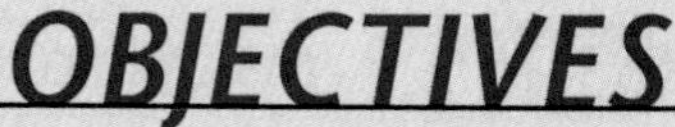

OBJECTIVES

ON COMPLETION OF THIS UNIT, YOU SHOULD BE ABLE TO:

- Briefly describe the cardiovascular system.
- Describe the primary functions of the various organs or structures of the cardiovascular system.
- Identify and give the meaning of the primary word elements for this unit.
- Analyze, build, spell, and pronounce selected medical words.
- Describe selected diseases/disorders of the cardiovascular system.
- List the primary pulse points and give their location.
- State the American Heart Association's warning signs of a heart attack.
- List some of the predisposing factors associated with heart disease.
- Describe blood pressure and name the equipment used to measure its reading.
- Describe selected drugs that are used for cardiovascular system diseases or disorders.
- Define selected abbreviations that pertain to the cardiovascular system.
- State the causes of a heart attack and list 10 possible risk factors for heart attack or stroke.
- Complete the Case Study on Angina Pectoris.
- Successfully complete the review section.

TECH LINK

CD-ROM Use the CD-ROM enclosed with your textbook to gain additional reinforcement through interactive word building exercises, spelling games, labeling activities, and additional quizzes.

www.prenhall.com/rice Use the above address to access the free, interactive Companion Website created specifically for this textbook. Get hints, instant feedback, and textbook references to chapter-related multiple choice and true/false questions, fill-in-the-blank, and labeling exercises. In addition, you will find an audio glossary, and essay questions.

The heart, arteries, veins, and capillaries make up the cardiovascular system. See Table 9–1. Through this system blood is circulated to all parts of the body by the action of the heart. The heart is a four-chambered, hollow muscular pump that circulates blood throughout the cardiovascular system. In an average, healthy adult the heart beats approximately 100,000 times a day.

The arteries constitute a branching system of vessels that transports blood from the right and left ventricles of the heart to all body parts. In a normal state, arteries are elastic tubes that recoil and carry blood in pulsating waves, known as the pulse.

The veins transport blood from peripheral tissues to the heart. In a normal state, veins have thin walls and valves that prevent the backflow of blood.

TABLE 9-1 THE CARDIOVASCULAR SYSTEM

Organ/Structure	Primary Functions
Heart	Hollow muscular pump that circulates blood throughout the cardiovascular system
Arteries	Branching system of vessels that transports blood from the right and left ventricles of the heart to all body parts
Veins	Vessels that transport blood from peripheral tissues to the heart
Capillaries	Microscopic blood vessels that connect arterioles with venules; facilitate passage of life-sustaining fluids containing oxygen and nutrients to cell bodies and the removal of accumulated waste and carbon dioxide

PRIMARY WORD ELEMENTS

The following word elements (prefixes, roots, combining forms, and suffixes) will be used to build medical terms that relate to this unit. Please commit these to memory.

PREFIX

PREFIX	MEANING	PREFIX	MEANING
a	without, lack of	**hyper**	above, excessive
brady	slow	**inter**	between
endo	within	**tachy**	fast

COMBINING FORM

COMBINING FORM / ROOT	MEANING	COMBINING FORM / ROOT	MEANING
ang / i, angi / o, vas / o	vessel	**log**	study
angin	to choke, quinsy	**man / o**	thin
arter	artery	**my / o**	muscle
arteri / o	artery	**phleb**	vein
ather / o	fatty substance, porridge	**phleb / o**	vein
card	heart	**pulmonar**	lung
card / i, cardi / o	heart	**rrhyth**	rhythm
electr / o	electricity	**scler**	hardening
embol	to cast, to throw	**sphygm / o**	pulse
erg / o	work	**steth / o**	chest
hem	blood	**tens**	tension
infarct	infarct (necrosis of an area)	**thromb**	clot
lipid	fat	**ven / i**	vein

SUFFIX

SUFFIX	MEANING	SUFFIX	MEANING
-al	pertaining to	**-logy**	study of
-dynia	pain	**-megaly**	enlargement, large
-emia	blood condition	**-meter**	instrument to measure, to measure
-gram	mark, record		
-graphy	recording	**-pathy**	disease
-ia, -ism, -osis, -y	condition of	**-puncture**	to pierce
-ion	process	**-scope**	instrument
-ist	one who specializes	**-tomy**	incision
-itis	inflammation	**-tripsy**	crushing

ANSWER COLUMN

9.1 ___________ means pertaining to the heart and blood vessels (arteries, veins, and capillaries).

cardiovascular
(car dee oh **VAS** kew lar)

9.2 ___________ means the study of the heart.
The word elements used to build this term are:
___________ combining form that means heart
___________ suffix that means study of

cardiology
(car dee **ALL** oh jee)
cardi / o
-logy

9.3 A ___________ is a physician who specializes in the study of the heart.
The word elements used to build this term are:
___________ combining form that means heart
___________ root that means study of
___________ suffix that means one who specializes

cardiologist
(car dee **ALL** oh jist)
cardi / o
log
-ist

EXPLANATION FRAME

The heart is a four-chambered, hollow muscular pump that circulates blood throughout the cardiovascular system. The heart is the center of the cardiovascular system from which the various blood vessels originate and later return. It is slightly larger than a man's fist and weighs approximately 300 grams in the average adult male. It lies slightly to the left of the midline of the body and is shaped like an inverted cone with its apex downward.

ANSWER COLUMN

9.4 The heart has three layers or linings and they are the:

__________ inner lining of the heart

__________ muscular, middle layer of the heart

__________ outer, membranous sac surrounding the heart

endocardium (en doh **CAR** dee um)
myocardium (my oh **CAR** dee um)
pericardium (pair ih **CAR** dee um)

9.5 The human heart acts as a double pump and is divided into the right and left heart by a partition called a __________.

septum (**SEP** tum)

9.6 Each side of the heart contains an upper and lower chamber. The __________ or upper chambers are separated by the interatrial septum. The __________ or lower chambers are separated by the interventricular septum. The prefix __________ means between and describes the location of the septum between the left atrium and the right atrium or between the left ventricle and the right ventricle.

atria (**AY** tree ah)
ventricles (**VEN** trik lz)
inter

EXPLANATION FRAME

The heartbeat is controlled by the autonomic nervous system. It is normally generated by specialized neuromuscular tissue of the heart that is capable of causing cardiac muscle to contract rhythmically. The neuromuscular tissue of the heart comprises the sinoatrial node, the atrioventricular (AV) node, and the atrioventricular bundle. Of these, the sinoatrial (SA) node is often called the pacemaker of the heart. See Figure 9–1.

9.7 The __________ __________ is often called the pacemaker of the heart.

sinoatrial node (sigh noh **AY** tree al node)

9.8 __________ are vessels that transport blood from the right and left __________ of the heart to all body parts. In a normal state, they are elastic tubes that recoil and carry blood in pulsating __________.

arteries (**AR** teh rees)
ventricles (**VEN** trik lz)
waves (**WAYVS**)

9.9 __________ means inflammation of an artery or arteries.

arteritis (ar teh **RYE** tis)

■ **FIGURE 9–1**

The conduction system of the heart. Action potentials for the SA and AV nodes, other parts of the conduction system, and the atrial and ventricular muscles are shown along with the correlation to recorded electrical activity (electrocardiogram-ECG/EKG).

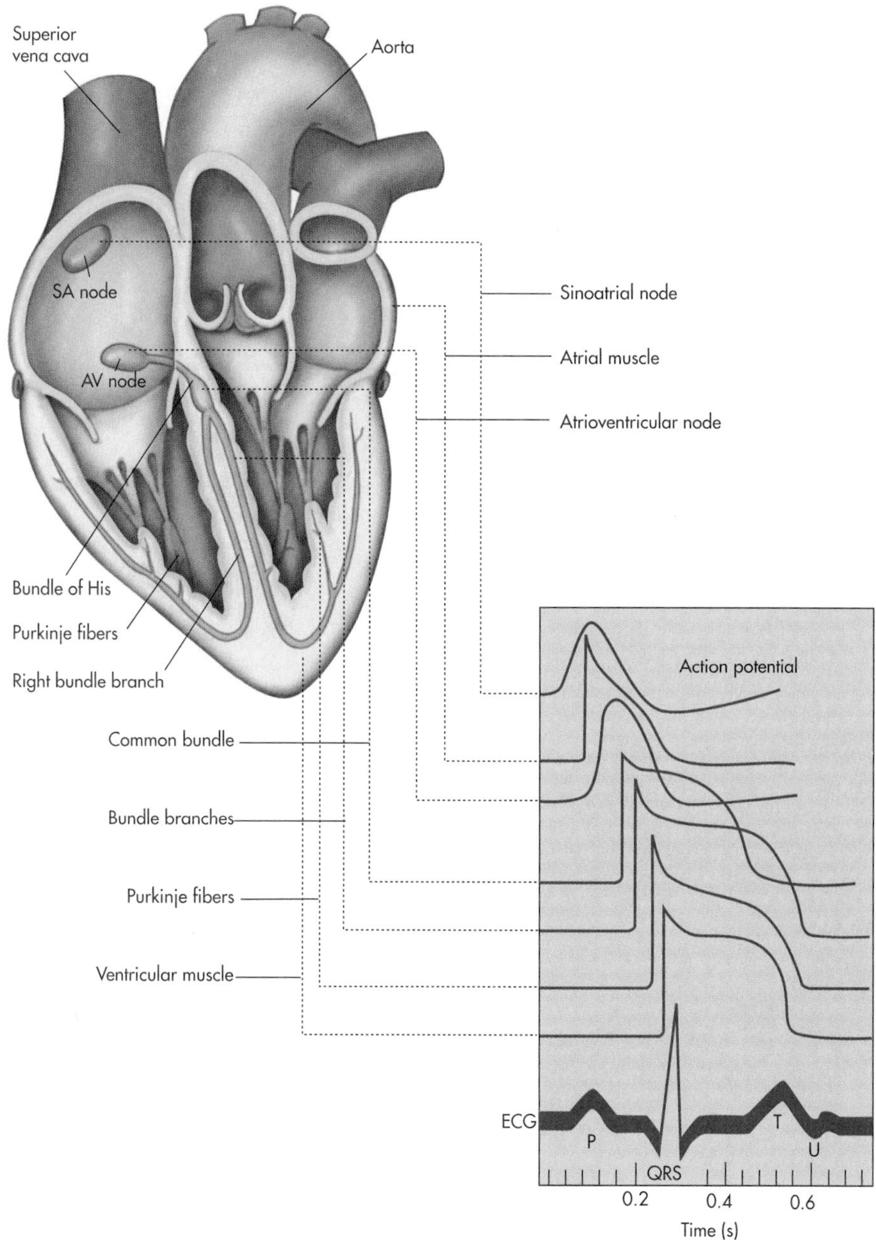

EXPLANATION FRAME

All arteries have a pulse reflecting the rhythmic beating of the heart; however, certain points are commonly used to check the rate, rhythm, and condition of the arterial wall. See Figure 9–2.

Some of these primary pulse points are:

PULSE	LOCATION
Radial	radial (thumb side) of the wrist
Brachial	antecubital space of the elbow
Carotid	neck
Temporal	temple
Femoral	groin

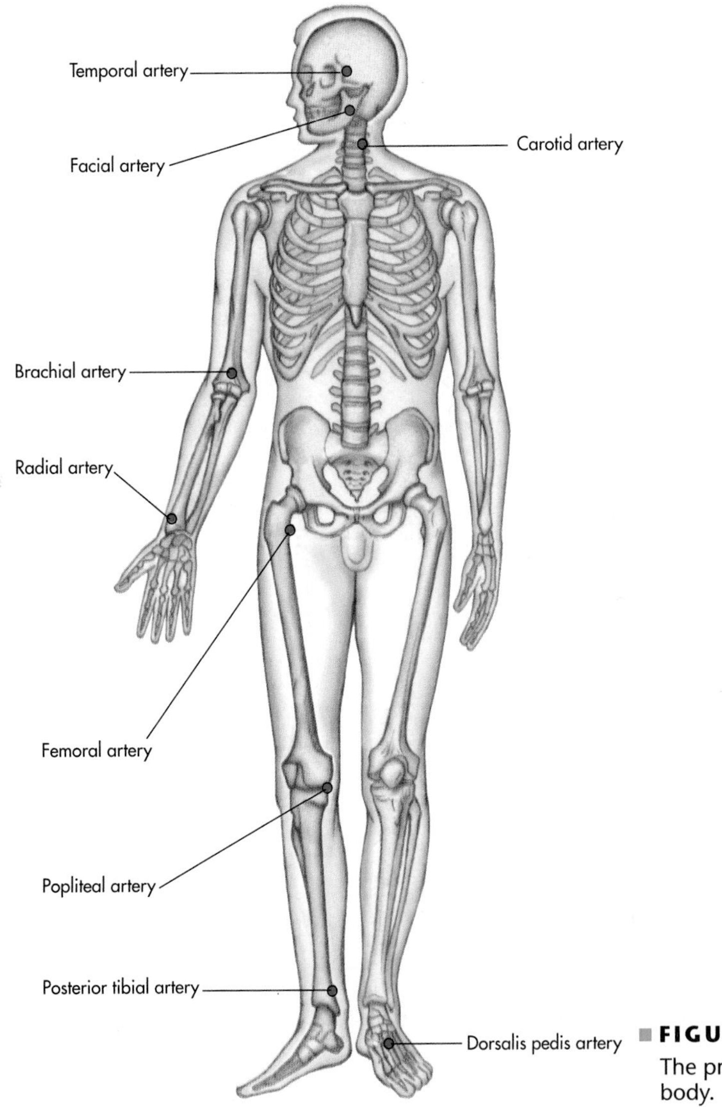

FIGURE 9–2
The primary pulse points of the body.

ANSWER COLUMN

9.10 The primary pulse point located on the thumb side of the wrist is known as the __________ point. It is the most common site for taking a patient's pulse.

radial (**RAY** dee al)

9.11 The primary pulse point located in the antecubital space of the elbow is known as the __________ point. It is the most common site that is used to check blood pressure.

brachial (**BRAY** kee al)

9.12 The primary pulse point located in the neck is known as the __________ point. It is the most readily accessible site to check for a pulse in an emergency, such as a cardiac arrest.

carotid (kah **ROT** id)

9.13 __________ is a medical term that is used to describe a condition of hardening of the arteries.

The word elements used to build this term are:

__________ combining form that means artery

__________ root that means hardening

__________ suffix that means condition of

*The patient with **arteri / o / scler / osis** has a condition in which there is __________ of an artery or arteries.*

arteriosclerosis (ar tee ree oh skleh **ROH** sis)

arteri / o

scler

-osis

hardening

9.14 __________ is a medical term that is used to describe a condition of hardening of the arteries with a buildup of fatty substance, porridge, within the arterial walls. See Figure 9–3.

The word elements used to build this term are:

__________ combining form that means fatty substance, porridge

__________ root that means hardening

__________ suffix that means condition of

atherosclerosis (ath er oh skleh **ROH** sis)

ather / o

scler

-osis

EXPLANATION FRAME

One should guard against confusing the terms arteriosclerosis and atherosclerosis. The patient with atherosclerosis has a condition characterized by a buildup of fatty substance(s) and the hardening of the walls of an artery or arteries. The buildup of fatty substances (usually cholesterol) is a contributing factor of heart disease. The patient with arteriosclerosis has a condition of hardening of the arteries that is usually associated with the aging process.

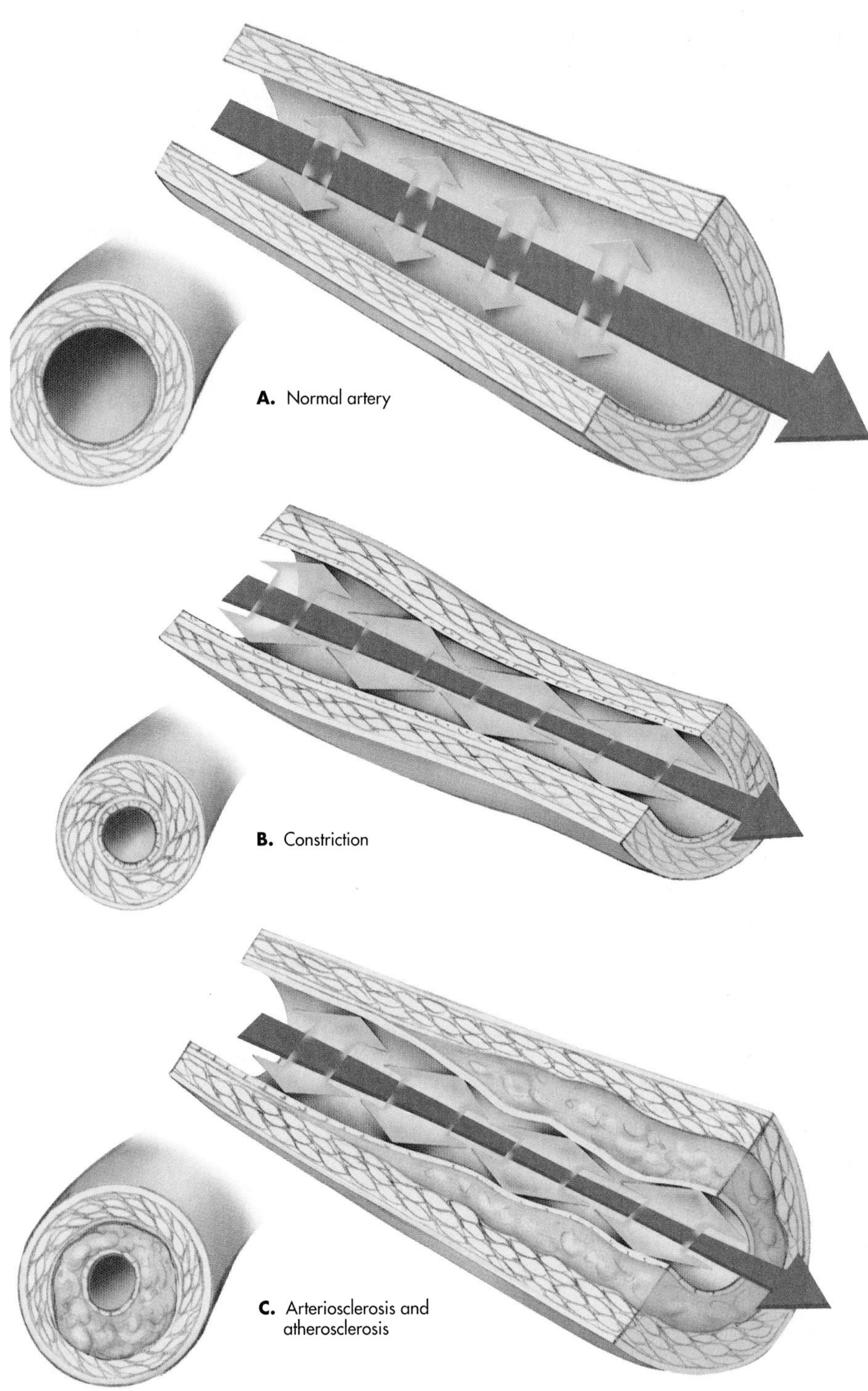

FIGURE 9–3
Blood vessels: (A) normal artery, (B) constriction, (C) arteriosclerosis and atherosclerosis.

Answer Column

9.15 ___________ is a waxy, fat-like substance in the bloodstream of all animals. *It is believed to be dangerous when it builds up on arterial walls and contributes to the risk of heart disease.*

cholesterol (koh **LES** ter all)

9.16 ___________ are lipids and protein molecules that are bound together. *They are classified as: VLDL—very-low-density lipoproteins; LDL—low-density lipoproteins; and HDL—high-density lipoproteins. High levels of VLDL and LDL are associated with cholesterol and triglyceride deposits in arteries, which could lead to coronary artery disease, hypertension, and* ***ather / o / scler / osis.***

lipoproteins (lip oh **PROH** teens)

EXPLANATION FRAME

In the United States, one out of four adults is at the risk of heart disease. Coronary heart disease is the number-one cause of death in the United States, outnumbering the deaths from cancer and accidents combined. It is said that every minute an American suffers a heart attack; 4.8 million Americans alive today have a history of heart attack, angina, or both; 1.5 million Americans will have a heart attack this year.

9.17 The American Heart Association lists the following as warning signs of heart attack:

___________, fullness, squeezing pain in the center of the chest that lasts 2 minutes or longer

___________ that spreads to the shoulders, neck, or arms

___________, fainting, sweating, nausea, or shortness of breath

pressure (**PRESH** ur)

pain (**PAYN**)

dizziness (**DIZ** ee nes)

9.18 ___________ ___________ can be caused by a variety of conditions, including angina, myocardial infarction, stress, anxiety, and gastrointestinal disorders. It is essential that the physician determine the cause of the pain and treat it appropriately.

chest pain (**CHEST PAYN**)

9.19 ___________ ___________ is defined as a severe pain and a sensation of constriction about the heart. It is caused by a decreased blood flow through the coronary arteries, usually due to atherosclerotic changes, that causes less oxygen to reach the myocardium. **Angina** means quinsy, to choke, and **pectoris** refers to the chest.

angina pectoris (an **JYE** nah **PEC** tor is)

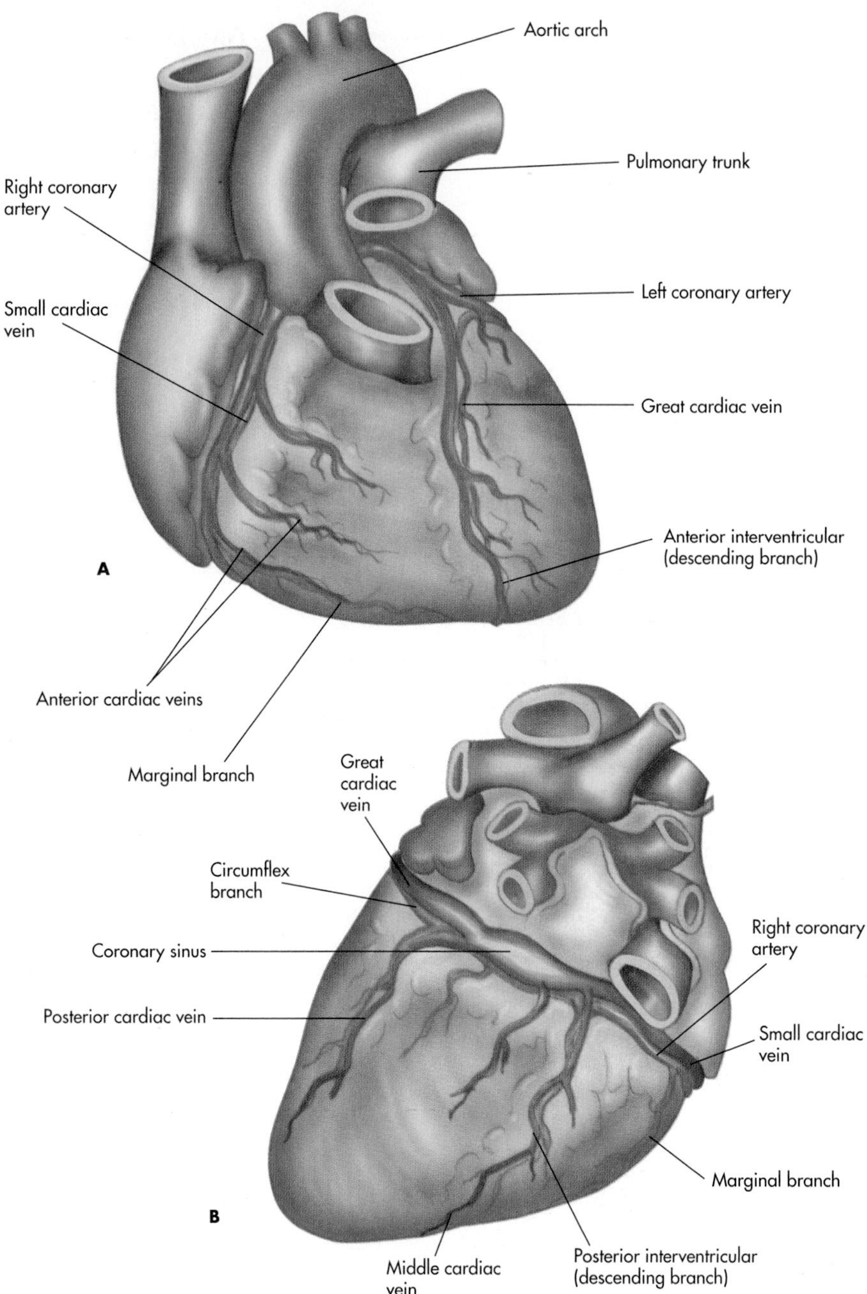

FIGURE 9–4

Coronary circulation. (A) Coronary vessels portraying the complexity and extent of the coronary circulation. (B) Coronary vessels that supply the anterior surface of the heart.

Answer Column

9.20 __________ means pain in the heart.
Cardi / o is a combining form that means heart and __________ is a suffix that means pain.

cardiodynia
(car dee oh **DIN** ee ah)
-dynia

9.21 __________ __________ is a condition caused by a partial or complete occlusion of a coronary artery or arteries. *The area involved becomes necrotic (infarct). It is typically called a "heart attack."*
The word elements used to build this term are:
__________ combining form that means muscle
__________ combining form that means heart
__________ suffix that means pertaining to
__________ root that means infarct (necrosis of an area)
__________ suffix that means process

myocardial infarction
(my oh **CAR** dee al in **FARC** shun)
my / o
card / i
-al
infarct
-ion

9.22 __________ is a condition in which a blood clot obstructs a blood vessel. *It is a moving blood clot and when it obstructs a coronary artery it can cause a heart attack.*
The word elements used to build this term are:
__________ root that means a throwing in
__________ suffix that means condition of

embolism
(**EM** boh lizm)
embol
-ism

9.23 __________ is a condition in which there is a blood clot within the vascular system. It is a stationary blood clot.
The word elements used to build this term are:
__________ root that means clot of blood
__________ suffix that means condition of

thrombosis
(throm **BOH** sis)
thromb
-osis

9.24 __________ __________ __________ is a drug that may be used within the first 6 hours of a myocardial infarction to dissolve fibrin clots. *It reduces the chance of dying after a myocardial infarction by 50%. Examples are Kabikinase (streptokinase) and Activase (alteplase recombinant).*

tissue plasminogen activator
(**TISH** oo plaz **MIN** oh jen **AK** tih vay tor)

9.25 __________ means enlargement of the heart. The combining form **cardi / o** means heart and the suffix __________ means enlargement.

cardiomegaly
(car dee oh **MEG** ah lee)
-megaly

Answer Column

9.26 ___________ is excessive lipids in the blood.
The word elements used to build this term are:
___________ prefix that means excessive
___________ root that means fat
___________ suffix that means blood

hyperlipidemia
(high per lip ih **DEE** mee ah)
hyper
lipid
-emia

EXPLANATION FRAME

Blood pressure, generally speaking, is the pressure exerted by the blood on the walls of the arteries. The term most commonly refers to the pressure exerted in large arteries at the peak of the pulse wave. This pressure is measured with a sphygmomanometer used in concert with a stethoscope. In an average adult, the systolic pressure usually ranges from 100 to 140 mm Hg and the diastolic from 60 to 90 mm Hg. A typical blood pressure reading showing systolic over diastolic is 120/80.

9.27 ___________ ___________ is the pressure exerted by the blood on the walls of the arteries.

blood pressure
(**BLUD PRESH** ur)

9.28 **Steth / o / scope** is a medical term. The combining form **steth / o** means ___________ and the suffix **-scope** means instrument.
A ___________ is an instrument used to listen to the sounds of the heart, lungs, and other internal organs.

chest (CHEST)
stethoscope
(**STETH** oh scope)

9.29 ___________ is a medical term. The combining form **sphygm / o** means pulse. See Figure 9–5.
Other word elements for the term **sphygm / o / man / o / meter** are:
___________ combining form that means thin
___________ suffix that means instrument to measure

sphygmomanometer
(sfig moh mah **NOM** eh ter)
man / o
-meter

9.30 ___________ blood pressure is referred to as the top reading. It occurs during the contraction phase of the heart cycle.

systolic
(sis **TOL** ik)

9.31 ___________ blood pressure is referred to as the bottom reading. It occurs during the relaxation phase of the heart cycle.

diastolic
(dye ah **STOL** ik)

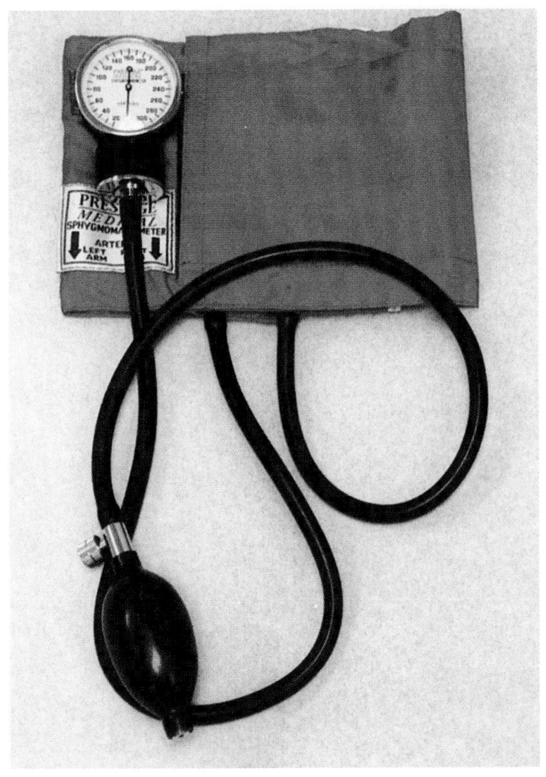

(A)

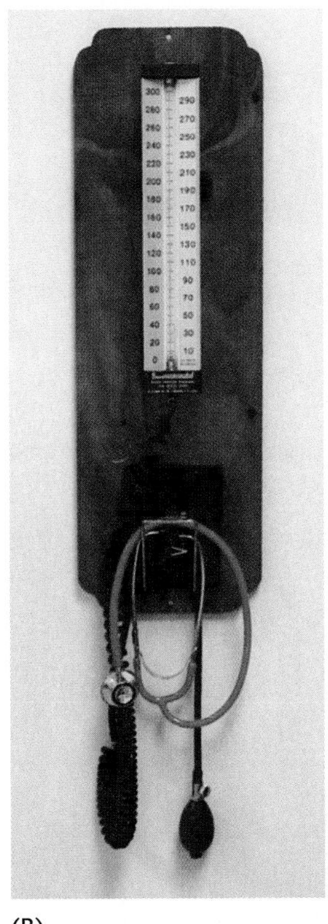

(B)

■ **FIGURE 9–5**
Sphygmomanometers: (A) aneroid type, (B) mercury type.

ANSWER COLUMN

9.32 Tapping sounds heard during auscultation of blood pressure are called ____________ ____________.

Auscultation is defined as a method of physical assessment using a stethoscope to listen to sounds within the chest, abdomen, and other parts of the body.

Korotkoff's sounds
(koh rot **KOFFS SOWNDS**)

9.33 The word for a method of physical assessment using a stethoscope to listen to sounds within the chest, abdomen, and other parts of the body is called ____________. The two heart sounds that can be heard with the use of a stethoscope are ____________.

auscultation
(oss kul **TAY** shun)
lubb-dupp (**LUB** dup)

9.34 ____________ is a medical term that is used to describe a blood pressure higher than normal: a systolic reading above 140 mm (millimeter) Hg (mercury) and a diastolic reading above 90 mm Hg. See Figure 9–6.

The word elements used to build this term are:

____________ prefix that means excessive, above
____________ root that means tension
____________ suffix that means process

hypertension
(high per **TEN** shun)

hyper
tens
-ion

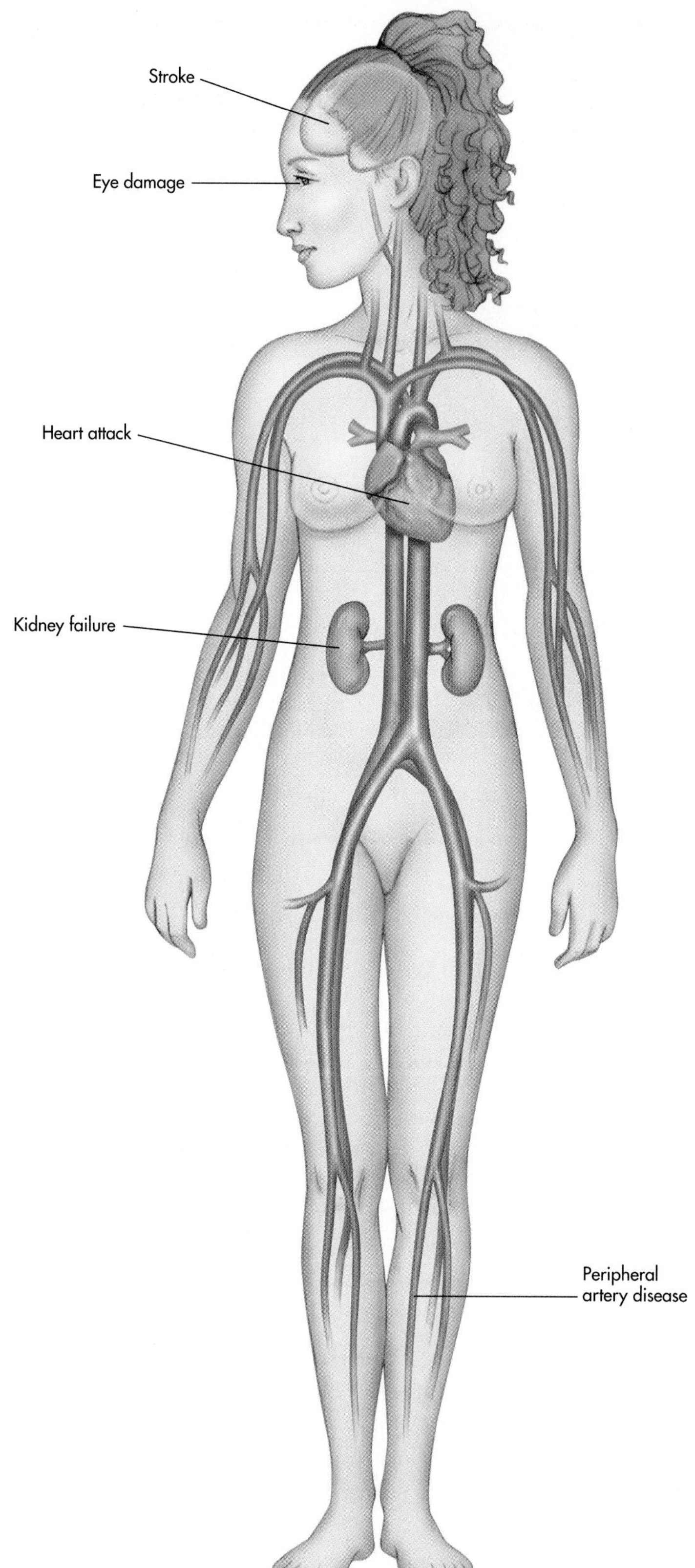

FIGURE 9–6

Uncontrolled hypertension can lead to kidney failure, stroke, heart attack, peripheral artery disease, and eye damage.

Answer Column

9.35 __________ is a medical term that is used to describe a blood pressure lower than normal: a systolic reading below 90 mm Hg and a diastolic reading below 60 mm Hg. The prefix __________ means deficient, below; the root **tens** means tension and the suffix __________ means process.

hypotension (high poh **TEN** shun)
hypo
-ion

9.36 A condition in which there is a lack of rhythm of the heartbeat is known as __________.

The word elements used to build this term are:

__________ prefix that means lack of
__________ root that means rhythm
__________ suffix that means condition of

arrhythmia (ah **RITH** mee ah)
a
rrhythm
-ia

EXPLANATION FRAME

Bradycardia and tachycardia are types of arrhythmias. Bradycardia is characterized by a pulse rate that is less than 60 beats per minute. Tachycardia is characterized by a pulse rate that is more than 100 beats per minute. Some arrhythmias do not require treatment while others may result in death if not treated by drug therapy or the use of an artificial pacemaker.

9.37 A slow heartbeat is called __________.

The word elements used to build this term are:

__________ prefix that means slow
__________ root that means heart
__________ suffix that means condition of

bradycardia (brad ee **CAR** dee ah)
brady
card
-ia

9.38 A fast heartbeat is called __________.

The word elements used to build this term are:

__________ prefix that means fast
__________ root that means heart
__________ suffix that means condition of

tachycardia (tak ee **CAR** dee ah)
tachy
card
-ia

9.39 An __________ pacemaker is an electronic device that stimulates impulse initiation within the heart. It can substitute for a defective natural pacemaker and control the heartbeat by a series of rhythmic electrical discharges. *If the device is placed on the outside of the chest it is called an external pacemaker. If it is placed within the chest wall it is called an internal pacemaker.*

artificial (ar tih **FISH** al)

Answer Column

9.40 ___________ is a medical term that means disease of the heart muscle. *The cause may be unknown or it may be caused by a viral infection, a parasitic infection, or overconsumption of alcohol. It may also be associated with congestive heart failure.*

cardiomyopathy (car dee oh my **OP** ah thee)

The word elements used to build this term are:

___________	combining form that means heart	**cardi / o**
___________	combining form that means muscle	**my / o**
___________	suffix that means disease	**-pathy**

9.41 When cardiomyopathy does not improve with treatment, then the patient may need a heart transplant. A heart transplant is the ___________ process of transferring the heart from a donor to a patient.

surgical (**SER** jih kal)

9.42 ___________ is the medical term that means to gather an organ and make it ready for transplantation.

harvest (**HAR** vest)

9.43 ___________ heart failure is the inability of the heart to pump sufficient blood to meet the needs of the tissues of the body. *The condition is characterized by weakness, breathlessness, abdominal discomfort, edema in lower extremities. It is also referred to as cardiac failure.*

congestive (kon **JESS** tiv)

EXPLANATION FRAME

A blood vessel may be an artery, vein, or capillary. Arteries transport blood away from the heart, veins transport blood to the heart, and capillaries connect arterioles (small arteries) to venules (small veins). In a normal state, arteries are elastic tubes that recoil and carry blood in pulsating waves (pulse). In a normal state, veins have thin walls and valves that prevent the backflow of blood. Capillaries are microscopic blood vessels with single-celled walls.

9.44 A tumor of a blood vessel is called ___________. See Figures 9–7 and 9–8.

hemangioma (hee man jee **OH** mah)

The word elements used to build this term are:

___________	root that means blood	**hem**
___________	combining form that means vessel	**ang / i**
___________	suffix that means tumor	**-oma**

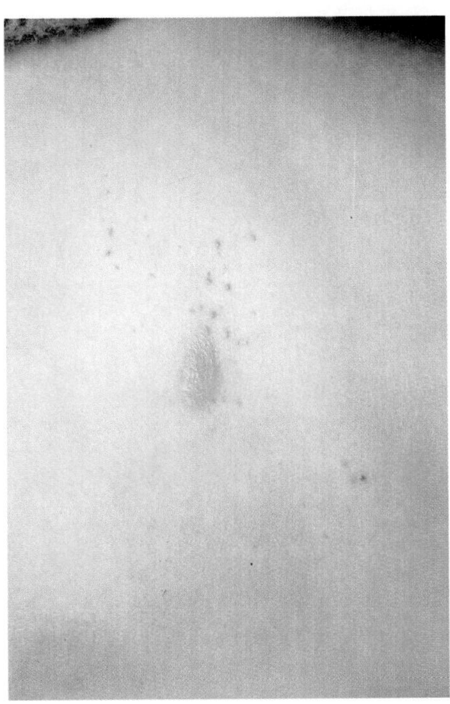

FIGURE 9–7
Hemangioma. *(Courtesy of Jason L. Smith, MD.)*

ANSWER COLUMN

9.45 An incision into a vein is known as __________.
The word elements used to build this term are:
__________ combining form that means vein
__________ suffix that means incision

phlebotomy
(fleh **BOT** oh mee)
phleb / o
-tomy

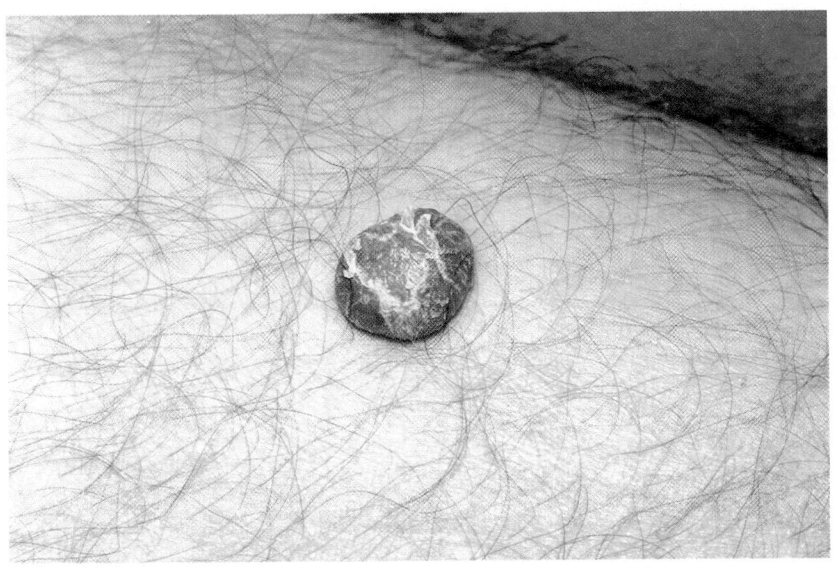

FIGURE 9–8
Sclerosing hemangioma. *(Courtesy of Jason L. Smith, MD.)*

Answer Column

9.46 ___________ is a medical term that means inflammation of a vein.
The word elements used to build this term are:
___________ root that means vein
___________ suffix that means inflammation

phlebitis
(fleh **BYE** tis)
phleb
-itis

9.47 ___________ is crushing of a blood vessel to stop hemorrhaging.
The word elements used to build this term are:
___________ combining form that means vessel
___________ suffix that means crushing

vasotripsy
(**VAS** oh trip see)
vas / o
-tripsy

9.48 ___________ is the medical term for puncturing a vein. The word venipuncture is usually associated with the piercing of a vein for the removal of a blood sample to be analyzed in a laboratory.
The word elements used to build this term are:
___________ combining form that means vein
___________ suffix that means to pierce

venipuncture
(**VEEN** ih punk cher)
ven / i
-puncture

9.49 The x-ray recording of a blood vessel after the injection of a radiopaque substance is called ___________.
The word elements used to build this term are:
___________ combining form that means vessel
___________ suffix that means recording

angiography
(an jee **OG** rah fee)
angi / o
-graphy

9.50 ___________ is the surgical repair of a blood vessel or vessels.

angioplasty
(**AN** jee oh plas tee)

9.51 ___________ **angioplasty** is the use of light beams to clear a path through a blocked artery.

laser
(**LAY** zer)

9.52 ___________ **transluminal coronary angioplasty** is the use of a balloon-tipped catheter to compress fatty plaques against an artery wall. *When successful, the plaques remain compresssed, and this permits more blood to flow through the artery, thereby relieving the symptoms of heart disease.*

percutaneous
(per kyoo **TAY** nee us)

Answer Column

9.53 ________ is the contraction or spasm of a blood vessel.

angiospasm (**AN** jee oh spazm)

9.54 ________ means the narrowing of a blood vessel.

vasoconstriction (vass oh con **STRIK** shun)

9.55 ________ means the widening of a blood vessel.

vasodilation (vas oh dye **LAY** shun)

9.56 A method of evaluating cardiovascular fitness that employs a treadmill and an electrocardiogram (ECG) monitoring is called a ________ ________. The ECG is monitored while the patient is subjected to increasing levels of work on a treadmill or ergometer. An **erg / o / meter** is an apparatus for measuring the amount of work done by a human or animal subject. **Erg / o** is a combining form that means work and **-meter** is a suffix that means instrument to measure, to measure.

stress test (**STRESS TEST**)

9.57 An ________ is a record of the electrical activity of the heart that shows certain waves called **P, Q, R, S,** and **T** waves. Sometimes a **U** wave is seen. See Figure 9–9.

The word elements used to build this term are:

________ combining form that means electricity

________ combining form that means heart

________ suffix that means record

electrocardiogram (ee lek troh **CAR** dee oh gram)

electr / o

cardi / o

-gram

9.58 ________ is a noninvasive ultrasound method for evaluating the heart for valvular defects and coronary artery disease.

echocardiography (ek oh car dee **OG** rah fee)

EXPLANATION FRAME

Cardiac catheterization is a test used in diagnosis of heart disorders. A tiny catheter is inserted into an artery in the groin area of the patient and is fed through this artery to the heart. Dye is then pumped through the catheter, enabling the physician to locate by x-ray any blockage in the arteries supplying the heart.

FIGURE 9–9
A normal electrocardiogram (ECG/EKG).

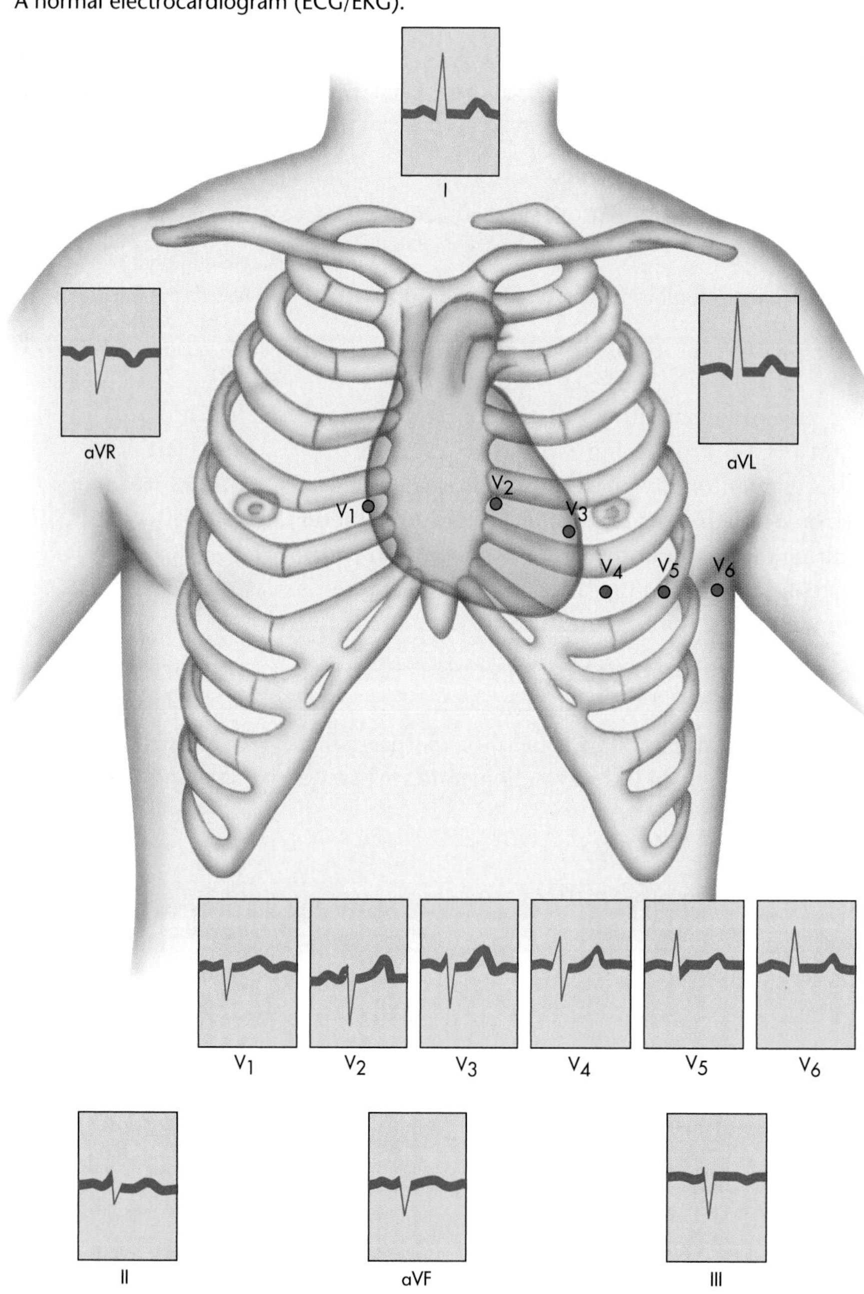

Answer Column

9.59 ___________ resuscitation (CPR) is a lifesaving skill that persons should learn in order to be prepared for an emergency situation involving a cardiac arrest.

The word elements used to build this term are:

___________ combining form that means heart

___________ root that means lung

___________ suffix that means pertaining to

cardiopulmonary (car dee oh **PULL** mon air ee)

cardi / o

pulmonar

-y

EXPLANATION FRAME

Drugs that are generally used for cardiovascular system diseases and disorders include digitalis, antiarrhythmics, vasopressors, nitrates, antihypertensives, anticoagulants, thrombolytics, and antilipemics.

9.60 ___________ is a cardiotonic drug that increases the tonicity of the heart. It is also referred to as having an inotropic effect, which influences the force of muscular contractility.

digitalis (dij ih **TAL** is)

9.61 ___________ agents are used to control cardiac arrhythmias.

antiarrhythmic (an tee ah **RITH** mik)

9.62 ___________ are drugs that cause contraction of the muscles associated with capillaries and arteries. They are used to elevate the blood pressure in shock and hypotension.

vasopressors (vas oh **PRESS** ors)

9.63 ___________ are classified as coronary vasodilators. They cause the relaxation of blood vessels and are used primarily for the treatment of angina pectoris.

nitrates (**NIGH** trayts)

9.64 ___________ agents are used in the treatment of hypertension.

antihypertensive (an tih high per **TEN** siv)

9.65 ______________ agents are used therapeutically to arrest or to prevent clotting.

anticoagulant (an tih koh **AG** yoo lant)

ANSWER COLUMN

9.66 ___________ agents act to dissolve existing thrombus when administered soon after its occurrence. Unless contraindicated they should be administered to a patient suffering a myocardial infarction within 6 hours of the onset of chest pain.

thrombolytic (throm boh **LIT** ik)

9.67 ___________ agents are used to lower abnormally high blood levels of fatty substances (lipids) when other treatment regimens fail.

antilipemic (an tih lih **PEE** mik)

9.68 ABBREVIATIONS

Write in the correct abbreviation for the following:

___________	arteriosclerotic heart disease	**ASHD**
___________	atrioventricular	**AV**
___________	blood pressure	**BP**
___________	coronary artery disease	**CAD**
___________	cardiac catheterization	**CC**
___________	congestive heart failure	**CHF**
___________	cardiomyopathy	**CMP**
___________	cardiopulmonary resuscitation	**CPR**
___________	electrocardiogram	**ECG, EKG**
___________	high-density lipoprotein	**HDL**
___________	mercury	**Hg**
___________	low-density lipoprotein	**LDL**
___________	myocardial infarction	**MI**
___________	millimeter	**mm**
___________	sinoatrial (node)	**S-A, SA**
___________	tissue plasminogen activator	**tPA, TPA**
___________	very-low-density lipoprotein	**VLDL**

IN THE SPOTLIGHT

HEART ATTACK

A heart attack occurs when the blood supply to part of the heart muscle (myocardium) is severely reduced or stopped. This occurs when one of the coronary arteries that supply blood to the heart muscle is blocked. The blockage is usually from the buildup of plaque (deposits of fat-like substances) due to atherosclerosis. The plaque can eventually tear or rupture, triggering a blood clot to form that blocks the artery and leads to a heart attack. Such an event is called a coronary thrombosis or coronary occlusion.

If the blood supply is cut off severely or for a long time, muscle cells suffer irreversible injury and die. Disability or death can result, depending on how much heart muscle is damaged.

Some heart attacks are sudden and intense, but most heart attacks start slowly, with mild pain or discomfort. Often the people affected are not sure of what is happening and wait too long before getting help. Heart attack and stroke are life-and-death emergencies and every second counts. Today heart attack and stroke victims can benefit from new medications and treatments. Clot-busting drugs can stop some heart attacks and strokes in progress, reducing disability and saving lives. But to be effective, these drugs must be given relatively quickly after heart attack or stroke symptoms first appear. Calling 911 is almost always the fastest way to get lifesaving treatment.

The American Heart Association gives the following as possible risk factors for heart attack or stroke:

- Man over 45 years of age
- Woman over 55 years of age or past menopause or following an oophorectomy and not taking estrogen
- Father or brother had a heart attack before age 55 or mother or sister had one before age 65
- Tobacco smoke
- Total cholesterol level is 240 mg/dL or higher
- HDL ("good") cholesterol level is less than 35 mg/dL
- LDL cholesterol level higher than 130
- Blood pressure 140/90 mm Hg or higher and not being treated or controlled
- Gets less than a total of 30 minutes of physical activity on most days
- 20 pounds or more overweight for height and build
- Diabetes or fasting blood sugar of 125 mg/dL or higher
- Coronary heart disease
- Previous heart attack
- Carotid artery disease
- Previous stroke or TIA (transient ischemic attack)
- Disease of the leg arteries

CASE STUDY

Please read the following case study and then work frames 9.69–9.73. Write in your answer in the answer column. Check your responses with the answers provided at the end of frame 9.73.

A 45-year-old male was seen by a cardiologist and the following is a synopsis of his visit.

PRESENT HISTORY: The patient states that during a workout session he felt a tightness in his chest, became short of breath, and felt very apprehensive. He states that this uncomfortable sensation went away after he stopped exercising.

SIGNS AND SYMPTOMS: Chief Complaints: tightness in his chest, dyspnea, apprehension.

DIAGNOSIS: Angina Pectoris. Diagnosis was determined by a complete physical examination, an electrocardiogram, and blood enzyme studies.

TREATMENT: Nitroglycerin Sublingual Tablets 0.4 mg as needed for chest pain. The patient is instructed to seek medical attention without delay if the pain is not relieved by three tablets, taken one every 5 minutes over a 15-minute period.

PREVENTION: Teach the patient to avoid situations that precipitate angina attacks. Proper rest and diet, stress management, lifestyle changes, avoidance of alcohol and tobacco are recommended.

9.69 Signs and symptoms of angina pectoris include tightness in the chest, ___________ (shortness of breath), and apprehension.

9.70 Give the abbreviation(s) for an electrocardiogram ___________.

9.71 The diagnosis of angina pectoris was determined by a complete physical examination, an ___________, and blood enzyme studies.

9.72 The medication regimen prescribed included ___________ 0.4 mg as needed for chest pain.

9.73 What should the patient do if the medication does not relieve the pain?

CASE STUDY ANSWERS

9.69 dyspnea
9.70 ECG, EKG
9.71 electrocardiogram
9.72 nitroglycerin
9.73 seek medical attention without delay

REVIEW A: WORD ELEMENTS

This review allows you to check your knowledge of some of the word elements presented in this unit. In the spaces provided, write the meaning of the word elements that are identified as **Prefix (P), Word Root (R), Combining Form (CF),** and/or **Suffix (S).**

MEDICAL WORD	*WORD ELEMENT*	*MEANING*
1. cardiology	cardi / o (CF)	____________
	-logy (S)	____________
2. arteriosclerosis	arteri / o (CF)	____________
	scler (R)	____________
	-osis (S)	____________
3. atherosclerosis	ather / o (CF)	____________
	scler (R)	____________
	-osis (S)	____________
4. cardiodynia	cardi / o (CF)	____________
	-dynia (S)	____________
5. myocardial	my / o (CF)	____________
	card (R)	____________
	-al (S)	____________
6. embolism	embol (R)	____________
	-ism (S)	____________
7. cardiomegaly	cardi / o (CF)	____________
	-megaly (S)	____________
8. electrocardiogram	electr / o (CF)	____________
	cardi / o (CF)	____________
	-gram (S)	____________
9. phlebotomy	phleb / o (CF)	____________
	-tomy (S)	____________

REVIEW B: MEDICAL TERMS

Please place the correct letter from column II on the appropriate line of column I.

COLUMN I		COLUMN II
______	1. endocardium	A. located on the thumb side of the wrist
______	2. atria	B. waxy, fat-like substance
______	3. ventricles	C. a moving blood clot
______	4. radial pulse point	D. the upper chambers of the heart
______	5. brachial pulse point	E. the inner lining of the heart
______	6. cholesterol	F. blood pressure higher than normal
______	7. embolism	G. lack of rhythm
______	8. hypertension	H. a fast heartbeat
______	9. arrhythmia	I. the lower chambers of the heart
______	10. tachycardia	J. located in the antecubital space of the elbow

REVIEW C: DISEASES AND DISORDERS

Please provide the correct disease or disorder for each of the following descriptions.

1. ______ ______ is a severe pain and sensation of constriction about the heart.
2. ______ ______ is typically called a "heart attack."
3. ______ is disease of the heart muscle.
4. ______ heart failure is the inability of the heart to pump sufficient blood to meet the needs of the tissues of the body.
5. ______ is a lack of rhythm of the heartbeat.

REVIEW D: UNSCRAMBLE THE WORDS

Unscramble the following medical terms and place the correct term on the line directly across from the scrambled word.

1. vestarh ______
2. iumdarcoym ______
3. putmes ______
4. tidorac ______
5. dyacdarrbia ______

REVIEW E: DRUGS USED FOR THE CARDIOVASCULAR SYSTEM

Please provide the correct answer for each of the following descriptions.

1. ____________ is a cardiotonic drug that increases the tonicity of the heart.
2. ____________ agents are used to control cardiac arrhythmias.
3. ____________ are drugs that cause contraction of the muscles associated with capillaries and arteries.
4. ____________ are classified as coronary vasodilators.
5. ____________ agents are used in the treatment of hypertension.
6. ____________ agents are used to arrest or to prevent clotting.
7. ____________ agents are used to lower abnormally high blood levels of lipids.

REVIEW F: ABBREVIATIONS

Please provide the correct abbreviation and/or meaning for the abbreviation.

1. ____________ blood pressure
2. CAD ____________
3. ________________ cardiomyopathy
4. CHF ____________
5. ____________ electrocardiogram
6. ____________ myocardial infarction

10 BLOOD, LYMPH, AND THE IMMUNE SYSTEM: HEMATOLOGY AND IMMUNOLOGY

LEARNING CONCEPTS

- essential terminology
- pronunciation guide
- word elements
- explanation frames
- blood
- formed elements
- anemias
- blood types: A, B, AB, and O
- plasma
- the lymphatic system
- immunity
- immunization
- selected diseases and disorders
- drugs used for blood, lymph, and the immune system
- abbreviations
- in the spotlight: immunization
- case study: AIDS
- review exercises

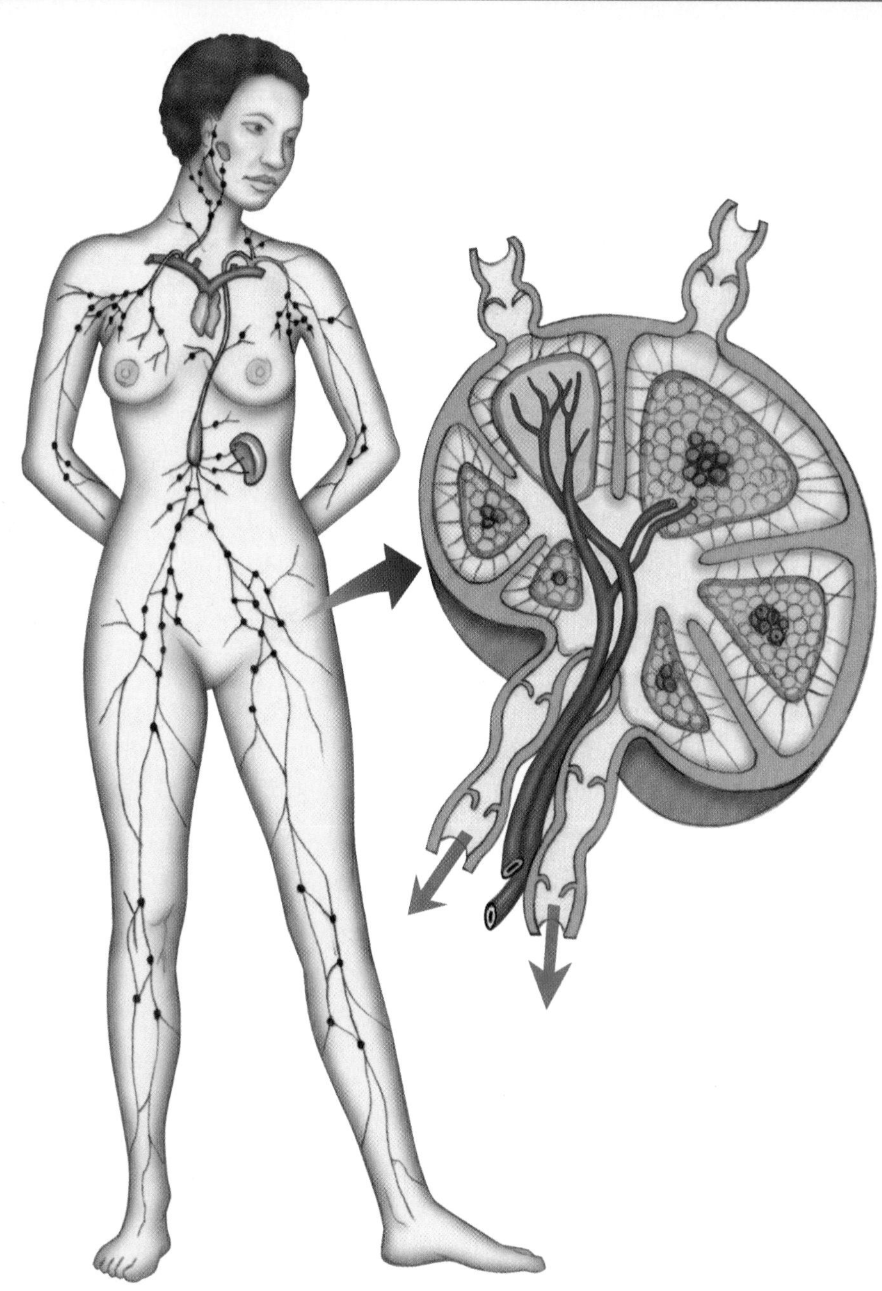

OBJECTIVES

ON COMPLETION OF THIS UNIT, YOU SHOULD BE ABLE TO:

- Briefly describe blood, lymph, and the immune system.
- Describe the primary functions of the various organs or structures of the blood and lymphatic system.
- Identify and give the meaning of the primary word elements for this unit.
- Analyze, build, spell, and pronounce selected medical words.
- Describe selected diseases/disorders of the blood, lymph, and immune system.
- Identify the various types of blood cells and give their function.
- Name the four recognized blood types.
- Describe immunity and immunization.
- Briefly describe acquired immunodeficiency syndrome (AIDS).
- Briefly describe hepatitis B.
- Describe selected drugs that are used for the blood, lymph, and the immune system diseases or disorders.
- Define selected abbreviations that pertain to the blood, lymph, and the immune system
- State the basis of recommendations for immunization of infants, children, and adults
- Name the committee and two academies that provide recommended immunization schedules
- State how to reduce the unnecessary occurrence of vaccine-preventable diseases.
- Complete the Case Study on AIDS.
- Successfully complete the review section.

TECH LINK

CD-ROM Use the CD-ROM enclosed with your textbook to gain additional reinforcement through interactive word building exercises, spelling games, labeling activities, and additional quizzes.

www.prenhall.com/rice Use the above address to access the free, interactive Companion Website created specifically for this textbook. Get hints, instant feedback, and textbook references to chapter-related multiple choice and true/false questions, fill-in-the-blank, and labeling exercises. In addition, you will find an audio glossary, and essay questions.

Blood and lymph are two of the body's main fluids. Blood is circulated by the action of the heart but lymph does not actually circulate. It is propelled in one direction, away from its source, through increasingly larger lymph vessels. Numerous valves within the lymph vessels permit one-directional flow. Blood is a fluid consisting of formed elements and plasma. The blood volume within an individual depends on body weight. An individual weighing 154 pounds (70 kg) has a blood volume of about 5 quarts or 5 liters.

The immune system consists of the tissues, organs, and physiologic processes used by the body to identify abnormal cells, foreign substances, and foreign tissue cells that may have been transplanted into the body.

It is composed of lymph capillaries, lymphatic vessels, lymphatic ducts, and lymph nodes. This system conveys lymph from the tissue to the blood. Lymph is clear, colorless, alkaline fluid that is about 95% water.

The accessory organs of the lymphatic system are the spleen, the tonsils, and the thymus. The spleen is a soft, dark-red oval body lying in the upper left quadrant of the abdomen. The spleen is the major site of erythrocyte destruction. It serves as a reservoir for blood. The spleen plays an essential role in the immune response and acts as a filter, removing microorganisms from the blood. The tonsils are lymphoid masses located in depressions of the mucous membranes of the face and pharynx. They consist of the palatine tonsil, the pharyngeal tonsil (adenoids), and the lingual tonsil. The tonsils filter bacteria and aid in the formation of white blood cells. The thymus is considered one of the endocrine glands, but because of its function and appearance, it is a part of the lymphoid system. It is located in the mediastinal cavity. The thymus plays an essential role in the formation of antibodies and the development of the immune response in the newborn. It manufactures infection-fighting T cells and helps distinguish normal T cells from those that attack the body's own tissue. T cells are important in the body's cellular immune response. See Table 10–1.

TABLE 10-1 BLOOD AND THE LYMPHATIC SYSTEM

Organ/Structure	Primary Functions
Blood	Fluid consisting of formed elements and plasma that transports respiratory gases (oxygen and carbon dioxide), chemical substances (foods, salts, hormones), and cells that act to protect the body from foreign substances
Lymphatic System	A vessel system composed of lymph capillaries, lymphatic vessels, lymphatic ducts, and lymph nodes that conveys lymph from the tissue to the blood. The three main functions of the lymphatic system are: 1. It transports proteins and fluids, lost by capillary seepage, back to the bloodstream 2. It protects the body against pathogens by phagocytosis and immune response 3. It serves as a pathway for the absorption of fats from the small intestines into the bloodstream
Spleen	Major site of erythrocyte destruction; serves as a reservoir for blood; acts as a filter, removing microorganisms from the blood
Tonsils	Filter bacteria and aid in the formation of white blood cells
Thymus	Essential role in the formation of antibodies and the development of the immune response in the newborn; manufactures infection-fighting T cells and helps distinguish normal T cells from those that attack the body's own tissue

PRIMARY WORD ELEMENTS

The following word elements (prefixes, roots, combining forms, and suffixes) will be used to build medical terms that relate to this unit. Please commit these to memory.

PREFIX

PREFIX	MEANING	PREFIX	MEANING
an	without, lack of	**poly**	many, much

COMBINING FORM

COMBINING FORM / ROOT	MEANING	COMBINING FORM / ROOT	MEANING
aden	gland	**log**	study
aden / o	gland	**lymph**	lymph, clear fluid
ang / i, angi / o	vessel	**lymph / o**	lymph, clear fluid
cyt	cell	**phag / o**	to eat
cyth	cell	**splen**	spleen
erythr / o	red	**splen / o**	spleen
glob	globe	**thromb**	clot
globin	globule	**thromb / o**	clot
hemat	blood	**thym**	thymus
hemat / o, hem / o	blood	**thym / o**	thymus
immun / o	immunity, safe	**tonsill**	tonsil
leuk / a, leuk / o	white		

SUFFIX

SUFFIX	MEANING	SUFFIX	MEANING
-blast	immature cell, germ cell	**-oma**	tumor
-cele	hernia, tumor, swelling	**-osis**	condition of
-crit	to separate	**-pathy**	disease
-cyte	cell	**-penia**	lack of, deficiency
-ectomy	surgical excision	**-pexy**	surgical fixation
-emia	blood condition	**-pheresis**	removal
-genic	formation, produce	**-philia**	attraction
-ist	one who specializes	**-phobia**	fear
-itis	inflammation	**-poiesis**	formation
-logy	study of	**-rrhage**	bursting forth
-lysis, -lyse	destruction, to separate	**-stasis**	control, stopping
-megaly	enlargement, large		

ANSWER COLUMN

10.1 __________ means the study of the blood.
The word elements used to build this term are:
__________ combining form that means blood
__________ suffix that means study of

hematology
(hee mah **TALL** oh jee)

hemat / o

-logy

ANSWER COLUMN

10.2 A __________ is a physician who specializes in the study of the blood. The word elements used to build this term are:

__________ combining form that means blood

__________ root that means study of

__________ suffix that means one who specializes

hematologist (hee mah **TALL** oh jist)
hemat / o
log
-ist

EXPLANATION FRAME

Blood is a fluid consisting of formed elements and plasma, both of which are continuously produced by the body for the purpose of transporting respiratory gases, chemical substances, and cells that act to protect the body from foreign substances.

10.3 The combining forms **hemat / o** and **hem / o** mean blood. Medical terms that begin with these word elements are:

__________ a blood cyst, hernia — **hematocele** (**HEE** mah toh seel)

__________ a blood test that separates solids from plasma in the blood by centrifuging the blood sample — **hematocrit** (hee **MAT** oh krit)

__________ a blood tumor (See Figure 10–1.) — **hematoma** (hee mah **TOH** mah)

__________ blood protein; the iron-containing pigment of red blood cells — **hemoglobin** (HEE moh **GLOH** bin)

__________ disease caused by or associated with abnormal hemoglobin — **hemoglobinopathy** (hee moh gloh bin **OP** ah thee)

__________ destruction of red blood cells — **hemolysis** (hee **MALL** ih sis)

__________ to produce hemolysis — **hemolyze** (**HEE** moh lize)

__________ is a hereditary blood disease characterized by prolonged clotting time and tendency to bleed; hemophilia A is due to a deficiency of blood coagulation factor VIII. *Hemophilia B refers to Christmas disease, a hemophilia-like disease caused by a lack of factor IX, a plasma thromboplastin component* — **hemophilia** (hee moh **FILL** ee ah)

__________ fear of blood — **hemophobia** (hee moh **FOH** bee ah)

__________ formation of blood cells — **hemopoiesis** (hee moh poy **EE** sis)

FIGURE 10–1
Traumatic hematoma. *(Courtesy of Jason L. Smith, MD.)*

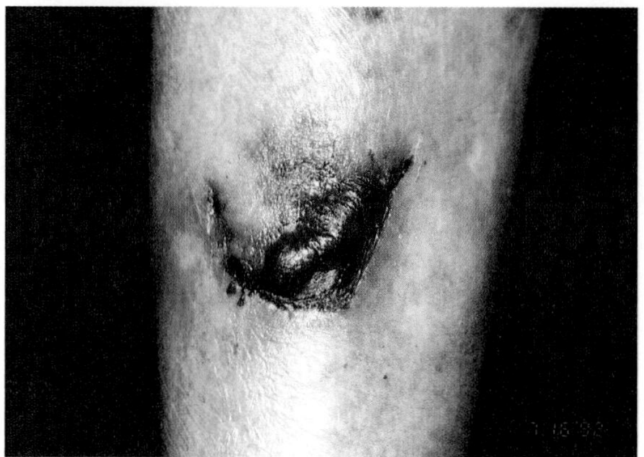

FIGURE 10–2
Hemorrhage, vein. *(Courtesy of Jason L. Smith, MD.)*

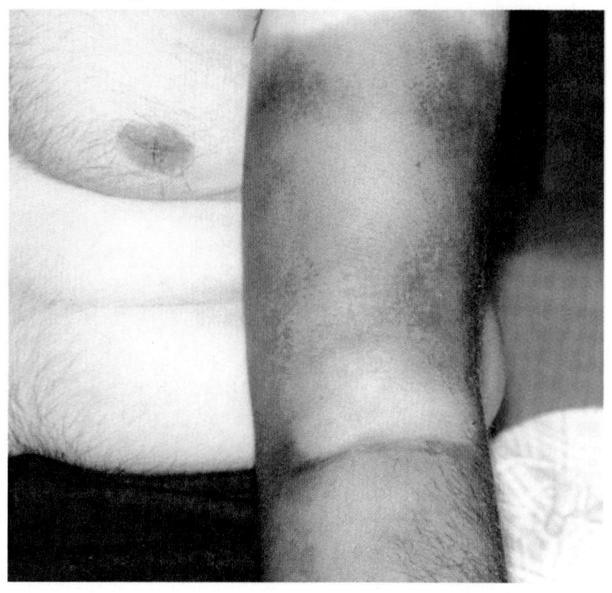

ANSWER COLUMN

continued

		Answer
___________	excessive bleeding (See Figure 10–2.)	**hemorrhage** (**HEM** eh rij)
___________	___________ an acute febrile disease; one type is dengue fever, which is transmitted by the mosquito	**hemorrhagic fever** (hem eh **RAJ** ik **FEE** ver)

10.4 The formed elements in blood are the red blood cells or ___________, platelets or **thrombocytes**, and white blood cells or **leukocytes**. *Formed elements comprise about 45% of the total volume of blood and are sometimes referred to as whole blood.* See Figure 10–3 and Table 10–2.

erythrocytes (eh **RITH** roh sights)

EXPLANATION FRAME

Erythrocytes or RBCs are doughnut-shaped cells without nuclei. They transport oxygen (most of which is bound to hemoglobin contained in the cell) and carbon dioxide. There are approximately 5 million erythrocytes per cubic millimeter of blood and they have a life span of 80 to 120 days. Erythrocytes are formed in the red bone marrow and are commonly called red blood cells.

FIGURE 10–3
The formed elements of blood: erythrocytes, leukocytes (neutrophils, eosinophils, basophils, lymphocytes, and monocytes), and thrombocytes (platelets).

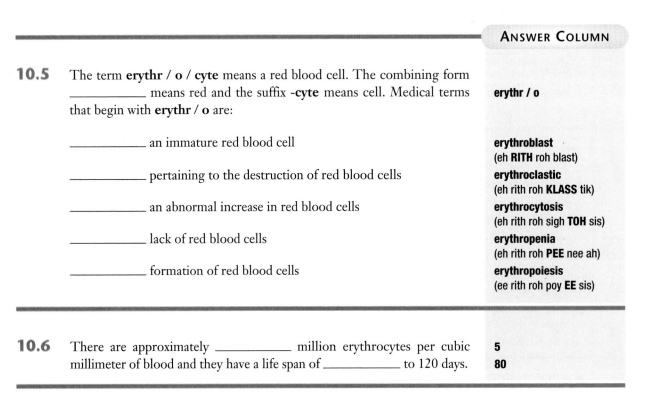

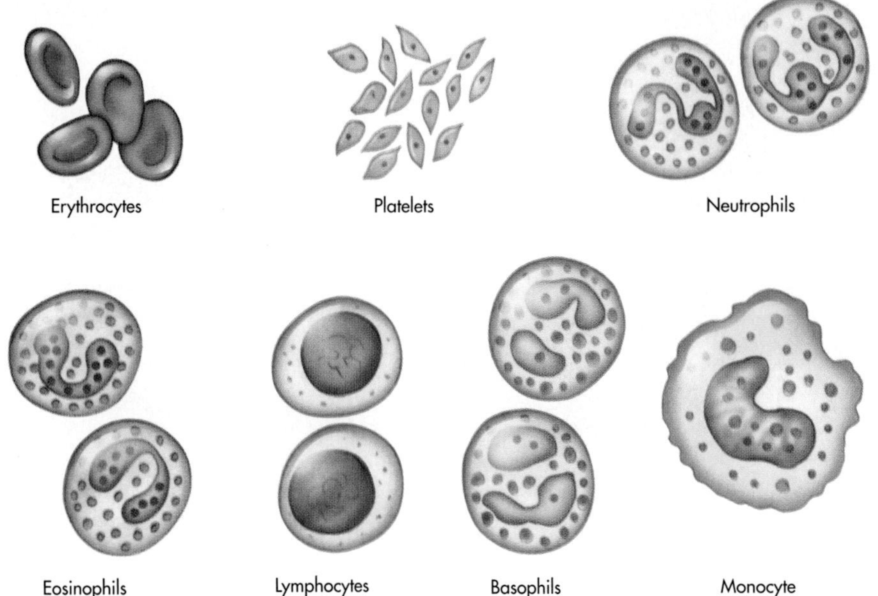

ANSWER COLUMN

10.5 The term **erythr / o / cyte** means a red blood cell. The combining form ___________ means red and the suffix **-cyte** means cell. Medical terms that begin with **erythr / o** are:

erythr / o

___________ an immature red blood cell

___________ pertaining to the destruction of red blood cells

___________ an abnormal increase in red blood cells

___________ lack of red blood cells

___________ formation of red blood cells

erythroblast
(eh **RITH** roh blast)
erythroclastic
(eh rith roh **KLASS** tik)
erythrocytosis
(eh rith roh sigh **TOH** sis)
erythropenia
(eh rith roh **PEE** nee ah)
erythropoiesis
(ee rith roh poy **EE** sis)

10.6 There are approximately ___________ million erythrocytes per cubic millimeter of blood and they have a life span of ___________ to 120 days.

5
80

TABLE 10-2 TYPES OF BLOOD CELLS AND FUNCTIONS

Blood Cell	Function
Erythrocyte (red blood cell)	Transports oxygen and carbon dioxide
Thrombocyte (platelet)	Blood clotting
Leukocyte (white blood cell)	Body's main defense against invasion of pathogens
Neutrophil	Protection against infection, phagocytosis
Eosinphil	Destroys parasitic organisms, plays a key role in allergic reactions
Basophil	Key role in releasing histamine and other chemicals that act on blood vessels, essential to nonspecific immune response to inflammation
Monocyte	One of the first lines of defense in the inflammatory process, phagocytosis
Lymphocyte	Provides the body with immune capacity
B lymphocyte	Identifies foreign antigens and differentiates into antibody-producing plasma cells (source for immunoglobulins–antibodies)
T lymphocyte	Essential for the specific immune response of the body

ANSWER COLUMN

10.7 ____________ literally means a lack of blood. *It is a reduction in the number of circulating red blood cells per cubic millimeter, the amount of hemoglobin per 100 mL, or the volume of packed red cells per 100 mL of blood.*

anemia
(ah **NEE** mee ah)

10.8 There are many types of anemias and the following are some of the types:

____________ anemia is caused by destruction of the bone marrow due to chemical agents such as certain drugs and/or physical factors such as x-rays.

aplastic
(ay **PLASS** tik)

____________ anemia is due to excessive blood loss.

blood loss

____________ anemia is also known as thalassemia. It is a hereditary anemia occurring in populations bordering the Mediterranean Sea and in Southeast Asia.

Cooley's
(**KOO** leez)

____________ ____________ anemia may be due to inadequate iron intake, malabsorption of iron, chronic blood loss, pregnancy and lactation, intravascular hemolysis, or a combination of these factors.

iron deficiency
(**EYE** ern dee **FISH** en see)

____________ anemia is due to megaloblasts found in the blood.

megaloblastic
(meg ah loh **BLAST** ik)

____________ anemia is due to a failure of the stomach to secrete enough intrinsic factor to ensure intestinal absorption of vitamin B_{12}, the extrinsic factor.

pernicious
(per **NISH** us)

____________ ____________ anemia is a hereditary, chronic, hemolytic anemia due to a defect in the hemoglobin molecule. It is characterized by the presence of large numbers of crescent-shaped or sickle-shaped red blood cells in the blood. It is most common among persons of African and Mediterranean descent.

sickle cell
(**SIK'L SELL**)

ANSWER COLUMN

10.9 ____________ is a medical term that means a condition of too many red blood cells.

The word elements used to build this term are:

____________ prefix that means many

____________ root that means cell

____________ suffix that means blood condition

polycythemia (pol ee sigh **THEE** mee ah)

poly

cyth

-emia

EXPLANATION FRAME

Thrombocytes or platelets are disk-shaped cells about half the size of erythrocytes. They play an important role in the clotting process by releasing thrombokinase, which, in the presence of calcium, reacts with prothrombin to form thrombin. There are approximately 200,000 to 500,000 thrombocytes per cubic millimeter of blood. Thrombocytes are fragments of certain giant cells called megakaryocytes, which are formed in the red bone marrow.

10.10 The term **thromb / o / cyte** refers to a clotting cell; a blood platelet.

The combining form ____________ and the root **thromb** mean clot and the suffix **-cyte** means cell.

thromb / o

10.11 A medical term that means an abnormal decrease in the number of platelets is ____________.

The word elements used to build this term are:

____________ combining form that means clot

____________ combining form that means cell

____________ suffix that means lack of, deficiency

thrombocytopenia (throm boh sigh toh **PEE** nee ah)

thromb / o

cyt / o

-penia

10.12 Build medical terms that begin with **thromb** or **thromb / o** and the following suffixes:

____________ that means surgical excision

____________ that means formation, produce

____________ that means destruction

____________ that means condition of

____________ surgical excision of a blood clot

____________ formation of a blood clot

-ectomy

-genic

-lysis

-osis

thrombectomy (throm **BEK** toh mee)

thrombogenic (throm boh **JEN** ik)

continued

		ANSWER COLUMN
___________	destruction of a blood clot	**thrombolysis** (throm **BOL** ih sis)
___________	condition of a blood clot formation	**thrombosis** (throm **BOH** sis)

10.13 There are approximately ___________ to 500,000 thrombocytes per cubic millimeter of blood. — **200,000**

EXPLANATION FRAME

Leukocytes are sphere-shaped cells containing nuclei of varying shapes and sizes. Leukocytes are the body's main defense against the invasion of pathogens (disease-producing microorganisms). There are approximately 8000 leukocytes per cubic millimeter of blood. There are five types of leukocytes: neutrophils, eosinophils, basophils, lymphocytes, and monocytes. Except for the lymphocytes, leukocytes are formed in the red bone marrow. Lymphocytes are formed in lymph nodes and other lymphatic tissue. Leukocytes are commonly called white blood cells.

10.14 The term **leuk / o / cyte** refers to a white blood cell. The combining forms **leuk / a** and ___________ and the root **leuk** mean white. The suffix **-cyte** means cell. — **leuk / o**

Medical terms that begin with **leuk, leuk / a,** or **leuk / o** are:

___________ removal of white blood cells from the circulation — **leukapheresis** (loo kah feh **REE** sis)

___________ a disease of the blood characterized by overproduction of leukocytes — **leukemia** (loo **KEE** mee ah)

___________ a lack of white blood cells — **leukocytopenia** (loo koh sigh toh **PEE** nee ah)

___________ is an increase in the number of leukocytes (above 10,000 per cubic millimeter) in the blood. It is generally caused by infection and is usually transient — **leukocytosis** (loo koh sigh **TOH** sis)

___________ is the formation and/or production of leukocytes — **leukopoiesis** (loo koh poy **EE** sis)

10.15 There are approximately ___________ leukocytes per cubic millimeter of blood. — **8000**

ANSWER COLUMN

EXPLANATION FRAME

There are four recognized blood types: **A, B, AB,** and **O.** Each is named for the antigens contained in the red cells. The presence of a substance called an agglutinogen in the red blood cells is responsible for what is known as the **Rh factor.** It was first discovered in the blood of the Rhesus monkey, from which the factor gets its name. About 85% of the population have the Rh factor and are called Rh positive. The other 15% lack the Rh factor and are designated Rh negative. Type O Rh negative is known as the universal donor and type AB Rh positive is known as the universal recipient.

10.16 **True or False**. There are four recognized blood types. These are types **A**, **B**, **AB**, and **O**.

true

EXPLANATION FRAME

The fluid part of the blood is called plasma. It comprises about 55% of the total volume of blood, is clear and somewhat straw-colored, and is composed of water (91%) and chemical compounds (9%). Plasma is the medium for circulation of blood cells. It provides nutritive substances to various body structures and removes waste products of metabolism from body structures. There are four major plasma proteins: albumin, globulin, fibrinogen, and prothrombin.

10.17 The fluid part of the blood is called ____________.

plasma
(**PLAZ** mah)

EXPLANATION FRAME

The lymphatic system is a vessel system apart from, but connected to, the circulatory system. It is composed of lymph capillaries, lymphatic vessels, lymphatic ducts, and lymph nodes. The system conveys lymph from the tissues to the blood. Lymph is a clear, colorless, alkaline fluid that is about 95% water. See Figure 10–4.

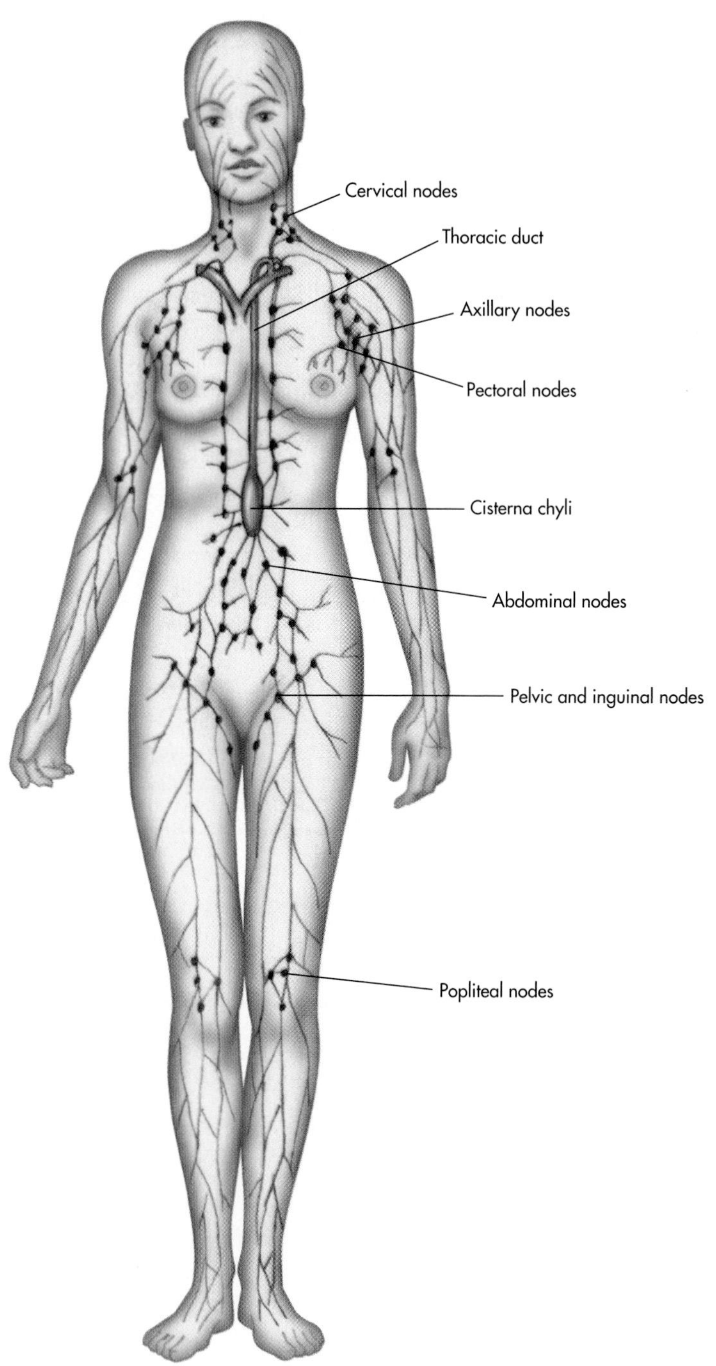

FIGURE 10–4
The lymphatic system.

ANSWER COLUMN

10.18 The combining form **lymph / o** and the root **lymph** mean lymph. Medical terms that begin with these word elements are:

		Answer
____________	inflammation of the lymph glands	**lymphadenitis** (lim fad en **EYE** tis)
____________	disease of the lymph glands	**lymphadenopathy** (lim fad eh **NOP** ah thee)
____________	incision into a lymph gland	**lymphadenotomy** (lim fad eh **NOT** oh mee)
____________	the study of the lymphatic vessels	**lymphangiology** (lim fan jee **ALL** oh jee)
____________	tumor of a lymph gland	**lymphangioma** (lim fan jee **OH** mah)
____________	resembling lymph	**lymphoid** (**LIM** foid)
____________	any neoplastic disorder of lymphoid tissue (See Figures 10–5 and 10–6.)	**lymphoma** (lim **FOH** mah)
____________	a malignant disease of lymphatic tissue	**lymphosarcoma** (lim foh sar **KOH** mah)
____________	control or stopping the flow of lymph	**lymphostasis** (lim **FOS** tah sis)

10.19 **True or False**. Lymph is a colorless, alkaline fluid that is about 95% water.

true

EXPLANATION FRAME

The spleen, the tonsils, and the thymus are closely related to the lymphatic system in their functions. See Figure 10–7. The spleen is the major site of erythrocyte destruction and serves as a reservoir for blood. It plays

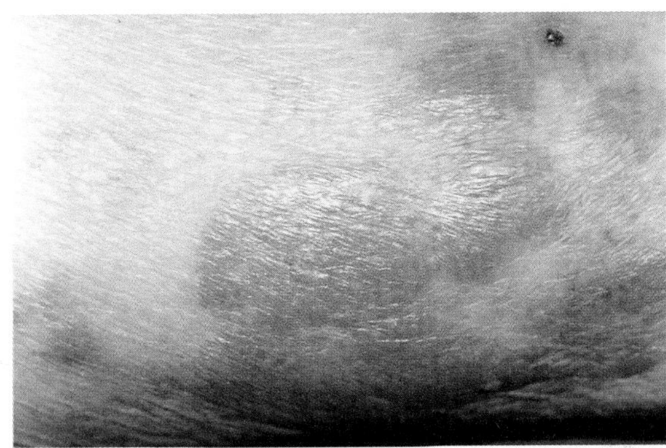

FIGURE 10–5
Lymphoma.
(Courtesy of Jason L. Smith, MD.)

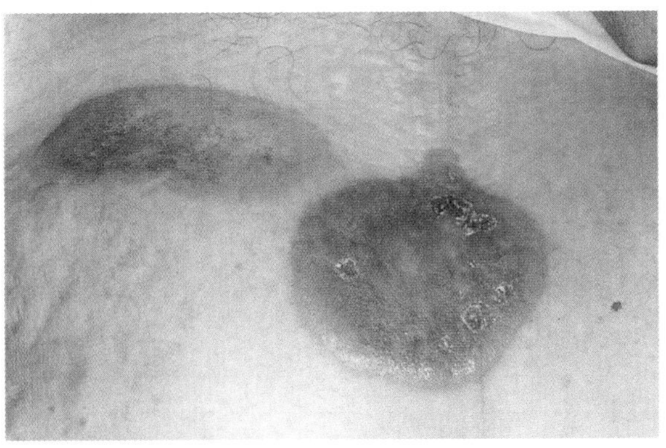

FIGURE 10–6
Cutaneous T-cell lymphoma.
(Courtesy of Jason L. Smith, MD.)

an essential role in the immune response and acts as a filter, removing microorganisms from the blood. The tonsils filter bacteria and aid in the formation of white blood cells. The thymus plays an essential role in the formation of antibodies and the development of the immune response in the newborn. It manufactures infection-fighting T cells. T cells are important in the body's cellular immune response.

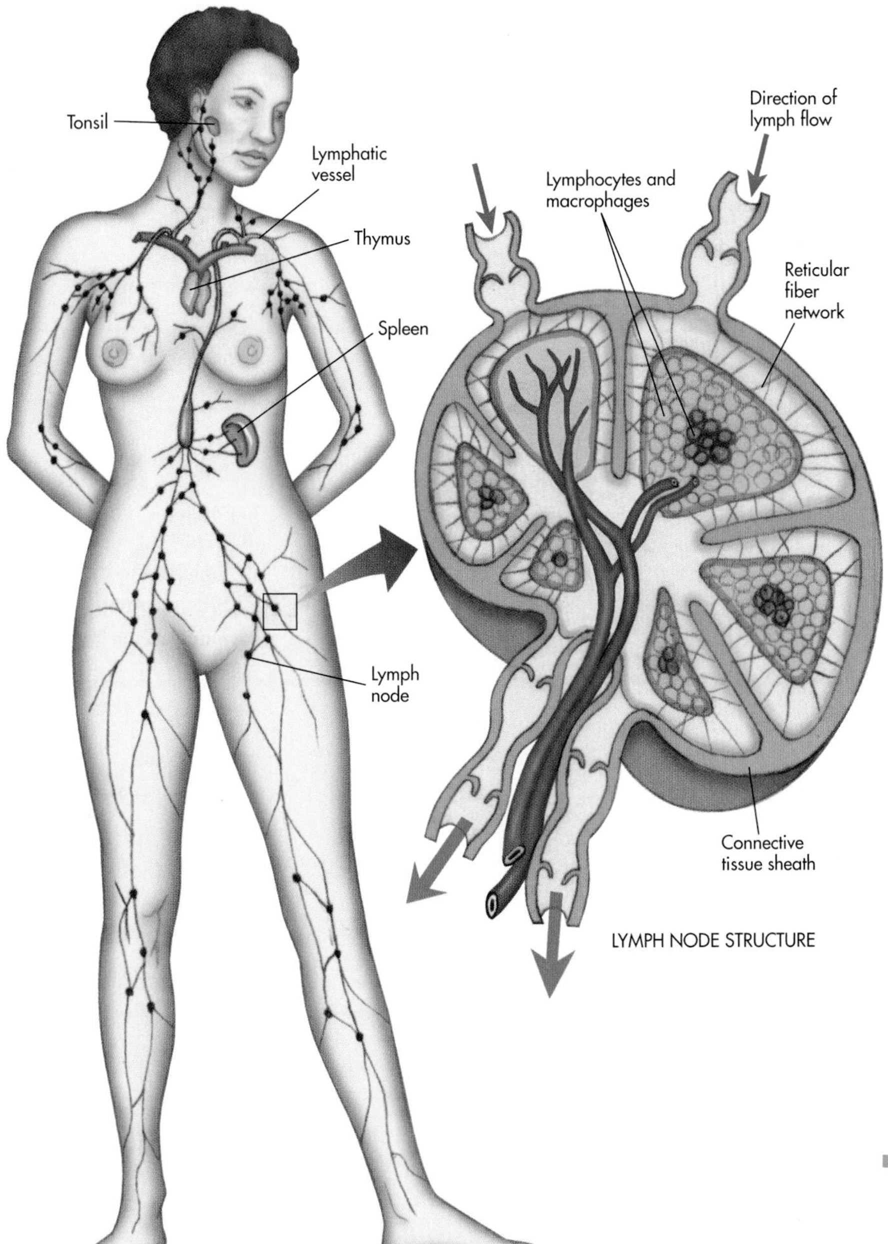

FIGURE 10–7

The tonsils, lymph nodes, thymus, spleen, and lymphatic vessels with an expanded view of a lymph node.

Answer Column

10.20 The __________, the __________, and the __________ are closely related to the lymphatic system in their functions.

spleen, tonsils, thymus (SPEEN, TON sulz, THIGH mus)

10.21 The combining form **splen / o** and the root **splen** mean spleen. Medical terms that begin with these word elements are:

__________ a condition in which the spleen is congested with blood

__________ enlargement of the spleen

__________ surgical fixation of a movable spleen

splenemia (splee **NEE** mee ah)
splenomegaly (splee noh **MEG** ah lee)
splenopexy (**SPLEE** noh pek see)

10.22 __________ is the inflammation of a tonsil or tonsils.

tonsillitis (ton sil **EYE** tis)

10.23 The combining form **thym / o** and the root **thym** mean thymus. Medical terms that begin with these word elements are:

__________ inflammation of the thymus

__________ a lymphocyte derived from the thymus

__________ tumor of the thymus

thymitis (thigh **MY** tis)
thymocyte (**THIGH** moh sight)
thymoma (thigh **MOH** mah)

10.24 The medical term __________ is defined as a condition of the engulfing and eating of bacteria by the phagocytes.
The word elements used to build this term are:

__________ combining form that means eat, engulf

__________ root that means cell

__________ suffix that means condition of

phagocytosis (fag oh sigh **TOH** sis)
phag / o
cyt
-osis

EXPLANATION FRAME

Immunity is the state of being protected from or resistant to a particular disease due to the development of antibodies. The mechanisms of immunity involve an antigen–antibody response. When an antigen enters the body, complex activities are set into motion. These activities involve chemical and mechanical forces that defend and protect the body's cells and tissues. Antibodies are formed and released from plasma cells after which they enter the body fluids where they react with the invading antigen.

		ANSWER COLUMN
10.25	The state of being protected from or resistant to a particular disease due to the development of antibodies is called ________.	**immunity** (im **YOO** nih tee)
10.26	An ________ is a protein substance produced in the body in response to an invading foreign substance (antigen).	**antibody** (**AN** tih bod ee)
10.27	An ________ is an invading foreign substance that induces the formation of antibodies.	**antigen** (**AN** tih jen)
10.28	________ is the study of immunity to diseases. The combining form **immun / o** means immunity and the suffix ________ means study of.	**immunology** (im yoo **NALL** oh jee) **-logy**
10.29	An ________ is a physician who specializes in immunology.	**immunologist** (im yoo **NALL** oh jist)
10.30	An ________ disease is one of a large group of diseases characterized by the alteration of the function of the immune system, resulting in the production of antibodies against the body's own cells.	**autoimmune** (aw toh ih **MYOON**)
10.31	________ is an abnormal condition in which the body reacts against constituents of its own tissues.	**autoimmunity** (aw toh ih **MYOON** ih tee)
10.32	________ blood transfusion is the use of the patient's own blood. The blood is donated by the patient prior to surgery or is collected from the patient during the surgical procedure.	**autologous** (aw **TALL** oh gus)
10.33	________ is the spread of an infection from its initial site to the bloodstream.	**sepsis** (**SEP** sis)
10.34	________ is a term denoting the process of inducing or providing immunity artificially by administering an immunobiologic (immunization agent).	**immunization** (im yoo nih **ZAY** shun)

	Answer Column
10.35 **True or False.** Immunization can be active or passive.	**true**

EXPLANATION FRAME

Acquired immunodeficiency syndrome (AIDS) is defined as the most severe form of a continuum of illnesses associated with human immunodeficiency virus (HIV) infection. This virus is most commonly transmitted through sexual contact, through exposure to infected blood or blood components, and perinatally from mother to infant. The virus may also be transmitted during breast-feeding to an infant by a woman infected with HIV.

The HIV virus invades the T4 lymphocytes and, as the disease progresses, the body's immune system becomes paralyzed. The patient becomes severely weakened and potentially fatal infections can occur. *Pneumocystis carinii* pneumonia (PCP) and Kaposi's sarcoma (KS) account for many of the deaths of AIDS patients. See Figures 10–8 and 10–9.

10.36 __________ is a disease caused by the human immunodeficiency virus (HIV). This virus is most commonly transmitted through sexual contact, through exposure to infected blood or blood components, and perinatally from mother to infant.	**AIDS**

EXPLANATION FRAME

Hepatitis B is a blood-borne viral disease. Over 300,000 cases occur annually in the United States. However, it can be prevented and a vaccine is available. About 50% of people who get hepatitis B do not have symptoms and unknowingly pass it on to others. Some of the possible symptoms include: nausea, loss of appetite, abdominal pain, jaundice, and skin rashes.

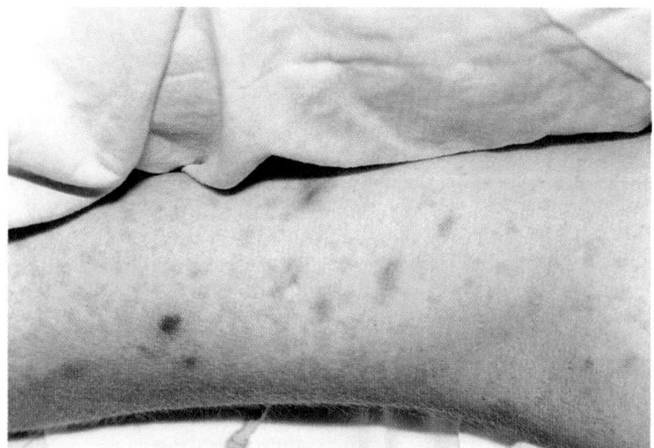

FIGURE 10–8
Kaposi's sarcoma. *(Courtesy of Jason L. Smith, MD.)*

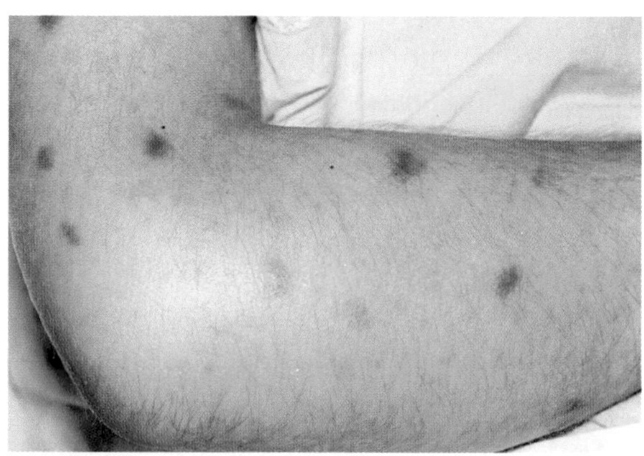

FIGUTE 10–9
Kaposi's sarcoma. *(Courtesy of Jason L. Smith, MD.)*

ANSWER COLUMN

10.37 **True or False.** Over 300,000 cases of hepatitis B occur annually in the United States.

true

EXPLANATION FRAME

Drugs that are generally used for the blood, lymph, and immune system include anticoagulants, the antiplatelet drug aspirin, thrombolytic agents, hemostatic agents, hematinic agents (irons), hemopoietin, folic acid, vitamin B_{12}, and immunizing agents. Antiretroviral drugs are used in treating AIDS.

10.38 ___________ are used to inhibit or prevent blood clot formation.

anticoagulants (an tih koh **AG** yoo lants)

10.39 The ___________ drug aspirin helps keep platelets from sticking together to form clots.

antiplatelet (an tih **PLAYT** let)

10.40 ___________ agents act to dissolve an existing thrombus when administered soon after its occurrence.

thrombolytic (throm boh **LIT** ik)

10.41 ___________ agents are used to control bleeding.

hemostatic (hee moh **STAT** ik)

10.42 ___________ agents are used to treat iron deficiency anemia.

hematinic (hee mah **TIN** ik)

10.43 ___________ ___________ is a genetically engineered hemopoietin that stimulates the production of red blood cells.

epoetin alfa (ee **POH** eh tin AL fah)

10.44 ___________ ___________ and vitamin B_{12} are used in treating megaloblastic anemias.

folic acid (**FOH** lik **ASS** id)

ANSWER COLUMN

10.45 ABBREVIATIONS

Write in the correct abbreviation for the following:

		Answer
____________	blood group	**ABO**
____________	acquired immunodeficiency syndrome	**AIDS**
____________	blood alcohol concentration	**BAC**
____________	hemoglobin	**Hb, Hgb, HGB**
____________	hematocrit	**Hct, HCT**
____________	human immunodeficiency virus	**HIV**
____________	Kaposi's sarcoma	**KS**
____________	*pneumocystis carinii* pneumonia	**PCP**
____________	red blood cell (count)	**RBC**
____________	Rhesus (factor)	**Rh**
____________	white blood cell (count)	**WBC**

IN THE SPOTLIGHT

IMMUNIZATION

Immunization is a term denoting the process of inducing or providing immunity artificially by administering an immunobiologic (immunization agent). Active immunization denotes the production of antibody or antitoxin in response to the administration of a vaccine or toxoid. Passive immunization denotes the provision of temporary immunity by the administration of preformed antitoxins or antibodies. The Centers for Disease Control and Prevention (CDC) recommend that children be vaccinated against diphtheria, polio, whooping cough (pertussis), mumps, rubella, hepatitis B, measles, *Haemophilus influenzae* type b, varicella zoster (chickenpox), and tetanus. Children need 12 shots by age 2. For more information you may call the CDC's 24-hour hot line at 404-332-4559.

The recommendations for immunization of infants, children, and adults are based on facts about immunobiologics and scientific knowledge about the principles of active and passive immunizations, and on judgments by public health officials and specialists in clinical and preventive medicine. Benefits and risks are associated with the use of all products—no vaccine is completely safe or completely effective. The benefits range from partial to complete protection from the consequences of disease, and the risks range from common, trivial, and inconvenient side effects to rare, severe, and life-threatening conditions.

Thus, recommendations on immunization practices balance scientific evidence of benefits, cost, and risks to achieve optimal levels of protection against infectious or communicable diseases. These recommendations may apply only in the United States, as epidemiological circumstances and vaccine may differ in other countries.

Immunization schedules are recommended by the CDC's Advisory Committee on Immunization Practices (ACIP), the American Academy of Pediatrics (AAP), and the American Academy of Family

Physicians (AAFP). These schedules are updated on a regular basis and recommendations for an immunization may change yearly.

The widespread and successful implementation of childhood immunization programs has greatly reduced the occurrence of many vaccine-preventable diseases. However, successful childhood immunization alone will not necessarily eliminate specific disease problems. A substantial proportion of the remaining morbidity and mortality from vaccine-preventable disease now occurs in older adolescents and adults. Persons who escaped natural infection or were not immunized with vaccine and toxoids against diphtheria, tetanus, measles, mumps, rubella, and poliomyelitis may be at risk of these diseases and their complications.

To further reduce the unnecessary occurrence of these vaccine-preventable diseases, all those who provide health care to older adolescents and adults should provide immunization as a routine part of their practice. In addition, the epidemiology of other vaccine-preventable diseases (e.g., hepatitis B, rabies, influenza, and pneumococcal disease) indicates that individuals who have special health problems are at increased risk of these illnesses and should be immunized. Travelers to some countries may be at increased risk of exposure to vaccine-preventable diseases and should be immunized.

CASE STUDY

Please read the following case study and then work frames 10.46–10.50. Write in your answer in the answer column. Check your responses with the answers provided at the end of frame 10.50.

A 52-year-old female was seen by a physician and the following is a synopsis of her visit. Note: More than 10% of all AIDS cases in the United States have occurred in persons age 50 or older.

PRESENT HISTORY: The patient states that several months after the death of her husband she became sexually involved with a younger man. She states that they didn't use condoms, as they were not concerned about pregnancy, and now she has found out that he has AIDS. She is most anxious and states that lately she has had "night sweats," weight loss for no apparent reason, constant fatigue, diarrhea, swollen lymph nodes, and unusual confusion.

SIGNS AND SYMPTOMS: Chief Complaints: Night sweats, weight loss, fatigue, diarrhea, swollen lymph nodes, and unusual confusion.

DIAGNOSIS: AIDS. Diagnosis was determined by a complete medical and social history, a physical examination, CD_4 lymphocyte count, which was 400 cells/mm^3 (normal is 800 to 1050 cells/mm^3), and laboratory evidence of immune dysfunction, identification of HIV antibodies, and signs and symptoms.

TREATMENT: The regimen includes treating any associated condition with proper medical intervention and starting the patient on a combination of antiretroviral therapy of three drugs: AZT-zidovudine, 3TC-lamivudine, and a protease inhibitor-Norvir-ritonavir. Drug therapy is carefully monitored for older adults, as they may have preexisting conditions, such as cardiac disease and/or renal insufficiency, that can make them less tolerant of drugs. Clinical

(*continued*)

evaluation and laboratory monitoring every 3 to 6 months and more frequently if needed. Provide for professional assistance as needed. Information on services available for the older adult with HIV infection and AIDS may be obtained by calling the CDC's AIDS Hot Line at 1-800-342-AIDS.

10.46 Signs and symptoms of AIDS include night sweats, weight loss, fatigue, ___________, swollen lymph nodes, and confusion.

10.47 What percentage of all AIDS cases in the United States have occurred in persons age 50 or older? ___________.

10.48 The diagnosis of AIDS was determined by a complete physical examination, laboratory evidence of ___________ dysfunction, and a CD4 lymphocyte count of 400 cells/mm^3.

10.49 ___________ is an antiretroviral drug that is combined with lamivudine and ritonavir in the treatment of AIDS.

10.50 For more information on HIV infection and AIDS one may call the CDC's AIDS Hot Line at ___________.

CASE STUDY ANSWERS

10.46 diarrhea
10.47 10%
10.48 immune
10.49 AZT and/or zidovudine
10.50 1-800-342-AIDS

REVIEW A: WORD ELEMENTS

This review allows you to check your knowledge of some of the word elements presented in this unit. In the spaces provided, write the meaning of the word elements that are identified as **Prefix (P), Word Root (R), Combining Form (CF),** and/or **Suffix (S).**

MEDICAL WORD	*WORD ELEMENT*	*MEANING*
1. hematology	hemat / o (CF)	__________
	-logy (S)	__________
2. hematologist	hemat / o (CF)	__________
	log (R)	__________
	-ist (S)	__________
3. erythrocyte	erythr / o (CF)	__________
	-cyte (S)	__________
4. polycythemia	poly (P)	__________
	cyth (R)	__________
	-emia (S)	__________
5. thrombectomy	thromb (R)	__________
	-ectomy (S)	__________
6. thrombolysis	thromb / o (CF)	__________
	-lysis (S)	__________
7. leukocyte	leuk / o (CF)	__________
	cyte (S)	__________
8. phagocytosis	phag / o (CF)	__________
	cyt (R)	__________
	-osis (S)	__________
9. immunology	immun / o (CF)	__________
	-logy (S)	__________

REVIEW B: MEDICAL TERMS

Please place the correct letter from column II on the appropriate line of column I.

COLUMN I		COLUMN II
________	1. hematocele	A. lack of red blood cells
________	2. hemolysis	B. the fluid part of the blood
________	3. hemophobia	C. resembling lymph
________	4. erythropenia	D. tumor of the thymus
________	5. thrombosis	E. enlargement of the spleen
________	6. plasma	F. protein substance
________	7. lymphoid	G. condition of a blood clot formation
________	8. splenomegaly	H. a fear of blood
________	9. thymoma	I. destruction of red blood cells
________	10. antibody	J. a blood cyst, hernia

REVIEW C: DISEASES AND DISORDERS

Please provide the correct disease or disorder for each of the following descriptions.

1. ________ is a hereditary blood disease characterized by prolonged clotting time and tendency to bleed.
2. ________ literally means a lack of blood.
3. ________ is a condition of too many red blood cells.
4. ________ is a disease of the blood characterized by overproduction of leukocytes.
5. ________ is a disease of the lymph glands.

REVIEW D: UNSCRAMBLE THE WORDS

Unscramble the following medical terms and place the correct term on the line directly across from the scrambled word.

1. genitan ________
2. binoglomeh ________
3. hagerromeh ________
4. nicierpous ________
5. miaekuel ________

REVIEW E: DRUGS USED FOR BLOOD, LYMPH, AND THE IMMUNE SYSTEM

Please provide the correct answer for each of the following descriptions.

1. ____________ are used to inhibit or prevent blood clot formation.
2. The ____________ drug aspirin helps keep platelets from sticking together to form clots.
3. ____________ agents act to dissolve an existing thrombus when administered soon after its occurrence.
4. ____________ agents are used to control bleeding.
5. ____________ agents are used to treat iron deficiency anemia.
6. ____________ ____________ is a genetically engineered hemopoietin that stimulates the production of red blood cells.
7. ____________ ____________ and vitamin B_{12} are used in treating megaloblastic anemias.

REVIEW F: ABBREVIATIONS

Please provide the correct abbreviation and/or meaning for the abbreviation.

1. ____________ blood group
2. AIDS ____________
3. ____________ red blood cell
4. KS ____________
5. ____________ hemoglobin
6. ____________ human immunodeficiency virus

11 THE DIGESTIVE SYSTEM: GASTROENTEROLOGY

LEARNING CONCEPTS

- the digestive system
- functions
- oral cavity
- the esophagus
- the stomach
- the small intestine
- the large intestine
- the liver
- the gallbladder
- the pancreas
- essential terminology
- pronunciation guide
- word elements
- explanation frames
- selected diseases and disorders
- drugs used for the digestive system
- abbreviations
- in the spotlight: hepatitis
- case study: acute gastric ulcer
- review exercises

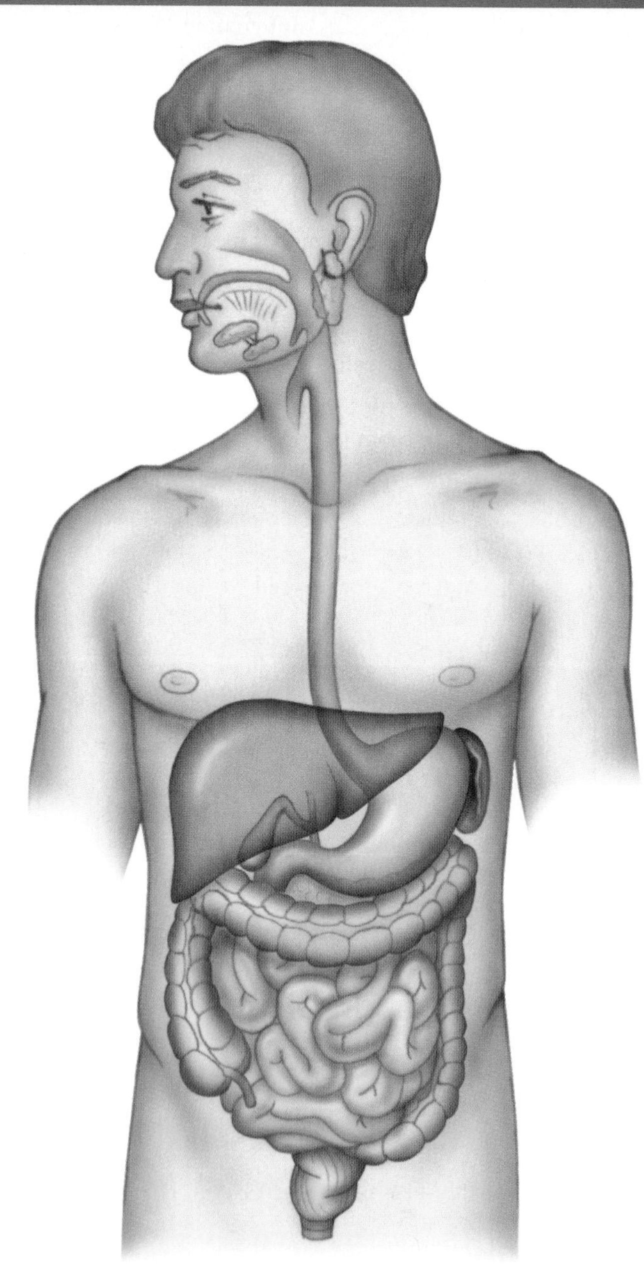

OBJECTIVES

ON COMPLETION OF THIS UNIT, YOU SHOULD BE ABLE TO:

- Briefly describe the digestive system.
- Describe the primary functions of the various organs or structures of the digestive system.
- Identify and give the meaning of the primary word elements for this unit.
- Analyze, build, spell, and pronounce selected medical words.
- Describe selected diseases/disorders of the digestive system.
- Describe selected drugs that are used for the digestive system diseases or disorders.
- Define selected abbreviations that pertain to the digestive system.
- Define hepatitis and describe the five main forms of hepatitis.
- Complete the Case Study on Acute Gastric Ulcer, Peptic Ulcer Disease (PUD).
- Successfully complete the review section.

TECH LINK

CD-ROM Use the CD-ROM enclosed with your textbook to gain additional reinforcement through interactive word building exercises, spelling games, labeling activities, and additional quizzes.

www.prenhall.com/rice Use the above address to access the free, interactive Companion Website created specifically for this textbook. Get hints, instant feedback, and textbook references to chapter-related multiple choice and true/false questions, fill-in-the-blank, and labeling exercises. In addition, you will find an audio glossary, and essay questions.

The digestive system is composed of the mouth, pharynx, esophagus, stomach, and small and large intestines. Its accessory organs are the salivary glands, liver, gallbladder, and pancreas. See Table 11–1.

The three main functions of the digestive system are digestion, absorption, and elimination. Digestion begins in the mouth, as food is broken apart by the action of the teeth, moistened and lubricated by saliva, and formed into a bolus. This bolus is then swallowed and passes down the pharynx and the esophagus and into the stomach. Food is stored in the stomach while it is reduced to a digestible state. Food is passed at intervals into the small intestine where digestion and absorption chiefly take place. In the large intestine digestion and absorption continue on a reduced scale. The waste products of digestion are eliminated from the body via the rectum and anus.

TABLE 11-1 THE DIGESTIVE SYSTEM

Organ	Functions
Mouth	Breaks food apart by the action of the teeth, moistens and lubricates food with saliva; food formed into a bolus
Pharynx	Common passageway for both respiration and digestion; muscular constrictions move the bolus into the esophagus
Esophagus	Peristalsis moves the food down the esophagus into the stomach
Stomach	Reduces food to a digestible state; converts food to a semiliquid form
Small Intestine	Digestion and absorption take place. Nutrients are absorbed into tiny capillaries and lymph vessels in the walls of the small intestine and transmitted to body cells by the circulatory system
Large Intestine	Removes water from the fecal material; stores and then eliminates waste from the body via the rectum and anus
Salivary Glands	Secrete saliva to moisten and lubricate food
Liver	Changes glucose to glycogen and stores it until needed; changes glycogen back to glucose; desaturates fats; assists in protein catabolism; manufactures bile, fibrinogen, prothrombin, heparin, and blood proteins; stores vitamins; produces heat; and detoxifies substances
Gallbladder	Stores and concentrates bile
Pancreas	Secretes pancreatic juice into the small intestine, contains cells that produce digestive enzymes, secretes insulin and glucagon

ANSWER COLUMN

11.1 The study of the stomach and the intestines is called ____________.
The word elements used to build this term are:
____________ combining form that means stomach
____________ combining form that means intestine
____________ suffix that means study of

gastroenterology
(gas troh en ter **ALL** oh jee)
gastr / o
enter / o
-logy

11.2 A ____________ is a physician who specializes in the study of the stomach and the intestines.
The word elements used to build this term are:
____________ combining form that means stomach
____________ combining form that means intestine
____________ root that means study of
____________ suffix that means one who specializes

gastroenterologist
(gas troh en ter **ALL** oh jist)
gastr / o
enter / o
log
-ist

PRIMARY WORD ELEMENTS

The following word elements (prefixes, roots, combining forms, and suffixes) will be used to build medical terms that relate to this unit. Please commit these to memory.

PREFIX

PREFIX	MEANING	PREFIX	MEANING
dys	bad, difficult, painful	**post**	after, behind
mega	large, great	**sub**	below, under
peri	around		

COMBINING FORM

COMBINING FORM / ROOT	MEANING	COMBINING FORM / ROOT	MEANING
append, appendic	appendix, hang to	**esophag / e, esophag / o**	esophagus
bucc	cheek	**gastr**	stomach
chol / e	gall, bile	**gastr / o**	stomach
cirrh	orange-yellow	**gingiv**	gums
col, colon	colon	**gloss / o**	tongue
col / i, col / o	colon	**hepat**	liver
cyst / o	bladder	**hepat / o**	liver
dent	tooth		
dent / i	tooth	**lingu**	tongue
duoden	duodenum	**pancreat**	pancreas
duoden / o	duodenum		
enter	intestine	**prand / i**	meal
enter / o	intestine	**proct / o**	anus, rectum
esophag	esophagus	**sigmoid / o**	sigmoid colon

SUFFIX

SUFFIX	MEANING	SUFFIX	MEANING
-al, -ic	pertaining to	**-oma**	tumor
-algia, -dynia	pain	**-paresis**	weakness
-ase	enzyme	**-pepsia**	to digest
-ectomy	surgical excision	**-plasty**	surgical repair
-gram	record	**-rrhexis**	rupture
-iasis, -osis	condition of	**-scope**	instrument
-ist	one who specializes	**-scopy**	to view, examine
-itis	inflammation	**-stalsis**	contraction
-logy	study of	**-stomy**	new opening
-megaly	enlargement, large		

ANSWER COLUMN

EXPLANATION FRAME

A general description of the digestive system is that of a continuous tube beginning with the mouth and ending at the anus. This tube is known as the alimentary canal and/or gastrointestinal tract. It measures about 30 feet in adults and contains both primary and accessory organs. The primary organs are the mouth, pharynx, esophagus, stomach, and small and large intestines. The accessory organs are the salivary glands, liver, gallbladder, and pancreas. The three main functions of the digestive system are digestion, absorption, and elimination. See Figure 11–1.

11.3 ____________ is the process by which food is changed in the mouth, stomach, and intestines by mechanical and chemical action so that it can be absorbed by the body.

digestion
(dye **JEST** shun)

11.4 ____________, as it relates to the digestive system, is the process whereby nutrient material is taken into the bloodstream or lymph.

absorption
(ab **SORP** shun)

11.5 ____________ is the process by which waste products are excreted from the body via the skin (perspiration), kidneys (urine), and intestines (feces).

elimination
(ee lim ih **NAY** shun)

EXPLANATION FRAME

The oral cavity is formed by the palate or roof, the lips and cheeks on the sides, and the tongue at its floor. Contained within are the teeth and salivary glands. The cheeks form the lateral walls and are continuous with the lips. The vestibule includes the space between the cheeks and the teeth. The gingivae (gums) surround the necks of the teeth. Digestion begins in the mouth as food is broken apart by the action of the teeth, moistened and lubricated by saliva, and formed into a bolus. See Figure 11–2.

11.6 A ____________ is a small mass of masticated (chewed) food ready to be swallowed.

bolus
(**BOH** lus)

11.7 ____________ is a medical term that means inflammation of the gums. The word root ____________ means gums and the suffix ____________ means inflammation.

gingivitis
(jin jih **VIGH** tis)
gingiv
-itis

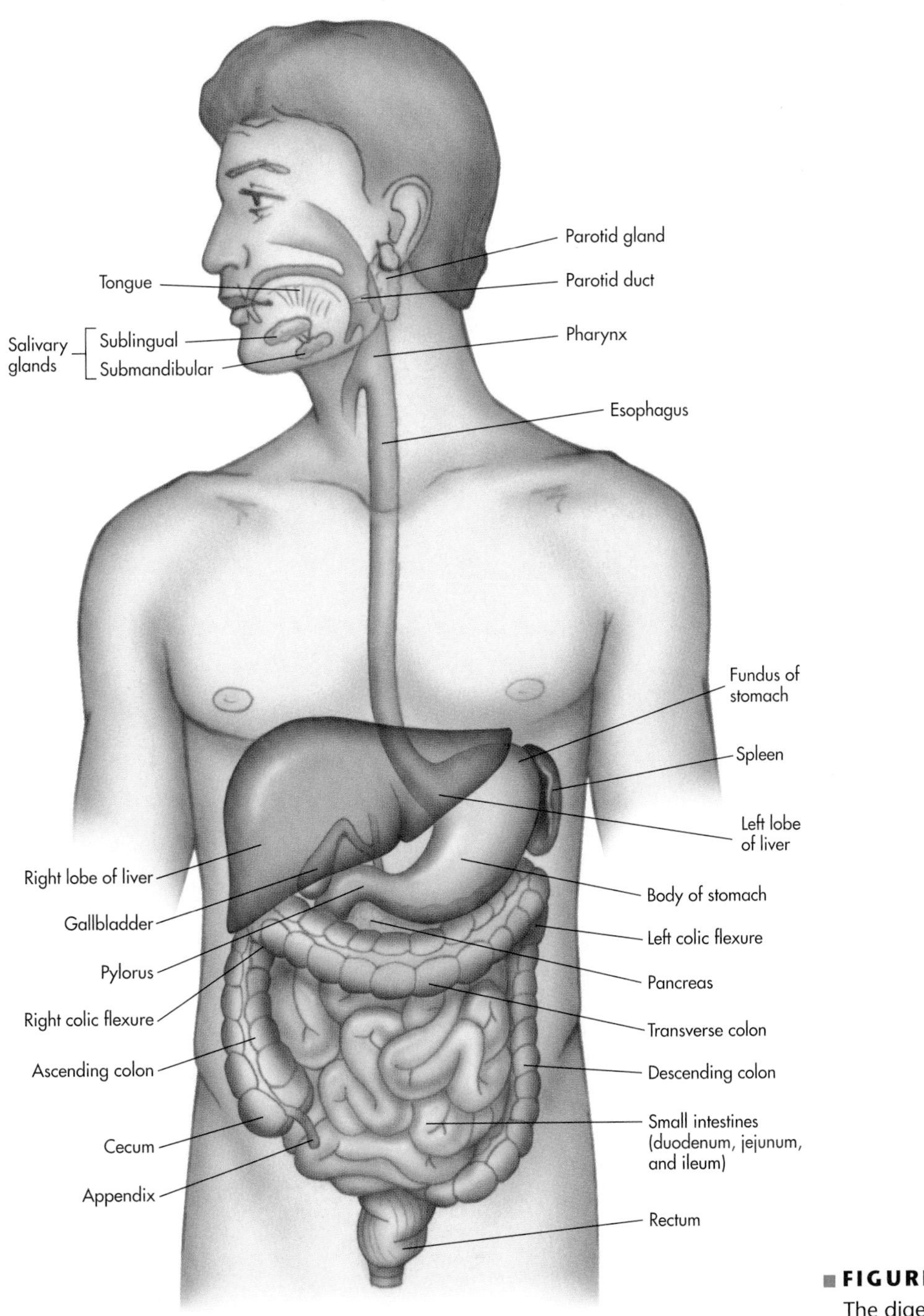

FIGURE 11–1
The digestive system.

ANSWER COLUMN

11.8 __________ is a medical term that means pertaining to the cheek. The word root __________ means cheek and the suffix __________ means pertaining to.

buccal (BUCK al)
bucc -al

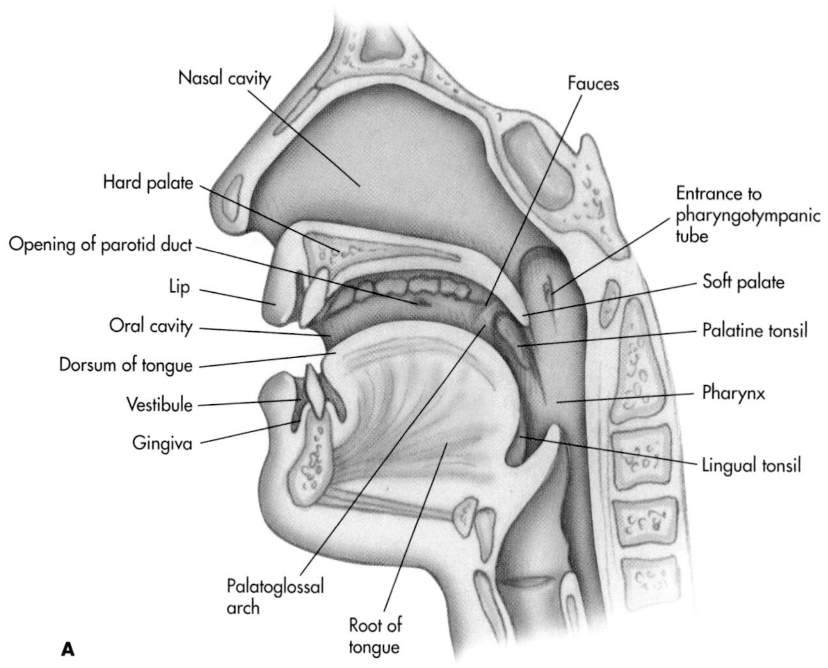

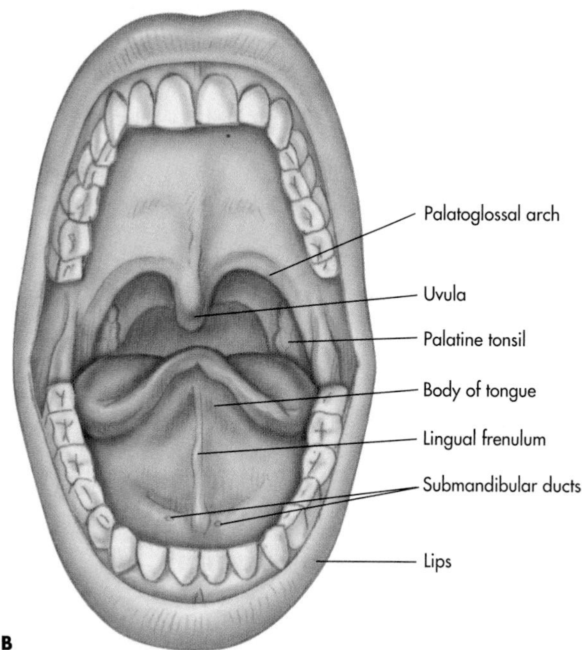

FIGURE 11–2
The oral cavity: (A) sagittal section, (B) anterior view as seen through the open mouth.

ANSWER COLUMN

11.9 The word root **lingu** and the combining form **gloss / o** mean tongue. Medical terms that contain these word elements are:

		Answer
__________	surgical repair of the tongue	**glossoplasty** (**GLOS** oh plas tee)
__________	incision into the tongue	**glossotomy** (glos **OT** oh mee)
__________	pertaining to the tongue	**lingual** (**LING** gwal)
__________	pertaining to under the tongue	**sublingual** (sub **LING** gwal)

11. 10 The word root **dent** and the combining form **dent / i** mean tooth. Medical terms that begin with these word elements are:

		Answer
__________	pain in a tooth; toothache	**dentalgia** (den **TAL** jee ah)
__________	pertaining to the teeth and the cheek	**dentibuccal** (den tih **BUCK** al)
__________	a physician who specializes in the teeth	**dentist** (**DEN** tist)

EXPLANATION FRAME

Just beyond the mouth, at the beginning of the esophagus, is the pharynx (throat). It serves as a common passageway for both respiration and digestion. Food that is swallowed passes through the pharynx into the esophagus. The esophagus is a collapsible tube about 10 inches long that leads to the stomach. Food is carried along the esophagus by a series of wave-like contractions called peristalsis. See Figure 11–1.

11.11 __________ contains two word elements:

		Answer
__________	(term)	**peristalsis** (pair ih **STALL** sis)
__________	prefix that means around	**peri**
__________	suffix that means contraction	**-stalsis**

Peristalsis is a series of wave-like contractions that occur involuntarily in hollow tubes of the body, especially the alimentary canal.

Answer Column

11.12 The word elements **esophag (R), esophag / e (CF),** and **esophag / o (CF)** mean esophagus. Medical terms that contain these word elements are:

		Answer Column
________	pertaining to the esophagus	**esophageal** (eh soff ah **JEE** al)
________ ________	tortuous dilated veins of the esophagus	**esophageal varices** (eh soff ah **JEE** al vair ih **SEEZ**)
________	an instrument used to examine the esophagus	**esophagoscope** (eh **SOFF** ah goh scope)
________	inflammation of the esophagus	**esophagitis** (eh soff ah **JIGH** tis)
________ ________	backward flow of gastric acid into the esophagus	**esophageal reflux** (eh soff ah **JEE** al **REE** fluks)

EXPLANATION FRAME

The stomach is a large sac-like organ into which food passes from the esophagus for storage while undergoing the early processes of digestion. In the stomach, food is further reduced to a digestible state. Hydrochloric acid and gastric juices convert the food to a semiliquid state, which is passed, at intervals, into the small intestine. See Figure 11–1.

11.13 The word elements **gastr (R)** and **gastr / o (CF)** mean stomach. Medical terms that begin with these word elements are:

		Answer Column
________	pertaining to the stomach	**gastric** (**GAS** trik)
________	inflammation of the stomach	**gastritis** (gas **TRY** tis)
________	pain in the stomach	**gastrodynia** (gas troh **DIN** ee ah)
________	inflammation of the stomach and intestines	**gastroenteritis** (gas troh en ter **EYE** tis)
________	inflammation of the stomach and duodenum	**gastroduodenitis** (gas troh doo od eh **NYE** tis)
________	inflammation of the stomach and esophagus	**gastroesophagitis** (gas troh eh soff ah **JYE** tis)
________	creation of a new opening into the stomach	**gastrostomy** (gas **TROSS** toh mee)
________	partial paralysis of the stomach	**gastroparesis** (gas troh pah **REE** sis)
________	an ulcer of the stomach; peptic ulcer	**gastric ulcer** (**GAS** trik **ULL** ser)
________ ________ ________	reflux of gastric contents into the esophagus	**gastroesophageal reflux disease** (gas troh eh soff ah **JEE** al **REE** fluks dih **ZEEZ**)

ANSWER COLUMN

EXPLANATION FRAME

The small intestine is about 21 feet long and 1 inch in diameter. It has three parts: the duodenum (first 12 inches, just beyond the stomach), the jejunum (next 8 feet), and the ileum (remaining 12 feet). Digestion and absorption take place chiefly in the small intestine. Nutrients are absorbed into tiny capillaries and lymph vessels in the walls of the small intestine and transmitted to body cells by the circulatory system. See Figure 11–1.

11.14 The __________ is the first portion of the small intestine.

duodenum (do oh **DEE** num or doo **OD** eh num)

11.15 An endoscopic examination of the esophagus, stomach, and small intestine is called __________.

This is an example of a really long word that might make you think that medical terminology is difficult. Not so! Let's break it down to smaller word elements: **esophag / o** plus **gastr / o** plus **duoden / o** plus **scopy**. **Esophag / o / gastr / o / duoden / o / -scopy** is simply three combining forms and a suffix:

__________ the esophagus
__________ the stomach
__________ the duodenum or first part of the intestine
__________ to view, examine

esophagogastroduodeno-scopy (eh soff ah goh gas troh doo od eh **NOS** koh pee)

esophag / o
gastr / o
duoden / o
-scopy

11.16 The word root **enter** and the combining form **enter / o** are often found when studying the digestive system, because they mean intestine, a major component of the gastrointestinal tract. Now, build some medical terms that use these word elements plus the suffixes **-ic** and **-itis.**

__________ pertaining to the intestine
__________ inflammation of the intestine; *regional enteritis is also called Crohn's disease*

enteric (en **TER** ik)
enteritis (en ter **EYE** tis)

11.17 __________ is inflammation of the intestines and the colon. *It is an acute, serious condition that requires immediate treatment. The treatment regimen consists of managing shock, regulation of electrolyte balance, and antibiotics.*

enterocolitis (en ter oh koh **LYE** tis)

ANSWER COLUMN

EXPLANATION FRAME

The large intestine is about 5 feet long and 2.5 inches in diameter. It is divided into the cecum, the colon, the rectum, and the anal canal. See Figure 11–1. The cecum is a pouchlike structure forming the beginning of the large intestine. It is about 3 inches long and has the appendix attached to it. The colon makes up the bulk of the large intestine and is divided into the ascending colon, transverse colon, descending colon, and sigmoid colon.

11.18 __________ is a combining form that means colon. **Col (R)** and **col / i (CF)** also are used to indicate the colon.

Medical terms that are built using these word elements are:

__________ inflammation of the colon

__________ puncture of the colon to relieve distention; SYN: colocentesis

__________ creation of a new opening into the colon

Answers: **col / o**; **colitis** (koh **LYE** tis); **colipuncture** (**KOH** lih pungk chur); **colostomy** (koh **LOSS** toh mee)

11.19 A condition in which the colon is extremely enlarged is called __________. **Mega** is a prefix that means great or large and __________ is a word root that means colon.

Answers: **megacolon** (**MEG** ah koh lon); **colon** (**KOH** lon)

11.20 __________ is the medical term that means inflammation of the appendix. The word root **appendic** means appendix, hang to and the suffix **-itis** means inflammation.

Answer: **appendicitis** (ah pen dih **SIGH** tis)

11.21 An __________ is the surgical excision of the appendix.

Answer: **appendectomy** (ah pen **DEK** toh mee)

11.22 __________ is the examination of the sigmoid colon. A physician may use a sigmoidoscope that is made of fine stainless steel or a flexible scope that utilizes fiberoptics.

Answer: **sigmoidoscopy** (sig moyd **OSS** koh pee)

ANSWER COLUMN

11.23 A **colonoscopy** is the examination of the upper portion of the rectum with an elongated speculum or a colonoscope. The word elements used to build **colon / o / scopy** are:

		Answer
___________	combining form that means colon	**colon / o**
___________	suffix that means to view, examine	**-scopy**

11.24 A physician who specializes in the study of the anus and the rectum is called a ___________. — **proctologist** (prock **TALL** oh jist)

The word elements used to build this term are:

		Answer
___________	combining form that means anus and/or rectum	**proct / o**
___________	word root that means study of	**log**
___________	suffix that means one who specializes	**-ist**

EXPLANATION FRAME

The liver weighs about 3 pounds and is located in the upper right part of the abdomen. The liver plays an essential role in the normal metabolism of carbohydrates, fats, and proteins. In carbohydrate metabolism, it changes glucose to glycogen and stores it until needed by body cells. It also changes glycogen back to glucose. In fat metabolism, the liver serves as a storage place and acts to desaturate fats before releasing them into the bloodstream. In protein metabolism, the liver acts as a storage place and assists in catabolism. See Figure 11–1.

11.25 The ___________ is the largest glandular organ in the body. — **liver** (**LIV** er)

11.26 The liver manufactures the following important substances:

	Answer
___________ a digestive juice	**bile** (**BYE** al)
___________ and ___________ coagulants essential for blood clotting	**fibrinogen** (fye **BRIN** oh jen) **prothrombin** (proh **THROM** bin)
___________ an anticoagulant that helps to prevent blood clotting	**heparin** (**HEP** er in)
___________ ___________ albumin, gamma globulin	**blood proteins** (**BLUD PROH** teens)

Answer Column

11.27 Additionally, the liver stores iron and vitamins B_{12}, A, D, E, and K. It also produces body heat and __________ many harmful substances such as drugs and alcohol.

detoxifies
(dee **TOK** sih fyes)

11.28 __________ is a chronic degenerative liver disease. *It is divided into three types: Laennec's portal cirrhosis (alcoholic, nutritional); postnecrotic cirrhosis (result of previous acute viral hepatitis); and biliary cirrhosis (result of chronic biliary obstruction and infection). Jaundice, a condition characterized by yellowness of skin, whites of the eyes, mucous membranes, and body fluids, is often a symptom of cirrhosis.*

Cirrh is a root that means orange-yellow and **-osis** is a suffix that means condition of.

cirrhosis
(sih **ROH** sis)

11.29 **Hepat (R)** and **hepat / o (CF)** are word elements used to indicate the liver. Medical terms that begin with these word elements are:

__________ inflammation of the liver

__________ a tumor of the liver

__________ rupture of the liver

__________ enlargement of the liver

hepatitis
(hep ah **TYE** tis)
hepatoma
(hep ah **TOH** mah)
hepatorrhexis
(hep ah toh **REK** sis)
hepatomegaly
(hep ah toh **MEG** ah lee)

EXPLANATION FRAME

The gallbladder is a membranous sac attached to the liver in which excess bile is stored and concentrated. Bile leaving the gallbladder is six to ten times as concentrated as that which comes to it from the liver. The gallbladder is referred to as **cholecyst.** The combining form **chol / e** means gall, bile and the root **cyst** means bladder; thus the combination means gallbladder. See Figure 11–1.

11.30 __________ is the surgical excision of the gallbladder.

The word elements used to build this term are:

__________ combining form that means gall, bile

__________ root that means bladder

__________ suffix that means surgical excision

cholecystectomy
(koh lee sis **TEK** toh mee)

chol / e

cyst

-ectomy

ANSWER COLUMN

EXPLANATION FRAME

A laparoscopic cholecystectomy is a surgical procedure in which the gallbladder is removed via a laparoscope. It is a less invasive procedure than a regular cholecystectomy because the abdomen does not have to be cut open.

11.31 ____________ is the medical term that means inflammation of the gallbladder. The word elements used to build this term are:

____________ combining form that means gall, bile

____________ root that means bladder

____________ suffix that means inflammation

cholecystitis
(koh lee sis **TYE** tis)
chol / e
cyst
-itis

11.32 ____________ is a radiographic picture of the gallbladder. The suffix **-gram** means a record.

cholecystogram
(koh lee **SIS** toh gram)

11.33 ____________ ultrasonography is a test used to visualize the gallbladder by using high-frequency sound waves. The echoes are recorded on an oscilloscope and film. See Figure 11–3. Abnormal results may indicate biliary obstruction, cholelithiasis, and acute cholecystitis.

gallbladder
(**GALL** blad er)

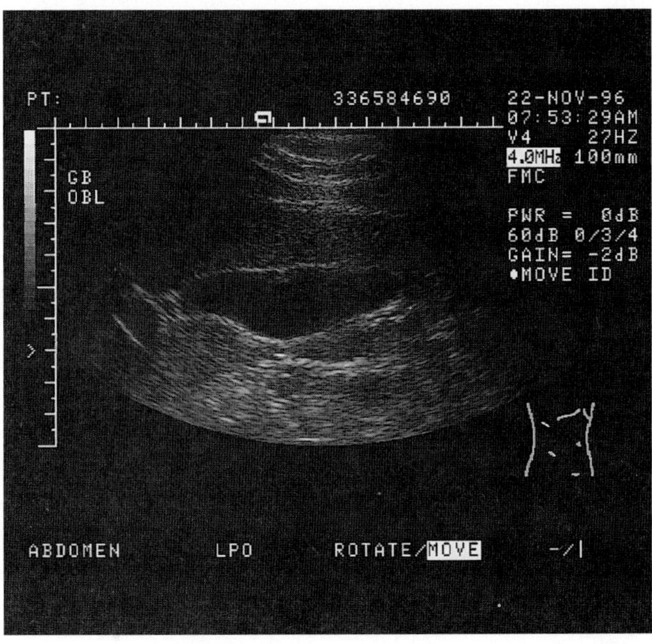

■ **FIGURE 11–3**
Gallbladder ultrasound. *(Courtesy of Teresa Resch.)*

Answer Column

11.34 ___________ is a medical term that means gallstones in the gallbladder. The root **lith** means stone and the suffix **-iasis** means condition.

cholelithiasis (koh lee lih **THIGH** ah sis)

EXPLANATION FRAME

The pancreas is a large, elongated gland situated behind the stomach and secreting pancreatic juice into the small intestine. It is 6 to 9 inches long and contains cells that produce digestive enzymes. Other cells in the pancreas secrete the hormones insulin and glucagon directly into the bloodstream. See Figure 11–1.

11.35 Inflammation of the pancreas is called ___________.

The word elements used to build this term are:

___________ root that means pancreas

___________ suffix that means inflammation

pancreatitis (pan kree ah **TYE** tis)

pancreat

-itis

EXPLANATION FRAME

Emesis is a medical term for vomiting. Hence, the medicine taken to induce vomiting is an emetic. A medication that prevents vomiting is called an antiemetic. You have learned that the prefix **anti** means against and that the suffix **-ic** means pertaining to. See how easy it is to understand medical terminology!

11.36 The act of vomiting is called ___________.

emesis (**EM** eh sis)

11.37 The medical term for indigestion is ___________.

The word elements used to build this term are:

___________ prefix that means difficult

___________ suffix that means to digest

dyspepsia (dis **PEP** see ah)

dys

-pepsia

11.38 ___________ is the medical term for belching.

eructation (eh ruk **TAY** shun)

11.39 The medical term for pertaining to after meals is called ___________.

Post is a prefix that means after, **prand / i** is a combining form that means ___________, and **-al** is a suffix that means pertaining to.

postprandial (post **PRAN** dee al)

meal

ANSWER COLUMN

EXPLANATION FRAME

An enzyme is a protein substance capable of causing chemical changes in other substances without being changed itself. Amylase (**amyl** is a word root that means starch) is an enzyme that breaks down starch. Lipase (**lip** is a word root that means fat) is an enzyme that breaks down lipids or fats.

11.40 The suffix -**ase** means ___________.

enzyme (EN zime)

11.41 An accumulation of serous fluid in the peritoneal cavity is called ___________.

ascites (ah **SIGH** teez)

11.42 ___________ is the twisting of the bowel upon itself that causes an obstruction. See Figure 11–4.

volvulus (**VOL** vyoo lus)

11.43 ___________ is the body waste expelled from the bowels; SYN: stool, excreta.

feces
(**FEE** seez)

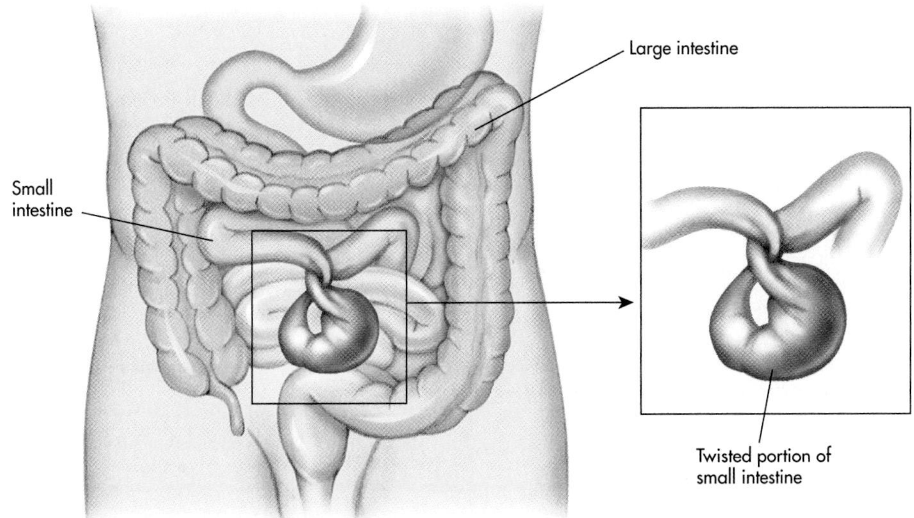

FIGURE 11–4
Volvulus.

ANSWER COLUMN

11.44 __________ is the medical term for heartburn.

pyrosis (pye **ROH** sis)

11.45 __________ means the frequent passage of unformed watery stools.

diarrhea (dye ah **REE** ah)

EXPLANATION FRAME

Dysentery is a medical term applied to various intestinal disorders, especially of the colon, marked by inflammation. It is characterized by abdominal pain, tenesmus (spasmodic contraction of anal sphincter with pain and persistent desire to empty the bowel), and diarrhea with passage of mucus or blood. It may be caused by bacterial or viral infection, infestation by protozoa or parasitic worms, or chemical irritants. Because of improved sanitary facilities throughout the world it is less prevalent today than in years past. It can be especially dangerous to infants, children, the elderly, and those whose immune system is compromised.

11.46 __________ is the infrequent passage of unduly hard and dry feces; difficult defecation.

constipation (kon stih **PAY** shun)

11.47 The medical term for gas in the stomach is __________.

flatus (**FLAY** tus)

11.48 __________ means chewing.

mastication (mas tih **KAY** shun)

11.49 __________ is the medical term for bad breath.

halitosis (hal ih **TOH** sis)

EXPLANATION FRAME

Drugs that are generally used for digestive system diseases and disorders include antacids, antacid mixtures, histamine H_2-receptor antagonists, mucosal protective medications and gastric pump inhibitors (proton pump inhibitors, PPIs), laxatives, antidiarrheal agents, and antiemetics.

11.50 __________ neutralize hydrochloric acid in the stomach.

antacids (ant **ASS** ids)

ANSWER COLUMN

11.51 ________ ________ combine aluminum (may cause constipation) and/or calcium compounds with magnesium (may cause diarrhea) salts. *These products provide the antacid action of both ingredients yet tend to counter the adverse effects of each other.*

antacid mixtures
(ant **ASS** id **MIKS** churs)

11.52 ________ ________ ________ ________ are used in the treatment of active duodenal ulcer. *They inhibit both daytime and nocturnal basal gastric acid secretion and inhibit gastric acid stimulated by food, histamine, caffeine, and other substances.*

histamine H_2-receptor antagonists
(**HISS** tah min / ree **SEP** tor / an **TAG** oh nists)

EXPLANATION FRAME

Mucosal protective medications protect the stomach's mucosal lining from acid, but they do not inhibit the release of acid. Two medications in this classification are sucralfate (Carafate) and misoprostol (Cytotec). Gastric acid pump inhibitors are anti-ulcer agents that suppress gastric acid secretion by specific inhibition of the H+/K+ATPase enzyme at the secretory surface of the gastric parietal cell. Because this enzyme system is regarded as the acid (proton) pump within the gastric mucosa, gastric acid pump inhibitors are so classified as they block the final step of acid production. Drugs included in this classification are omeprazole (Prilosec), rabeprazozle sodium (Aciphex), lansoprazole (Prevacid), and pantoprazole (Protonix).

11.53 ________ are used to relieve constipation and to facilitate the passage of feces through the lower gastrointestinal tract.

laxatives
(**LACK** sah tivs)

11.54 ________ agents are used to treat diarrhea.

antidiarrheal
(an tih dye ah **REE** al)

11.55 ________ prevent or arrest vomiting.

antiemetics
(an tih ee **MET** iks)

11.56 ABBREVIATIONS

Write in the correct abbreviation for the following:

________	before meals (ante cibum)	**ac**
________	bowel movement	**BM**
________	bowel sounds	**BS**
________	food (cibus)	**cib**
________	chronic ulcerative colitis	**CUC**
________	esophagogastroduodenoscopy	**EGD**

continued

		ANSWER COLUMN
___________	gallbladder	**GB**
___________	gastroesophageal reflux disease	**GERD**
___________	gastrointestinal	**GI**
___________	hepatitis A virus	**HAV**
___________	hepatitis B virus	**HBV**
___________	after meals (post cibum)	**pc**
___________	postprandial (after meals)	**PP**
___________	peptic ulcer disease	**PUD**
___________	proton pump inhibitors	**PPIs**

IN THE SPOTLIGHT

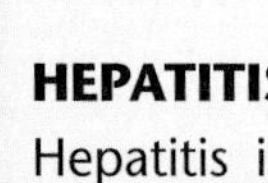

HEPATITIS

Hepatitis is defined as an inflammation of the liver. There are five main forms of hepatitis and each form is named after the virus causing the disease: hepatitis A (HAV), hepatitis B (HBV), hepatitis C (HCV), hepatitis D (HDV), and hepatitis E (HEV). With hepatitis A there may be no symptoms or one may have light stools, dark urine, fatigue, fever, nausea, vomiting, abdominal pain, and jaundice. With the other four forms of hepatitis there may be no symptoms, or a person may have flu-like symptoms, dark urine, light stools, jaundice, fatigue, and fever.

Hepatitis A (HAV) does not lead to chronic liver disease. It is transmitted by the fecal/oral route, through close person-to-person contact or ingestion of contaminated food and water. The incubation period is 2 to 7 weeks. There is a vaccine for hepatitis A with two doses of vaccine for anyone 2 years of age or older. Each year an estimated 180,000 HAV infections occur in the United States. Approximately 100 Americans die each year from hepatitis A. In the United States, the annual cost associated with hepatitis A is estimated to be $200 million.

Hepatitis B (HBV) can cause liver cell damage, leading to cirrhosis and cancer. It is spread by contact with infected blood, seminal fluid, vaginal secretions, and contaminated needles, including tattoo and body-piercing tools. It can be transmitted from mother to newborn, through sexual contact, and/or by human bite. The incubation period is 6 to 23 weeks. There is a vaccine for hepatitis B with three doses of vaccine for persons of any age. This vaccine can provide immunity in over 95% of young healthy adults. An estimated 350 million people worldwide are infected with HBV. The hepatitis B virus can live on a dry surface for at least 7 days. Household bleach (10 parts water to 1 part bleach) can kill the HBV. Every year 5000 Americans die from cirrhosis and 1000 from liver cancer due to HBV infections.

Hepatitis C (HCV) can cause liver cell damage, leading to cirrhosis and cancer. It is spread by contact with infected blood, contaminated IV needles, razors, and tattoo or body-piercing tools. It can be transmitted from mother to newborn. It is not easily spread by sexual contact. The incubation period is 2 to 25 weeks. Approximately 3% of the world population is infected with HCV or about 170 million people.

Hepatitis D (HDV) infects only those persons with hepatitis B. It is spread by contact with infected blood, contaminated needles, and sexual contact with an HDV-infected person. The incubation period is 2 to 8 weeks. The hepatitis B vaccine prevents hepatitis D.

Hepatitis E (HEV) is rare in the United States. It is transmitted through the fecal/oral route. Outbreaks are associated with contaminated water supply in other countries.

CASE STUDY

Please read the following case study and then work frames 11.57–11.62. Write in your answer in the answer column. Check your responses with the answers provided at the end of frame 11.62.

A 35-year-old male was seen by a physician and the following is a synopsis of the visit.

PRESENT HISTORY: The patient states that he has been under a lot of pressure at work lately and that he has noticed a dull, aching pain in his stomach and back. He states that he has heartburn and "belches" a lot.

SIGNS AND SYMPTOMS: Dull, gnawing pain and a burning sensation in the midepigastrium. Pyrosis (heartburn) and sour eructation (belching).

DIAGNOSIS: Acute gastric ulcer, peptic ulcer disease (PUD). Diagnosis determined by a gastrointestinal (GI) series, gastric analysis, and histology with culture to determine presence of *H. pylori*. No *Helicobacter pylori* were found in the culture. See Figures 11–5 and 11–6.

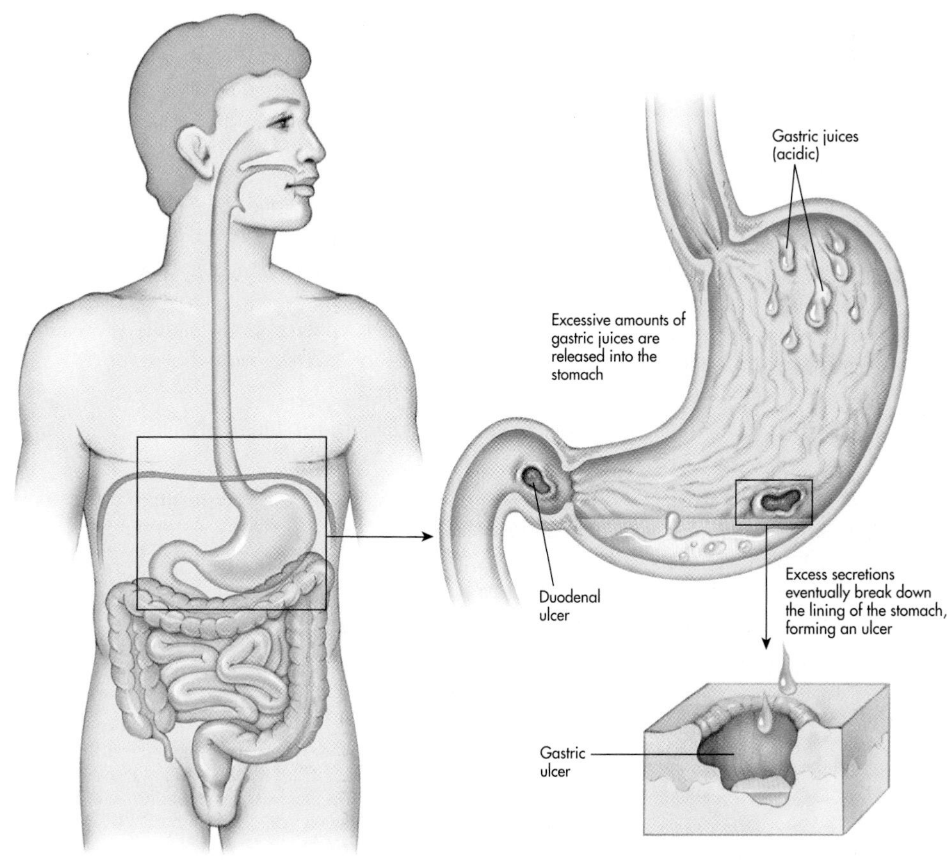

■ **FIGURE 11–5**
Peptic ulcer disease.

(*continued*)

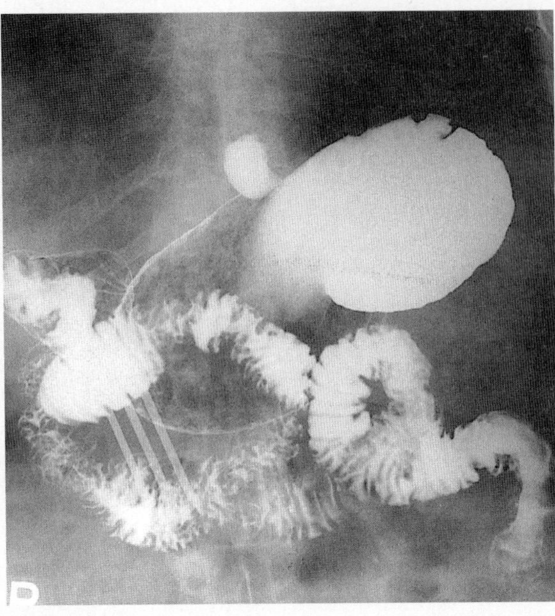

■ **FIGURE 11-6**
Upper GI series. *(Courtesy of Teresa Resch.)*

TREATMENT: Goal is to manage and reduce gastric acidity. This may be accomplished through various treatment regimens such as stress management; rest; diet; avoidance of tobacco, caffeine, and alcohol; and medication. The patient is placed on Mylanta 2 tablets every 2 to 4 hours between meals and at bedtime, and Zantac 300 mg at bedtime.

PREVENTION: Avoid substances that produce gastric acidity. Stress management; rest; diet; and avoidance of tobacco, caffeine, and alcohol are recommended.

11.57 Signs and symptoms of a gastric ulcer include a dull, gnawing pain and a burning sensation in the midepigastrium. Other indications are: ____________, which is heartburn, and sour eructation.

11.58 To help reduce gastric acidity the patient should avoid tobacco, caffeine, and ____________.

11.59 The diagnosis of acute gastric ulcer was determined by a gastric analysis and a ____________ series.

11.60 The goal of treatment for acute gastric ulcer is to manage and reduce gastric ____________.

11.61 The medication regimen prescribed included ____________ 2 tablets every 2 to 4 hours between meals and at bedtime and

11.62 Zantac ____________ mg at bedtime.

CASE STUDY ANSWERS

11.57 pyrosis
11.58 alcohol
11.59 gastrointestinal
11.60 acidity
11.61 Mylanta
11.62 300

REVIEW A: WORD ELEMENTS

This review allows you to check your knowledge of some of the word elements presented in this unit. In the spaces provided, write the meaning of the word elements that are identified as **Prefix (P), Word Root (R), Combining Form (CF),** and/or **Suffix (S).**

MEDICAL WORD	*WORD ELEMENT*	*MEANING*
1. gastroenterology	gastr / o (CF)	____________
	enter / o (CF)	____________
	-logy (S)	____________
2. gingivitis	gingiv (R)	____________
	-itis (S)	____________
3. peristalsis	peri (P)	____________
	-stalsis (S)	____________
4. enteritis	enter (R)	____________
	-itis (S)	____________
5. appendicitis	appendic (R)	____________
	-itis (S)	____________
6. proctologist	proct / o (CF)	____________
	log (R)	____________
	-ist (S)	____________
7. cholecystectomy	chol / e (CF)	____________
	cyst (R)	____________
	-ectomy (S)	____________
8. pancreatitis	pancreat (R)	____________
	-itis (S)	____________
9. dyspepsia	dys (P)	____________
	-pepsia (S)	____________

REVIEW B: MEDICAL TERMS

Please place the correct letter from column II on the appropriate line of column I.

COLUMN I		COLUMN II
________	1. buccal	A. inflammation of the esophagus
________	2. lingual	B. pertaining to the stomach
________	3. dentalgia	C. pertaining to the intestine
________	4. esophagitis	D. the act of vomiting
________	5. gastric	E. pertaining to the cheek
________	6. duodenum	F. gas in the stomach
________	7. enteric	G. pertaining to the tongue
________	8. emesis	H. bad breath
________	9. flatus	I. toothache
________	10. halitosis	J. first portion of the small intestine

REVIEW C: DISEASES AND DISORDERS

Please provide the correct disease or disorder for each of the following descriptions.

1. ________ ________ are tortuous dilated veins of the esophagus.
2. ________ ________ is the backward flow of gastric acid into the esophagus.
3. ________ disease is also known as regional enteritis.
4. ________ is a chronic degenerative liver disease.
5. ________ is the twisting of the bowel upon itself that causes an obstruction.

REVIEW D: UNSCRAMBLE THE WORDS

Unscramble the following medical terms and place the correct term on the line directly across from the scrambled word.

1. hearraid ________
2. cesfe ________
3. zymeen ________
4. horricsis ________
5. viler ________

REVIEW E: DRUGS USED FOR THE DIGESTIVE SYSTEM

Please provide the correct answer for each of the following descriptions.

1. ____________ are agents that neutralize hydrochloric acid in the stomach.
2. ____________ are used to relieve constipation.
3. ____________ agents are used to treat diarrhea.
4. ____________ prevent or arrest vomiting.

REVIEW F: ABBREVIATIONS

Please provide the correct abbreviation and/or meaning for the abbreviation.

1. ____________ bowel movement
2. GB ____________
3. ____________ gastrointestinal
4. HAV____________
5. ____________ after meals (post cibum)
6. ____________ postprandial

12 THE RESPIRATORY SYSTEM: PULMONARY MEDICINE

LEARNING CONCEPTS

- the respiratory system
- essential terminology
- pronunciation guide
- word elements
- explanation frames
- respiratory rates
- selected types of respiration
- selected types of breathing patterns
- selected diseases and disorders
- drugs used for the respiratory system
- abbreviatons
- in the spotlight: tuberculosis
- case study: pulmonary tuberculosis
- review exercises

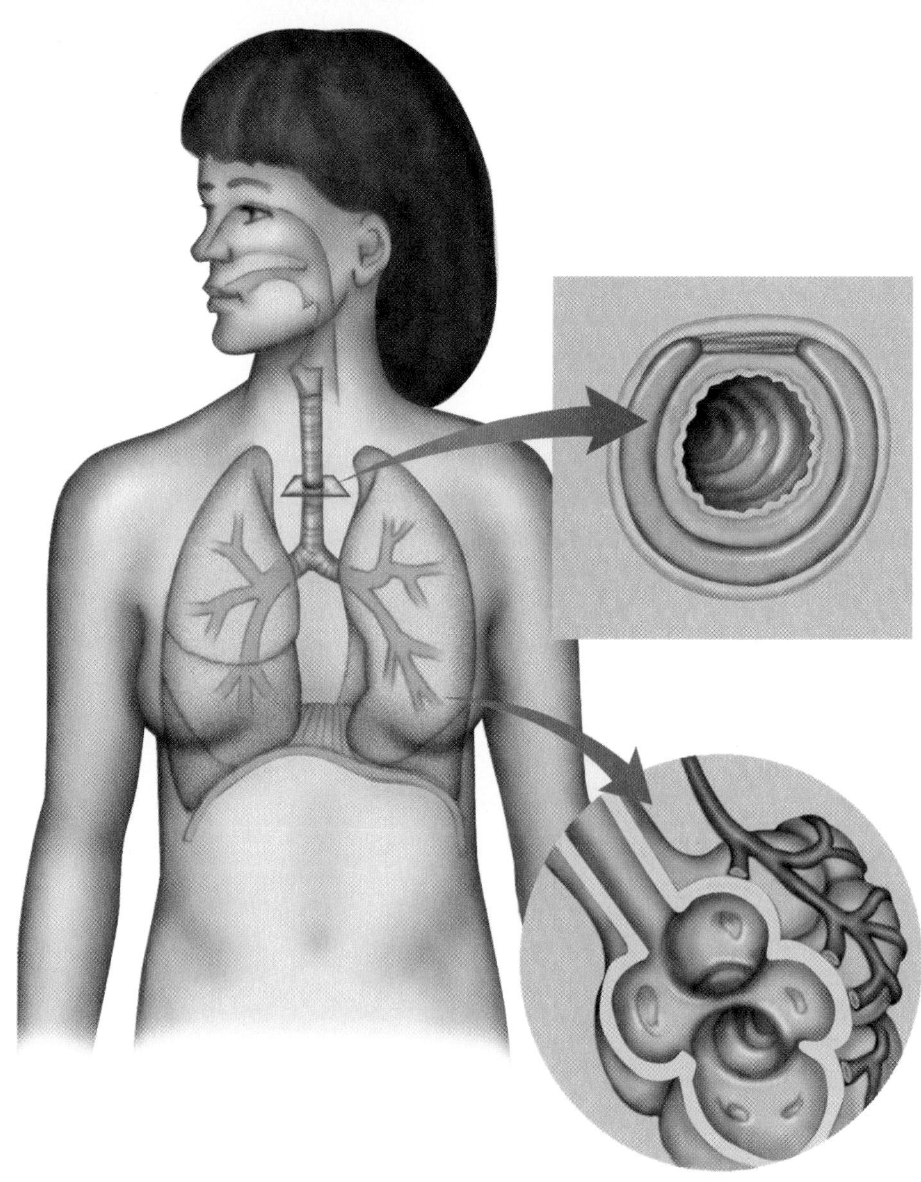

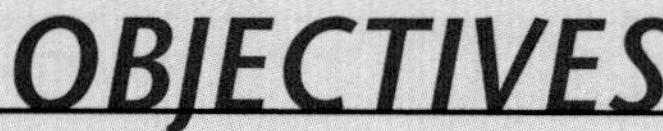

OBJECTIVES

ON COMPLETION OF THIS UNIT, YOU SHOULD BE ABLE TO:

- Briefly describe the respiratory system.
- Describe the primary functions of the various organs or structures of the respiratory system.
- Identify and give the meaning of the primary word elements for this unit.
- Analyze, build, spell, and pronounce selected medical words.
- Describe selected diseases/disorders of the respiratory system.
- State the respiratory rates for selected age groups.
- Describe selected drugs that are used for the respiratory system diseases or disorders.
- Define selected abbreviations that pertain to the respiratory system.
- Briefly describe tuberculosis.
- List the symptoms of tuberculosis of the lungs.
- List other symptoms of tuberculosis.
- Explain how tuberculosis is diagnosed.
- Complete the Case Study on Pulmonary Tuberculosis.
- Successfully complete the review section.

The respiratory system consists of the nose, pharynx, larynx, trachea, bronchi, and lungs. See Table 12–1. The primary function of the respiratory system is to furnish oxygen for use by individual tissue cells and to take away their gaseous waste product, carbon dioxide. This process is accomplished through the act of respiration.

Respiration consists of external and internal processes. External respiration is the process whereby the lungs are ventilated and oxygen and carbon dioxide are exchanged between the air in the lungs and the blood within capillaries of the alveoli. The lungs contain around 300 million alveoli, and if they were opened up and spread out flat, they would cover an area equal to approximately eight room-size carpets. Internal respiration is the process whereby oxygen and carbon dioxide are exchanged between the blood in tissue capillaries and the cells of the body.

TECH LINK

CD-ROM Use the CD-ROM enclosed with your textbook to gain additional reinforcement through interactive word building exercises, spelling games, labeling activities, and additional quizzes.

www.prenhall.com/rice Use the above address to access the free, interactive Companion Website created specifically for this textbook. Get hints, instant feedback, and textbook references to chapter-related multiple choice and true/false questions, fill-in-the-blank, and labeling exercises. In addition, you will find an audio glossary, and essay questions.

TABLE 12-1 THE RESPIRATORY SYSTEM

Organ/Structure	Primary Functions
The Nose	Serves as an air passageway; warms and moistens inhaled air; its cilia and mucous membrane trap dust, pollen, bacteria, and other foreign matter; contains olfactory receptors, which sort out odors; aids in phonation and the quality of voice
The Pharynx	Serves as a passageway for air and for food; aids in phonation by changing its shape
The Larynx	Production of vocal sounds
The Trachea	Provides an open passageway for air to the lungs
The Bronchi	Provide a passageway for air to and from the lungs
The Lungs	Bring air into intimate contact with blood so that oxygen and carbon dioxide can be exchanged in the alveoli

PRIMARY WORD ELEMENTS

The following word elements (prefixes, roots, combining forms, and suffixes) will be used to build medical terms that relate to this unit. Please commit these to memory.

PREFIX

PREFIX	MEANING	PREFIX	MEANING
a	without, lack of	**hyp**	below, deficient
dys	bad, difficult, painful	**hyper**	above, excessive
epi	upon, over, above	**tachy**	fast
eu	good, normal		

COMBINING FORM

COMBINING FORM / ROOT	MEANING	COMBINING FORM / ROOT	MEANING
anthrac	coal	**orth / o**	straight
atel	imperfect	**ox**	oxygen
bronch, bronch / i, bronch / o	bronchi	**pharyng**	pharynx
		pneum / o, pulm / o	air, lung
con / i	dust	**pneumon, pulmon, pulmon / o**	lung
cyan	dark blue		
laryng, laryng / e	larynx	**pollen**	dust
laryng / o	larynx	**rhin, rhin / o**	nose
ment	chin	**sinus**	a hollow curve
myc	fungus	**trache**	trachea
nas / o, rhin / o	nose	**trache / o**	trachea

SUFFIX

SUFFIX	MEANING	SUFFIX	MEANING
-al, -ary	pertaining to	**-pnea**	breathing
-algia	pain	**-rrhagia**	bursting forth
-ectasis	dilation, distention	**-rrhea**	flow, discharge
-ia, -osis	condition of	**-scope**	instrument
-itis	inflammation	**-staxis**	dripping, trickling
-meter	instrument to measure, measure	**-stomy**	new opening
		-tomy	incision
-plasty	surgical repair		

Answer Column

12.1 __________ medicine involves the study of diseases/disorders of the lungs and the respiratory system.

pulmonary
(**PULL** mon air ee)

12.2 A __________ is a physician who specializes in the study of the lungs and the respiratory system.

pulmonologist
(pull moh **NOL** oh jist)

EXPLANATION FRAME

The respiratory system consists of the nose, pharynx, larynx, trachea, bronchi, and lungs. See Figure 12–1. The nose is the projection in the center of the face and consists of an external and internal portion. See Figure 12–2. Five functions have been attributed to the nose.

- It serves as an air passageway.
- It warms and moistens inhaled air.
- Its cilia and mucous membrane trap dust, pollen, bacteria, and other foreign matter.
- It contains olfactory receptors, which sort out odors.
- It aids in phonation and quality of voice.

12.3 The combining forms **nas / o** and **rhin / o** and the root **rhin** mean nose. Medical terms that begin with these word elements are:

__________ pertaining to the nose and chin — **nasomental** (nay zoh **MEN** tal)

__________ inflammation of the nose and pharynx — **nasopharyngitis** (nay zoh fair in **JYE** tis)

__________ inflammation of the nose — **rhinitis** (rye **NYE** tis)

__________ surgical repair of the nose — **rhinoplasty** (**RYE** noh plas tee)

__________ the bursting forth of blood from the nose — **rhinorrhagia** (rye noh **RAH** jee ah)

__________ discharge from the nose — **rhinorrhea** (riye noh **REE** ah)

__________ narrowing of the nasal passages — **rhinostenosis** (rye noh steh **NOH** sis)

__________ incision of the nose — **rhinotomy** (rye **NOT** oh me)

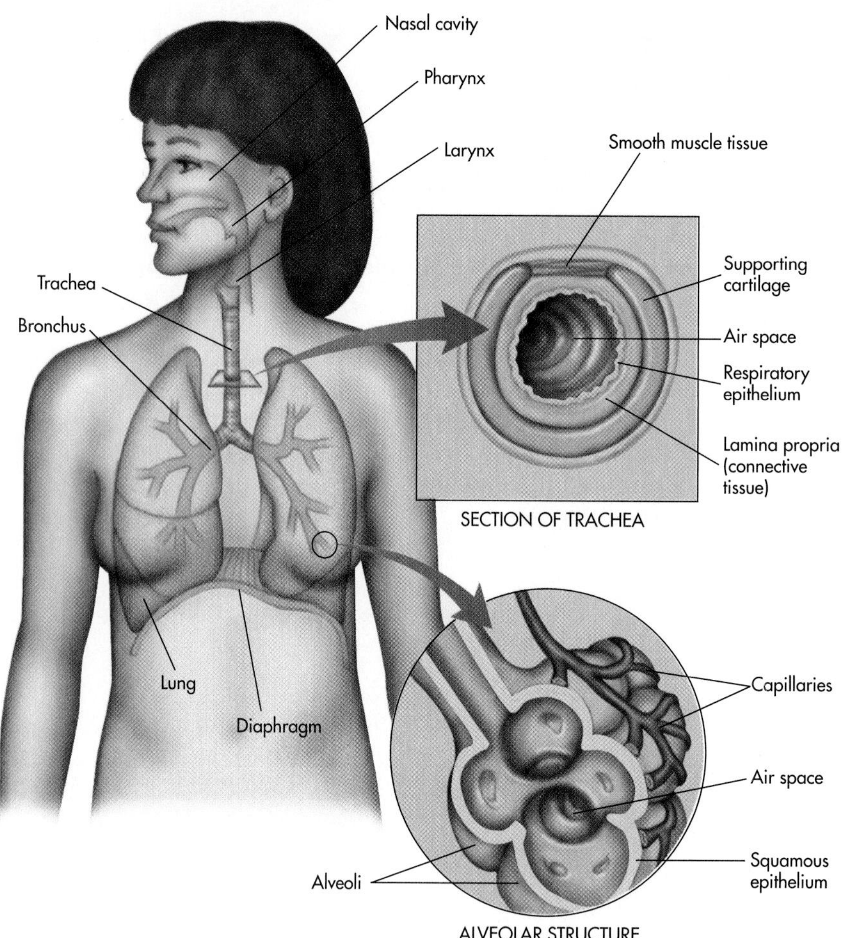

FIGURE 12–1

The respiratory system: nasal cavity, pharynx, larynx, trachea, bronchus, and lung with expanded views of the trachea and alveolar structure.

EXPLANATION FRAME

The pharynx or throat is a musculomembranous tube about 5 inches long. See Figure 12–1. It extends from the base of the skull, lies anterior to the cervical vertebrae, and becomes continuous with the esophagus. See Figure 12–2.

The functions of the pharynx are:

- It serves as a passageway for air.
- It serves as a passageway for food and liquids.
- It aids in phonation by changing its shape.

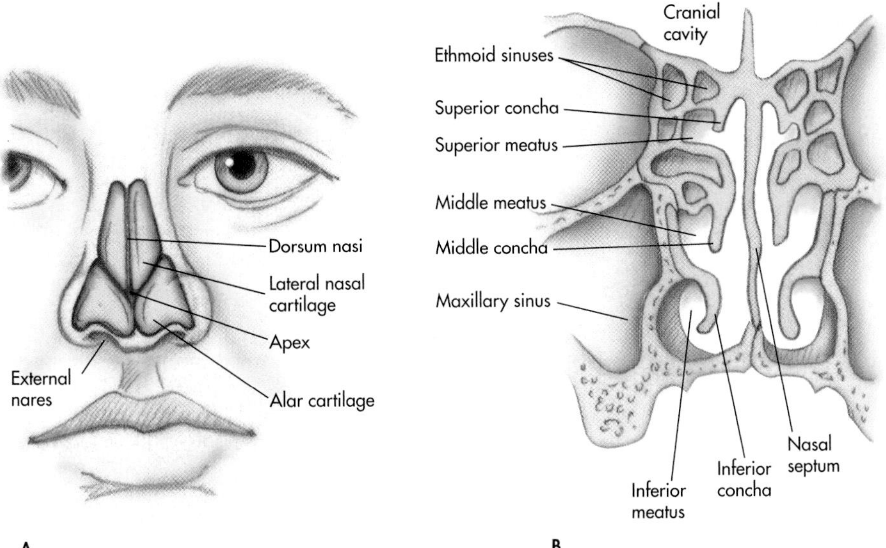

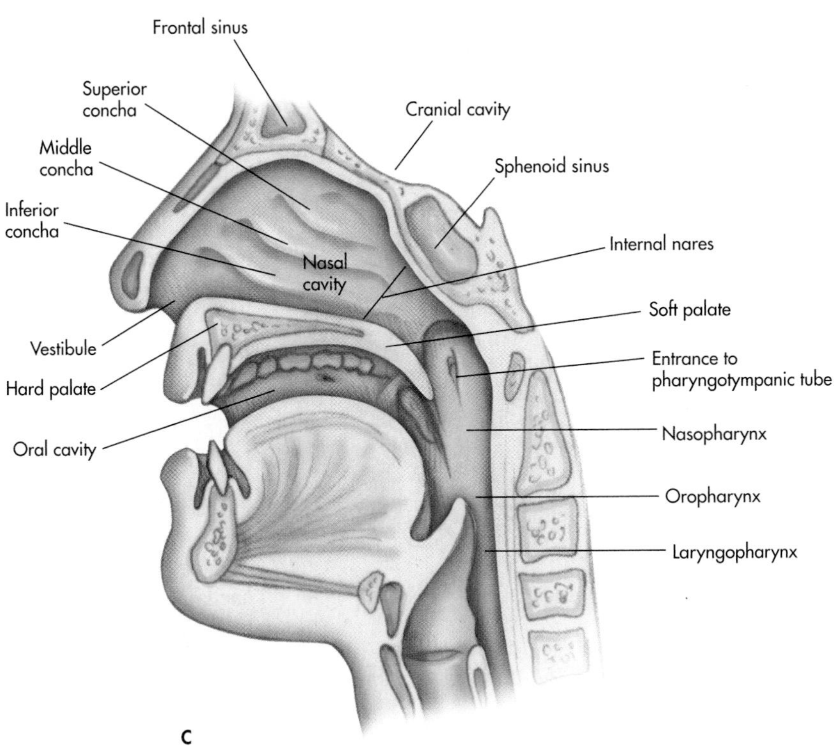

FIGURE 12–2

The nose, nasal cavity, and pharynx: (A) nasal cartilages and external structures, (B) meatuses and positions of the entrance to the ethmoid and maxillary sinuses, (C) sagittal section of the nasal cavity and pharynx.

ANSWER COLUMN

12.4 The root **pharyng** means pharynx.
Medical terms that begin with this word element are:

_________ pain in the pharynx

_________ inflammation of the pharynx

pharyngalgia
(fair in **GAL** jee ah)
pharyngitis
(fair in **JYE** tis)

EXPLANATION FRAME

The larynx or voicebox is a muscular, cartilaginous structure lined with mucous membrane. See Figure 12–1. It is the enlarged upper end of the trachea below the root of the tongue and hyoid bone. The larynx is composed of nine cartilages bound together by muscles and ligaments. The function of the larynx is the production of vocal sounds.

12.5 The epiglottic cartilage is a small cartilage attached to the superior border of the thyroid cartilage. It is known as the _________ and it covers the entrance of the larynx. During swallowing, it acts as a lid to prevent aspiration of food into the trachea. *When the epiglottis fails to cover the entrance to the larynx, food or liquid intended for the esophagus may enter, causing irritation, coughing, or in extreme cases, choking.*

epiglottis
(ep ih **GLOT** iss)

12.6 The combining forms **laryng / e** and **laryng / o** and the root **laryng** mean larynx.
Medical terms that begin with these word elements are:

_________ pertaining to the larynx

_________ surgical excision of the larynx

_________ inflammation of the larynx

_________ surgical repair of the larynx

_________ an instrument used to examine the larynx

_________ a new opening into the larynx

laryngeal
(lah **RIN** jee al)
laryngectomy
(lair in **JEK** toh mee)
laryngitis
(lair in **JYE** tis)
laryngoplasty
(lair **RING** goh plas tee)
laryngoscope
(lair **RING** goh scope)
laryngostomy
(lair in **GOSS** toh mee)

ANSWER COLUMN

EXPLANATION FRAME

The trachea or windpipe is a cylindrical cartilaginous tube that is the air passageway extending from the pharynx and larynx to the main bronchi. See Figure 12–1 and Figure 12–3. It is about 1 inch wide and 4 inches long. Mucous membrane lining the trachea contains cilia, which sweep foreign matter out of the passageway. The function of the trachea is to provide an open passageway for air to the lungs.

12.7 The combining form **trache / o** and the root **trache** mean trachea.
Medical terms that begin with these word elements are:

		Answer
____________	pertaining to the trachea	**tracheal** (**TRAY** kee al)
____________	pain in the trachea	**trachealgia** (tray kee **AL** jee ah)
____________	inflammation of the trachea	**tracheitis** (tray kee **EYE** tis)
____________	incision into the larynx and trachea	**tracheolaryngotomy** (tray kee oh lair in **GOT** oh mee)
____________	new opening into the trachea	**tracheostomy** (tray kee **OSS** toh mee)

EXPLANATION FRAME

The bronchi are the two main branches of the trachea, which provide the passageway for air to the lungs. See Figure 12–1 and Figure 12–3. The function of the bronchi is to provide a passageway for air to and from the lungs.

12.8 The combining forms **bronch / i** and **bronch / o** and the root **bronch** mean bronchi.
Medical terms that begin with these word elements are:

		Answer
____________	dilation of the bronchi	**bronchiectasis** (brong kee **EK** tah sis)
____________	inflammation of the bronchi	**bronchitis** (brong **KIGH** tis)
____________	a fungus condition of the bronchi	**bronchomycosis** (brong koh my **KOH** sis)
____________	surgical repair of the bronchi	**bronchoplasty** (**BRONG** koh plas tee)
____________	an instrument used to examine the bronchi	**bronchoscope** (**BRONG** koh scope)

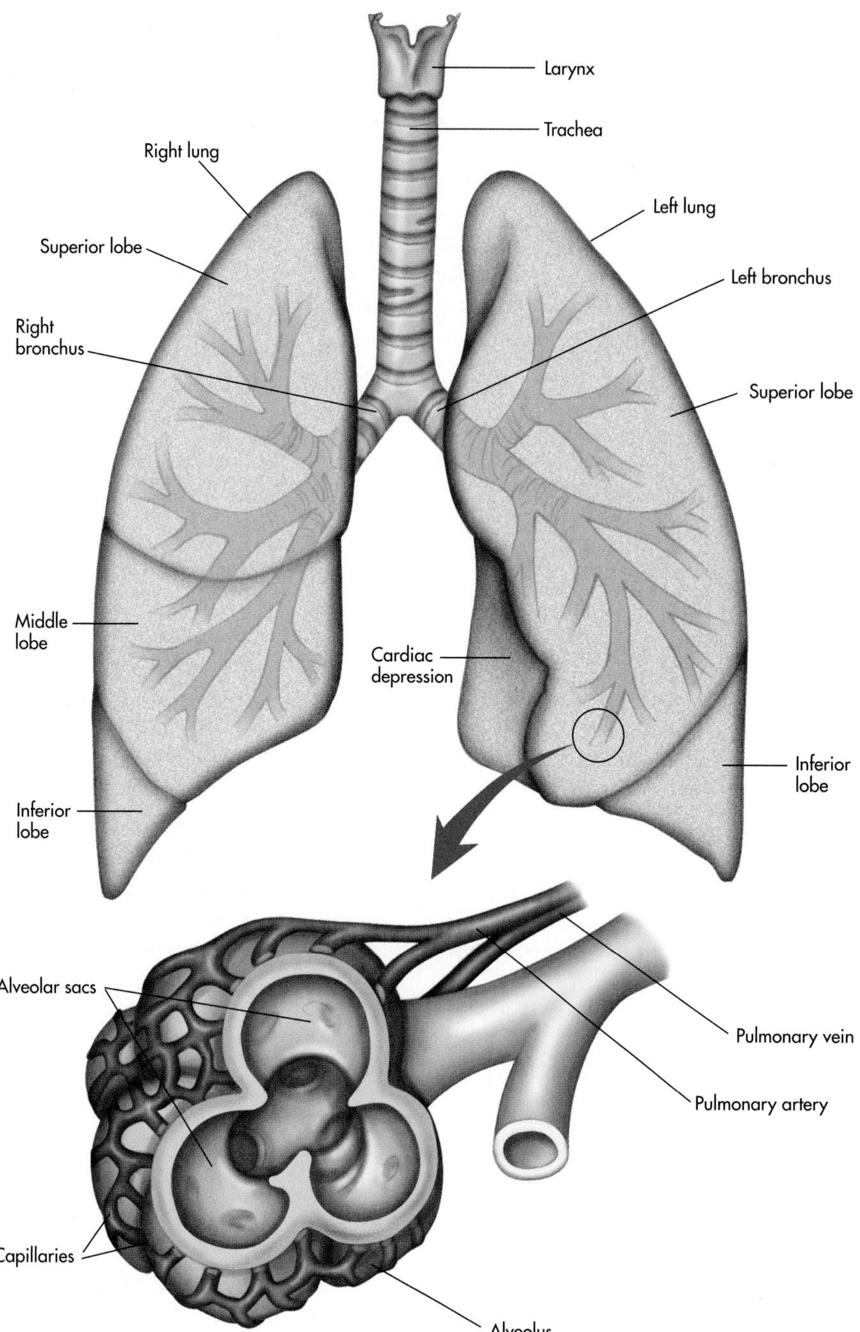

FIGURE 12–3

The larynx, trachea, bronchi, and lungs with an expanded view showing the structures of an alveolus and the pulmonary blood vessels.

ANSWER COLUMN

EXPLANATION FRAME

The lungs are cone-shaped, spongy organs of respiration lying on either side of the heart within the pleural cavity of the thorax. See Figure 12–1 and Figure 12–3. The lungs consist of elastic tissue filled with interlacing networks of tubes and sacs that carry air. The lungs are divided into lobes with the right lung having three lobes and the left lung having only two lobes. The lungs contain around 300 million alveoli, which are the air cells where the exchange of oxygen and carbon dioxide takes place. The main function of the lungs is to bring air into intimate contact with blood so that oxygen and carbon dioxide can be exchanged in the alveoli.

12.9 The combining forms **pneum /o** and **pulm / o** and the roots **pneumon** and **pulmon** mean lung.

Medical terms that begin with these word elements are:

___________ a lung condition caused by inhalation of dust (**con / i** is a combining form that means dust)

pneumoconiosis (noo moh koh nee **OH** sis)

___________ inflammation of the lung caused by bacteria, viruses, or chemical irritants

pneumonia (new **MOH** nee ah)

___________ inflammation of the lung; SYN: pulmonitis

pneumonitis (noo moh **NYE** tis)

___________ is the collection of air or gas in the pleural cavity as the result of a perforation through the pleura covering the lung. It may be caused by injury, rupture of an emphysematous bleb, lung abscess, or tuberculosis abscess. SYN: aeropleura, aerothorax, or pneumatothorax

pneumothorax (new moh **THOH** raks)

___________ an instrument used to measure lung capacity

pulmometer (pull **MOM** eh ter)

___________ pertaining to the lung

pulmonary (**PULL** mon air ee)

___________ surgical excision of the lung or part of a lung; SYN: pneumonectomy

pulmonectomy (pull moh **NEK** toh mee)

EXPLANATION FRAME

Individuals of different ages breathe at different respiratory rates. Respiratory rate is regulated by the respiratory center located in the medulla oblongata. The following are respiratory rates for some different age groups:

- Newborn 30–80 per minute
- 1st year 20–40 per minute
- 5th year 20–25 per minute
- 15th year 15–20 per minute
- Adult 12–20 per minute

Answer Column

12.10 __________ is defined as the interchange of gases between an organism and its environment. Selected types of respiration are:

__________ walls of the chest are nearly at rest and chiefly the diaphragm exerts itself

__________ process of using artificial means to cause air to flow into and out of an individual's lungs when breathing is inadequate or ceases

__________ __________ a rhythmic cycle of breathing with a gradual increase in respiration followed by apnea (which may last from 10 to 60 seconds), then a repeat of the same cycle

__________ a distressing, deep gasping type of breathing associated with metabolic acidosis and coma; also called air hunger

respiration (res pir **AY** shun)

abdominal (ab **DOM** ih nal)

artificial (ar tih **FISH** al)

Cheyne-Stokes (CHAIN STOHKS)

Kussmaul's (**KOOS** mowlz)

12.11 Respiratory distress syndrome, also known as __________ membrane disease, is a condition that may occur in a premature infant. The lungs have not matured to the point of manufacturing lecithin, a pulmonary surfactant. This results in collapse of the alveoli, which leads to cyanosis and hypoxia.

hyaline (**HIGH** ah leen)

12.12 __________ is a dark blue condition of the skin and mucous membranes caused by oxygen deficiency.

The word elements used to build this term are:

__________ root that means dark blue

__________ suffix that means condition of

cyanosis (sigh ah **NOH** sis)

cyan

-osis

12.13 __________ is a condition of deficient amounts of oxygen in the inspired air. The word elements used to build this term are:

__________ prefix that means deficient

__________ root that means oxygen

__________ suffix that means condition of

hypoxia (high **POX** ee ah)

hyp

ox

-ia

12.14 Medical terms that describe breathing use the suffix **-pnea** which means breathing, and various prefixes such as **a**—lack of, **dys**—difficult, **eu**—normal, **hyper**—excessive, **tachy**—fast, and a combining form **orth / o**—straight.

__________ is a temporary cessation of breathing.

Sleep apnea is a disorder characterized by cessation of breathing during sleep. In order to be so classified, the apnea lasts for at least 10 seconds and occurs 30 or more times during a 7-hour period of sleep.

apnea (**AP** nee ah)

	Answer Column
continued	
__________ difficulty in breathing	**dyspnea** (**DISP** nee ah)
__________ good or normal breathing	**eupnea** (yoop **NEE** ah)
__________ excessive or rapid breathing	**hyperpnea** (high per **NEE** ah)
__________ inability to breathe unless in an upright or straight position	**orthopnea** (or **THOP** nee ah)
__________ fast breathing	**tachypnea** (tak ip **NEE** ah)
12.15 __________ is a lung condition caused by inhalation of coal dust and silica. It is also called "black lung" disease.	**anthracosis** (an thrah **KOH** sis)
12.16 __________ is a condition of imperfect dilation of the lungs. In this condition the lungs are collapsed or airless.	**atelectasis** (at eh **LEK** tah sis)
The word elements used to build this term are:	
__________ root that means imperfect	**atel**
__________ suffix that means dilation	**-ectasis**
12.17 __________ is a disease of the bronchi characterized by wheezing, dyspnea, and a feeling of constriction in the chest.	**asthma** (**AZ** mah)
12.18 __________ is a chronic pulmonary disease in which the bronchioles become obstructed with mucus.	**emphysema** (em fih **SEE** mah)
12.19 __________ is pus in a body cavity, especially the pleural cavity.	**empyema** (em pye **EE** mah)
12.20 __________ is the medical term for nosebleed.	**epistaxis** (ep ih **STAKS** is)
12.21 __________ is the medical term for the common cold. It is characterized by sneezing, nasal discharge, coughing, and malaise.	**coryza** (kor **RYE** zuh)

Answer Column

12.22 __________ is inflammation of a sinus. A sinus is a cavity within certain bones. The paranasal sinuses are the frontal, maxillary, ethmoidal, and sphenoidal.

sinusitis (sigh nus **EYE** tis)

12.23 __________ is an acute, infectious disease characterized by coryza, an explosive paroxysmal cough ending in a "crowing" or "whooping" sound; also called whooping cough.

pertussis (per **TUH** sis)

12.24 __________ is an allergic reaction to pollen or pollens. It is also known as hay fever, which is characterized by nasal congestion of mucous membranes.

pollinosis (pol ih **NOH** sis)

12.25 __________ is inflammation of the pleural cavity caused by injury, infection, or a tumor. This condition is generally very painful.

pleurisy (**PLOOR** ih se)

12.26 __________ is a substance coughed up from the lungs that may be watery, thick, purulent, clear, or bloody and may contain microorganisms.

sputum (**SPEW** tum)

EXPLANATION FRAME

Drugs that are generally used for diseases and disorders of the respiratory system include antihistamines, antibiotics, decongestants, antitussives, expectorants, mucolytics, bronchodilators, inhalational corticosteroids, and antituberculosis agents.

12.27 __________ act to counter the effects of histamine by blocking histamine-1 receptors. They are used in the control of allergy symptoms or for preventing or controlling motion sickness and, in combination with cold remedies, to decrease mucus secretion and to produce bedtime sedation.

antihistamines (an tih **HISS** tah meens)

12.28 __________ are used to treat infectious diseases. They are natural or synthetic substances that inhibit the growth of or destroy microorganisms, especially bacteria.

antibiotics (an tih bye **OT** iks)

Answer Column

12.29 __________ act to constrict dilated arterioles in the nasal mucosa. Decongestants are used for the temporary relief of nasal congestion associated with the common cold, hay fever, other upper respiratory allergies, and sinusitis.

decongestants (dee kon **JESS** tants)

12.30 __________ act to reduce the cough reflex.

antitussives (an tih **TUSS** ivs)

12.31 __________ promote and facilitate the removal of mucus from the lower respiratory tract.

expectorants (ek **SPEK** toh rants)

12.32 __________ break chemical bonds in mucus, thereby lowering its thickness.

mucolytics (myoo koh **LIT** iks)

12.33 __________ are used to improve pulmonary airflow.

bronchodilators (brong koh **DYE** lay tors)

12.34 Inhalational __________ are used in the treatment of bronchial asthma and in seasonal or perennial allergic condition when other forms of treatment are not effective.

corticosteroids (kor tih koh **STAIR** oydz)

12.35 __________ agents are used in the long-term treatment of tuberculosis. They are often used in combination of two or more drugs.

antituberculosis (an tih too ber kyoo **LOH** sis)

12.36 ABBREVIATIONS

Write in the correct abbreviation for the following:

		Answer
__________	acute respiratory disease	**ARD**
__________	acute respiratory distress syndrome	**ARDS**
__________	carbon dioxide	**CO_2**
__________	chronic obstructive lung disease	**COLD**
__________	chronic obstructive pulmonary disease	**COPD**
__________	hyaline membrane disease	**HMD**
__________	oxygen	**O_2**
__________	postnasal drip	**PND**

continued

		ANSWER COLUMN
____________	purified protein derivative (TB test)	**PPD**
____________	respiration	**R**
____________	respiratory disease	**RD**
____________	sudden infant death syndrome	**SIDS**
____________	shortness of breath	**SOB**
____________	tuberculosis	**TB**
____________	upper respiratory infection	**URI**

IN THE SPOTLIGHT

TUBERCULOSIS

Tuberculosis is a contagious disease caused by the bacillus *Mycobacterium tuberculosis*. This bacillus is carried in airborne particles, known as droplets. An infected person releases large and small droplets through talking, coughing, sneezing, laughing, or singing. The large droplets settle, while the small droplets remain suspended in the air and can be inhaled by a susceptible person.

Treatment of TB requires long-term drug therapy (9 to 12 months), often using a regimen that includes a combination of antituberculosis agents. The use of multiple drugs is indicated in all but a few active cases, because any large population of *Mycobacterium tuberculosis* will have naturally occurring mutants that are resistant to each of the drugs administered. Diet and rest are important aspects of the treatment of TB. The primary drug regimen for active tuberculosis combines the drugs rifampin, isoniazid, and ethambutol.

Tuberculosis, once called consumption, is not a new disease. At one time it was the number-one killer in the United States. It is still a major cause of death worldwide, killing 2 million people each year. An estimated 10 million Americans are infected with the TB bacterium.

At the present time TB occurs primarily among AIDS patients, the homeless, drug abusers, prison inmates, and immigrants. Health officials are concerned about the rapid spread of this disease and the risks for the general public. Virtually anyone who comes in contact with an infected person is at risk of contracting TB. Studies show that exposure to an infected person in confined quarters such as homes and classrooms increases an individual's risk.

Symptoms of TB depend on where in the body the TB bacteria are growing. TB bacteria usually grow in the lungs and symptoms include a chronic cough, hemoptysis, and in the early stages, scanty, whitish or grayish-yellow frothy sputum. Other symptoms are fatigue, low-grade fever, night sweats, weakness, chills, anorexia, and weight loss.

To determine a diagnosis of tuberculosis, a careful history is taken and a complete physical examination is performed. After evaluation of the patient, the physician may order a tuberculin test, chest x-ray, bronchoscopy, or sputum culture for a positive diagnosis. A sputum culture is essential to confirming a diagnosis, determining an infection's susceptibility to drugs, and assessing response to treatment. If the TB bacteria become resistant to two of the drugs that are used to treat tuberculosis, then MDR TB (multidrug-resistant tuberculosis) is suspected. Appropriate measures must be instituted promptly to treat and prevent the spread of MDR TB.

CASE STUDY

Please read the following case study and then work frames 12.37–12.40. Write in your answer in the answer column. Check your responses with the answers provided at the end of frame 12.40.

A 28-year-old male was seen by a physician and the following is a synopsis of the visit.

PRESENT HISTORY: The patient states that he has had a persistent cough for the past three weeks, is very tired, has lost 8 pounds recently, doesn't have an appetite, and that he wakes up in the middle of the night soaked in sweat.

SIGNS AND SYMPTOMS: Chief Complaints: chronic cough, fatigue, night sweats, weakness, anorexia, and weight loss.

DIAGNOSIS: Pulmonary Tuberculosis. The diagnosis was determined by a physical examination, a sputum culture that was positive for *Mycobacterium tuberculosis*, a positive PPD (purified protein derivative) test, and a chest x-ray that revealed lesions in the upper right lobe.

TREATMENT: The physician ordered a regimen of diet, rest, and a combination of three antituberculosis agents: isoniazid, rifampin, and ethambutol. The medication is to be taken as ordered for 9 months. A follow-up visit was scheduled for 2 weeks.

PREVENTION: Avoid exposure to *Mycobacterium tuberculosis* bacillus. The Centers for Disease Control and Prevention has published a booklet on *Guidelines for Preventing the Transmission of Tuberculosis in Health-Care Settings*. The following are specific actions to reduce the risk of tuberculosis transmission:

- Screening patients for active TB and TB infection
- Providing rapid diagnostic services
- Prescribing an appropriate curative and preventive therapy
- Maintaining physical measures to reduce microbial contamination of the air
- Providing isolation rooms for persons with, or suspected of having, infectious TB
- Screening health-care-facility personnel for TB infection
- Promptly investigating and controlling outbreaks

12.37 Signs and symptoms of pulmonary tuberculosis include a chronic cough, fatigue, night sweats, weakness, ____________, and weight loss.

12.38 Give the abbreviation for purified protein derivative ____________.

12.39 The diagnosis was determined by a physical examination, a positive PPD test, and a positive sputum culture for ____________ ____________ bacillus.

12.40 Treatment included diet, rest, and a medication regimen of three antituberculosis agents: ____________, rifampin, and ethambutol.

CASE STUDY ANSWERS

12.37 anorexia

12.38 PPD

12.39 *Mycobacterium tuberculosis*

12.40 isoniazid

REVIEW A: WORD ELEMENTS

This review allows you to check your knowledge of some of the word elements presented in this unit. In the spaces provided, write the meaning of the word elements that are identified as **Prefix (P), Word Root (R), Combining Form (CF),** and/or **Suffix (S).**

MEDICAL WORD	*WORD ELEMENT*	*MEANING*
1. nasopharyngitis	nas / o (CF)	__________
	pharyng (R)	__________
	-itis (S)	__________
2. rhinoplasty	rhin / o (CF)	__________
	-plasty (S)	__________
3. pharyngalgia	pharyng (R)	__________
	-algia (S)	__________
4. laryngectomy	laryng (R)	__________
	-ectomy (S)	__________
5. laryngostomy	laryng / o (CF)	__________
	-stomy (S)	__________
6. tracheitis	trache (R)	__________
	-itis (S)	__________
7. bronchoscope	bronch / o (CF)	__________
	-scope (S)	__________
8. pneumonitis	pneumon (R)	__________
	-itis (S)	__________
9. pulmonary	pulmon (R)	__________
	-ary (S)	__________
10. cyanosis	cyan (R)	__________
	-osis (S)	__________
11. hypoxia	hyp (P)	__________
	ox (R)	__________
	-ia (S)	__________
12. dyspnea	dys (P)	__________
	-pnea (S)	__________

REVIEW B: MEDICAL TERMS

Please place the correct letter from column II on the appropriate line of column I.

COLUMN I		COLUMN II
______	1. epiglottis	A. dilation of the bronchi
______	2. laryngitis	B. excessive or rapid breathing
______	3. tracheolaryngotomy	C. nosebleed
______	4. bronchiectasis	D. inflammation of a sinus
______	5. pneumoconiosis	E. inflammation of the larynx
______	6. hyperpnea	F. "whooping cough"
______	7. epistaxis	G. acts as a lid to prevent aspiration of food into the trachea
______	8. sinusitis	H. hay fever
______	9. pertussis	I. a lung condition caused by inhalation of dust
______	10. pollinosis	J. incision into the larynx and trachea

REVIEW C: DISEASES AND DISORDERS

Please provide the correct disease or disorder for each of the following descriptions.

1. ____________ is a disease of the bronchi characterized by wheezing, dyspnea, and a feeling of constriction in the chest.
2. ____________ is the medical term for the common cold.
3. ____________ is a chronic pulmonary disease in which the bronchioles become obstructed with mucus.
4. ____________ is pus in a body cavity, especially the pleural cavity.
5. ____________ is a condition of imperfect dilation of the lungs.

REVIEW D: UNSCRAMBLE THE WORDS

Unscramble the following medical terms and place the correct term on the line directly across from the scrambled word.

1. monulpary ___________
2. neuiamonp ___________
3. lineayh ___________
4. neapothor ___________
5. isyruelp ___________
6. tumups ___________
7. culertubosis ___________
8. ialcifitar ___________

REVIEW E: DRUGS USED FOR THE RESPIRATORY SYSTEM

Please provide the correct answer for each of the following descriptions.

1. ___________ promote the removal of mucus from the lower respiratory tract.
2. ___________ break chemical bonds in mucus, thereby lowering its thickness.
3. ___________ act to constrict dilated arterioles in the nasal mucosa.
4. ___________ act to reduce the cough reflex.

REVIEW F: ABBREVIATIONS

Please provide the correct abbreviation and/or meaning for the abbreviation.

1. ___________ acute respiratory disease
2. COPD ___________
3. ___________ postnasal drip
4. R ___________
5. ___________ shortness of breath
6. TB ___________

13 THE URINARY SYSTEM: UROLOGY

LEARNING CONCEPTS

- the urinary system
- essential terminology
- pronunciation guide
- word elements
- explanation frames
- terminology that refers to abnormal urine and/or urination
- urinalysis as a diagnostic tool
- abnormal constituents that may be found in urine
- selected diseases and disorders
- drugs used for the urinary system
- abbreviations
- in the spotlight: cystitis
- case study: acute cystitis
- review exercises

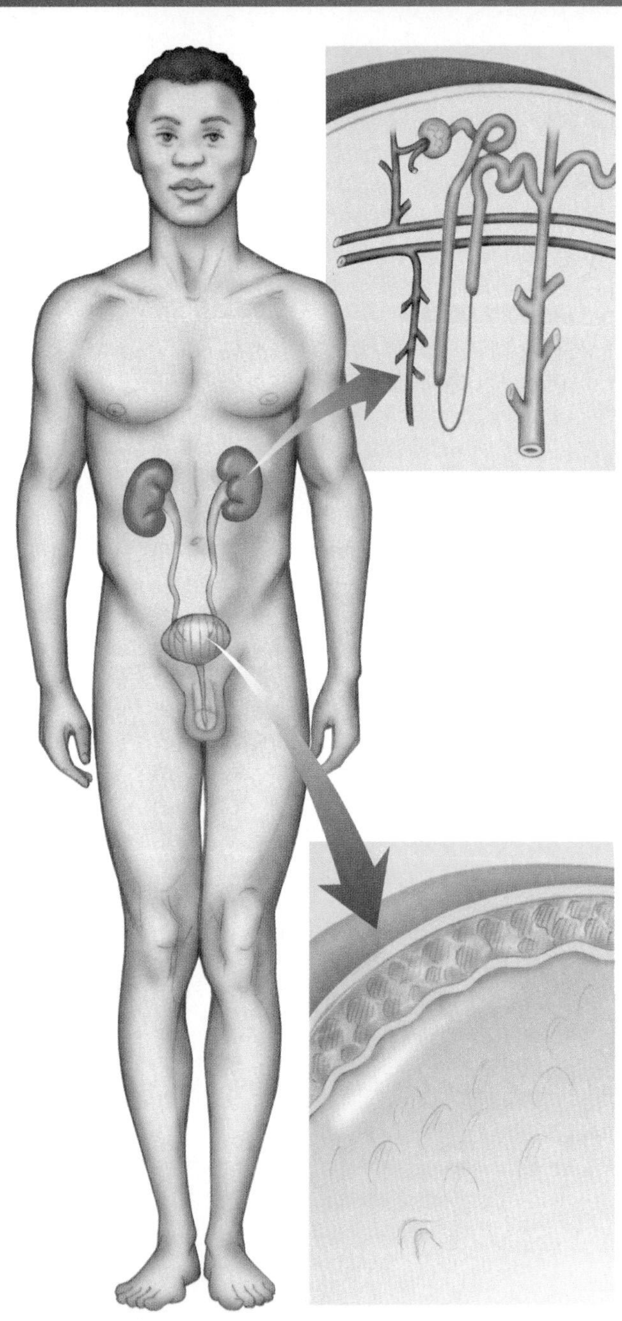

OBJECTIVES

ON COMPLETION OF THIS UNIT, YOU SHOULD BE ABLE TO:

- Briefly describe the urinary system.
- Describe the primary functions of the various organs or structures of the urinary system.
- Identify and give the meaning of the primary word elements for this unit.
- Analyze, build, spell, and pronounce selected medical words.
- Describe selected diseases/disorders of the urinary system.
- Briefly describe urinalysis.
- Describe some abnormal constituents that may be found in urine during a chemical examination.
- Describe selected drugs that are used for the urinary system diseases or disorders.
- Define selected abbreviations that pertain to the urinary system.
- Describe cystitis, giving the cause, how it is diagnosed, the symptoms, and treatment.
- Complete the Case Study on Acute Cystitis.
- List five guidelines to help avoid cystitis in the female.
- Successfully complete the review section.

The urinary system consists of two kidneys, two ureters, one bladder, and one urethra. See Table 13–1. It is referred to as the excretory system, genitourinary system, or urogenital system. The vital function of the urinary system is extraction of certain wastes from the bloodstream, conversion of these materials to urine, transport of the urine from the kidneys via the ureters to the bladder, and elimination of it at appropriate intervals via the urethra.

Urine consists of 95% water and 5% solid substances. It is stored in the bladder before being discharged from the body. An average normal adult feels the need to void when the bladder contains about 300 to 350 mL of urine. An average of 1000 to 1500 mL of urine is voided daily. Normal urine is clear, yellow to amber in color, and has a faintly aromatic odor, a specific gravity of 1.015 to 1.025, and a slightly acid pH.

Approximately 1000 to 1200 mL of blood passes through the kidney per minute. At a rate of 1000 mL of blood per minute about 1.5 million mL pass through the kidney in each 24-hour day.

TECH LINK

CD-ROM Use the CD-ROM enclosed with your textbook to gain additional reinforcement through interactive word building exercises, spelling games, labeling activities, and additional quizzes.

www.prenhall.com/rice Use the above address to access the free, interactive Companion Website created specifically for this textbook. Get hints, instant feedback, and textbook references to chapter-related multiple choice and true/false questions, fill-in-the-blank, and labeling exercises. In addition, you will find an audio glossary, and essay questions.

TABLE 13-1 THE URINARY SYSTEM

Organ/Structure	Primary Functions
Kidneys	Produce urine and help regulate body fluids
Ureters	Transport urine from the kidneys to the bladder
Urinary Bladder	Serves as a reservoir for urine
Urethra	Conveys urine to the outside of the body; in the male conveys both urine and semen

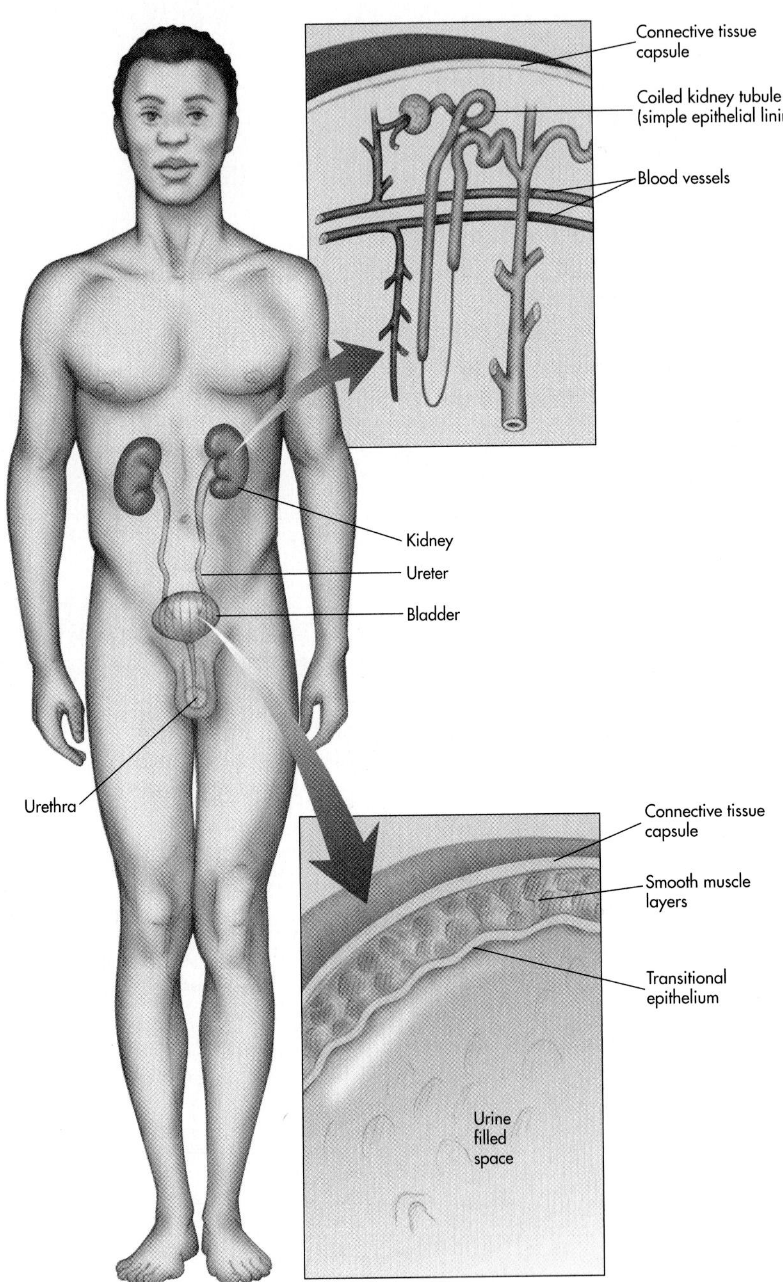

■ **FIGURE 13–1**
The urinary system: kidneys, ureters, bladder, and urethra with expanded views of a nephron and the urine filled space within a bladder.

PRIMARY WORD ELEMENTS

The following word elements (prefixes, roots, combining forms, and suffixes) will be used to build medical terms that relate to this unit. Please commit these to memory.

PREFIX

PREFIX	MEANING	PREFIX	MEANING
an	without, lack of	**in**	in, into, not
di(a)	through	**olig**	little, scanty
dys	bad, difficult, painful	**poly**	many, much
en	within		

COMBINING FORM

COMBINING FORM / ROOT	MEANING	COMBINING FORM / ROOT	MEANING
albumin	protein	**nephr / o, ren / o**	kidney
bacter / i	bacteria	**noct**	night
calc / i	calcium	**penile**	penis
col / o	colon	**py**	pus
cyst, vesic	bladder	**pyel / o**	renal pelvis
cysti / i, cyst / o	bladder	**sten**	narrowing
glomerul	glomerulus, little ball	**ureter / o**	ureter
glomerul / o	glomerulus, little ball	**urethr**	urethra
glyc/ os	sweet, sugar	**urethr/ o**	urethra
hemat	blood	**urin**	urine
keton	ketone	**urin / o**	urine
lith / o	stone	**ur / o**	urine
nephr, ren	kidney		

SUFFIX

SUFFIX	MEANING	SUFFIX	MEANING
-al, -ar	pertaining to	**-oma**	tumor
-algia	pain	**-pexy**	surgical fixation
-cele	hernia, tumor, swelling	**-phraxis**	to obstruct
-ectasy	dilation	**-plasty**	surgical repair
-ectomy	surgical excision	**-ptosis**	drooping
-ist	one who specializes	**-rrhaphy**	suture
-itis	inflammation	**-scope**	instrument
-logy	study of	**-staxis**	dripping, trickling
-malacia	softening	**-tripsy**	crushing
-megaly	enlargement, large	**-uria**	urine
-meter	instrument to measure, measure		

ANSWER COLUMN

13.1 __________ is the study of the urinary system.

urology
(yoo **RALL** oh jee)

13.2 A __________ is a physician who specializes in the study of the urinary system.

urologist
(yoo **RALL** oh jist)

EXPLANATION FRAME

The kidneys are purplish-brown bean-shaped organs located at the back of the abdominal cavity (retroperitoneal area). They lie, one on each side of the spinal column, just above the waistline, against the muscles of the back. See Figure 13–2 and Figure 13–3. The kidneys form urine from blood plasma. They are the major regulators of the water, electrolyte, and acid-base content of the blood.

13.3 The combining form **nephr / o** and the roots **nephr** and **ren** mean kidney. Medical terms that begin with these word elements are:

			Answer
__________	surgical excision of the kidney		**nephrectomy** (neh **FREK** toh mee)
__________	inflammation of the kidney		**nephritis** (neh **FRYE** tis)
__________	kidney tumor		**nephroma** (neh **FROH** mah)
__________	softening of the kidney		**nephromalacia** (nef roh mah **LAY** she ah)
__________	enlargement of the kidney		**nephromegaly** (nef roh **MEG** ah lee)
__________	disease of the kidney		**nephropathy** (neh **FROP** ah thee)
__________	surgical fixation of a floating kidney		**nephropexy** (**NEF** roh pek see)
__________	prolapse of the kidney		**nephroptosis** (nef rop **TOH** sis)
__________	pertaining to the kidney		**renal** (**REE** nal)
__________	__________	a kidney stone	**renal calculus** (**REE** nal **KAL** kew lus)
__________	__________	an acute pain that occurs in the kidney area	**renal colic** (**REE** nal **KOL** ik)
__________	__________	cessation of proper functioning of the kidney	**renal failure** (**REE** nal **FAIL** yoor)
__________	__________	to transfer a kidney from a donor to a patient	**renal transplant** (**REE** nal **TRANS** plant)

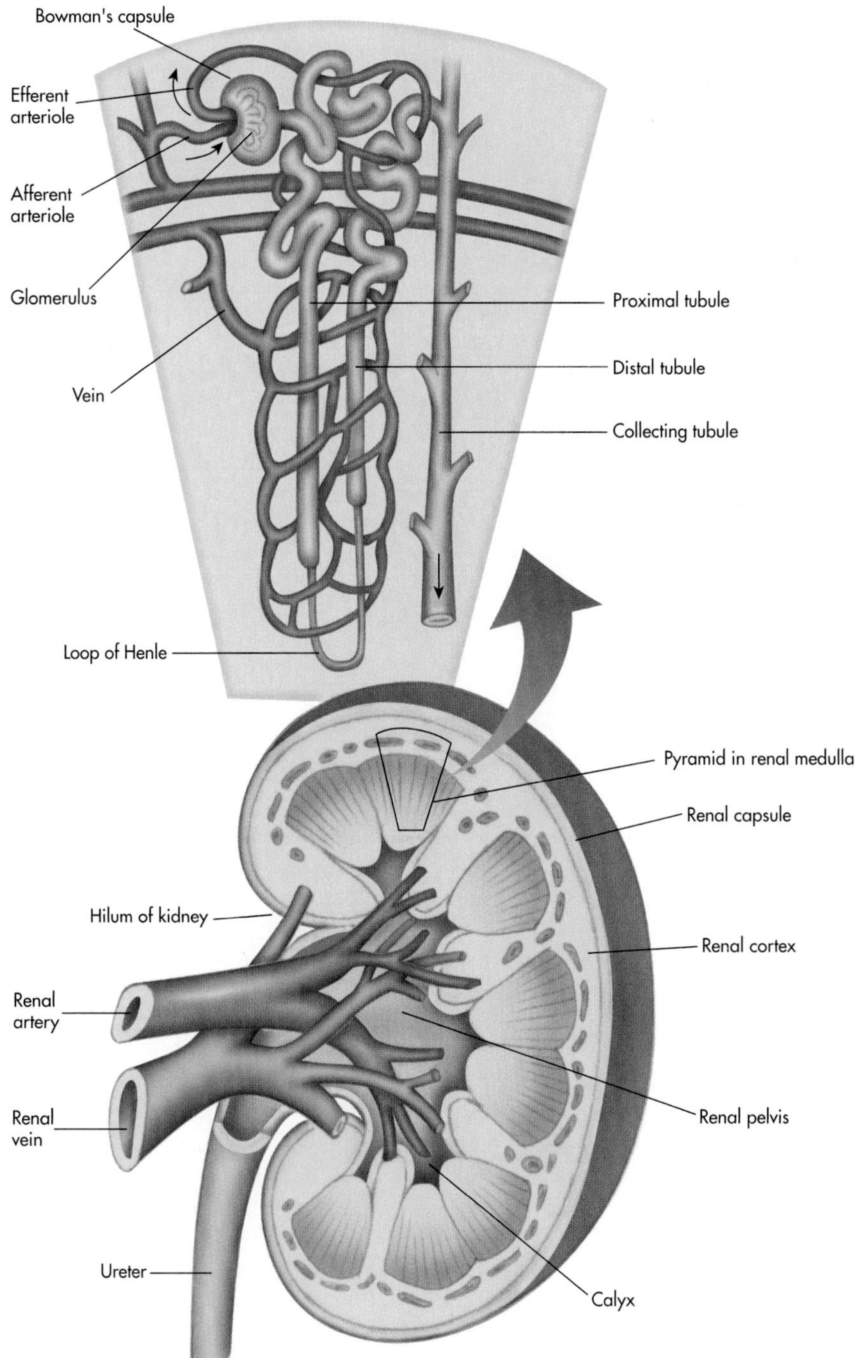

FIGURE 13–2
The kidney with an expanded view of a nephron.

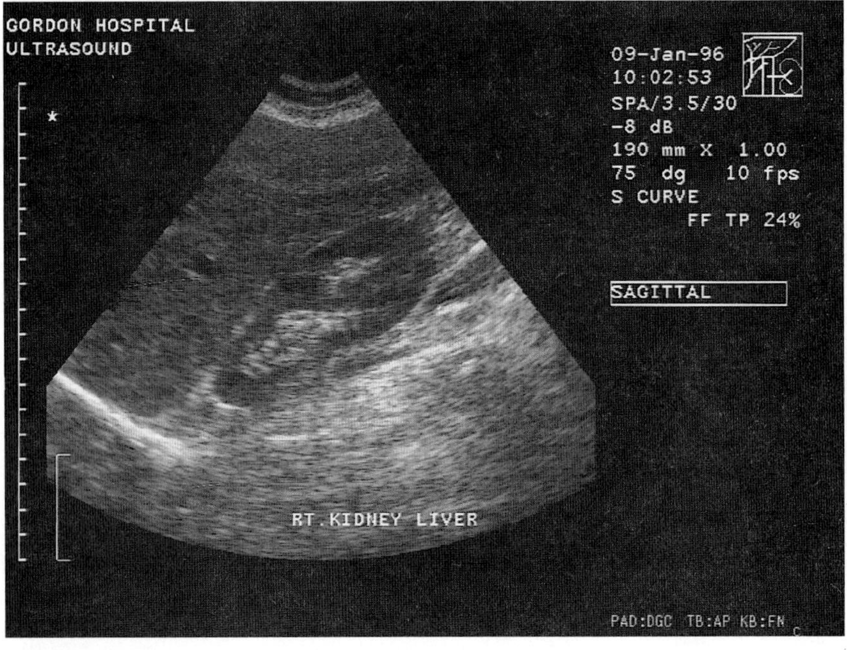

FIGURE 13–3
Ultrasound liver and right kidney. *(Courtesy of Teresa Resch.)*

ANSWER COLUMN

EXPLANATION FRAME

There are two ureters, one for each kidney. See Figure 13–1 and Figure 13–4. They are narrow, muscular tubes that transport urine from the kidneys to the bladder. The walls of the ureters consist of three layers: an inner coat of mucous membrane, a middle coat of smooth muscle, and an outer coat of fibrous tissue.

13.4 The narrow, muscular tubes that transport urine from the kidneys are known as the ____________.

ureters
(yoo **REE** ters)

13.5 The combining form **ureter / o** means ureter.
Medical terms that begin with this word element are:

____________ surgical implantation of the ureter into the colon

ureterocolostomy
(yoo ree ter oh koh **LOS** toh mee)

____________ surgical excision of a kidney and its ureter

ureteronephrectomy
(yoo ree ter oh neh **FREK** toh mee)

____________ surgical repair of the ureter

ureteroplasty
(yoo **REE** ter oh plas tee)

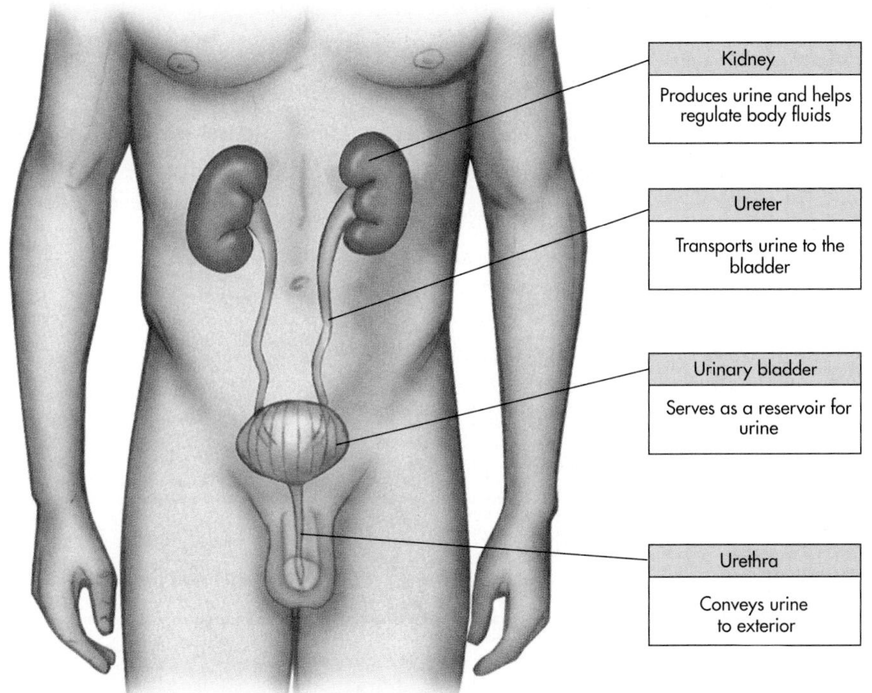

FIGURE 13–4
The organs of the urinary system with major functions.

continued

		ANSWER COLUMN
__________	suture of the ureter	**ureterorrhaphy** (yoo ree ter **OR** ah fee)
__________	a condition of narrowing of the ureter	**ureterostenosis** (yoo ree ter oh sten **OH** sis)
__________	pertaining to a connection between the ureter and bladder	**ureterovesical** (yoo ree ter oh **VES** ih kal)

EXPLANATION FRAME

The ureter enters the kidney through the hilum (a notch in the concave border of the kidney) into a sac-like collecting portion called the renal pelvis.

13.6 The combining form **pyel / o** means renal pelvis.
Medical terms that begin with this word element are:

__________	inflammation of the bladder and renal pelvis	**pyelocystitis** (pye eh loh sis **TYE** tis)
__________	establishing a surgical opening between the renal pelvis and bladder	**pyelocystostomosis** (pye eh loh sis tos toh **MOH** sis)

continued

		Answer Column
___________	surgical incision into the renal pelvis for removal of a stone	**pyelolithotomy** (pye eh loh lih **THOT** oh mee)
___________	inflammation of the kidney and renal pelvis	**pyelonephritis** (pye eh loh neh **FRYE** tis)

EXPLANATION FRAME

Microscopic examination of the kidney reveals about 1 million nephrons, which are the structural and functional units of the organ. Each nephron consists of a renal corpuscle and tubule. The renal corpuscle or Malpighian corpuscle consists of a glomerulus and Bowman's capsule. See Figure 13–2.

13.7 The structural and functional units of the kidney are called ________.

Answer: **nephrons** (**NEF** rons)

13.8 The combining form **glomerul / o** and the root **glomerul** mean glomerulus, little ball.

Medical terms that begin with these word elements are:

		Answer
___________	pertaining to the glomerulus	**glomerular** (glom **AIR** yoo lar)
___________	inflammation of the renal glomeruli	**glomerulitis** (gloh mer yoo **LYE** tis)
___________	inflammation of the kidney involving primarily the glomeruli	**glomerulonephritis** (gloh mair yoo loh neh **FRYE** tis)

EXPLANATION FRAME

The urinary bladder is the muscular, membranous sac that serves as a reservoir for urine. See Figure 13–1 and Figure 13–4. It is located in the anterior portion of the pelvic cavity and consists of a lower portion, the neck, which is continuous with the urethra; and an upper portion, the apex, which is connected with the umbilicus by the median umbilical ligament. The trigone is a small, triangular area near the base of the bladder.

13.9 Urine is stored in a reservoir commonly referred to as the urinary ___________.

Answer: **bladder** (**BLAD** er)

Answer Column

13.10 The combining forms **cyst / o** and **cyst / i** and the root **cyst** mean bladder. Medical terms that begin with these word elements are:

		Answer
____________	dilation of the bladder	**cystectasy** (sis **TEK** tah see)
____________	surgical excision of the bladder or part of the bladder	**cystectomy** (sis **TEK** toh mee)
____________	oozing of blood from the mucous membrane into the bladder	**cystistaxis** (sis tih **STAK** sis)
____________	inflammation of the bladder	**cystitis** (sis **TYE** tis)
____________	hernia of the bladder that protrudes into the vagina	**cystocele** (**SIS** toh seel)
____________	an x-ray record of the bladder	**cystogram** (**SIS** toh gram)
____________	an instrument used for examination of the bladder	**cystoscope** (**SIS** toh scope)

EXPLANATION FRAME

The urethra is a musculomembranous tube extending from the bladder to the outside of the body. See Figure 13–1 and Figure 13–4. The external urinary opening is the urinary meatus. The male urethra is approximately 8 inches long and conveys both urine and semen. The female urethra is approximately 1.5 inches long. The urinary meatus of the female is situated between the clitoris and the opening of the vagina. The female urethra conveys urine to the exterior of the body.

13.11 The combining form **urethr / o** and the root **urethr** mean urethra. Medical terms that begin with these word elements are:

		Answer
____________	pain in the urethra	**urethralgia** (yoo ree **THRAL** jee ah)
____________	relating to the urethra and penis	**urethropenile** (yoo ree throh **PEE** nile)
____________	surgical fixation of the urethra	**urethropexy** (yoo ree throh **PEK** see)
____________	obstruction of the urethra	**urethrophraxis** (yoo ree throh FRAK sis)
____________	urethral spasm	**urethrospasm** (yoo **REE** throh spazm)
____________	pertaining to the urethra and vagina	**urethrovaginal** (yoo ree throh **VAJ** ih nal)

ANSWER COLUMN

EXPLANATION FRAME

Urine consists of 95% water and 5% solid substances. It is secreted by the kidneys and transported by the ureters to the bladder, where it is stored before being discharged from the body via the urethra. An average normal adult feels the need to **void** when the bladder contains around 300 to 350 mL of urine. An average of 1000 to 1500 mL of urine is voided daily. Normal urine is clear, yellow to amber in color, and has a faintly aromatic odor, a specific gravity of 1.015 to 1.025, and a slightly acid pH.

13.12 Urine consists of ________% water and ________% solid substances.

95 5

13.13 An average daily urinary output is approximately ___________.

1000–1500 mL

EXPLANATION FRAME

The vital function of the urinary system is extraction of certain wastes from the bloodstream, conversion of these materials to urine, transport of the urine from the kidneys via the ureters to the bladder, and elimination of it at appropriate intervals via the urethra. Through this vital function, homeostasis of body fluids is maintained.

13.14 The part of the urinary system that carries urine from the bladder to the exterior is the ___________.

urethra (yoo **REE** thrah)

13.15 Medical terms that are used to describe the emptying of the bladder are:

____

____

____

void
(VOYD)
urination
(yoo rih **NAY** shun)
micturition
(mik too **RIH** shun)

13.16 Medical terms that are used to describe various types of abnormal urine and/or urination are:

___________ presence of serum protein in the urine

___________ lack of urine or without the formation of urine

albuminuria
(al byoo min **YOO** ree ah)
anuria (an **YOO** ree ah)

continued

		ANSWER COLUMN
________	presence of bacteria in the urine	**bacteriuria** (back tee ree **YOO** ree ah)
________	presence of calcium in the urine	**calciuria** (kal see **YOO** ree ah)
________	a condition of increased flow of urine	**diuresis** (dye yoo **REE** sis)
________	difficult or painful urination	**dysuria** (dis **YOO** ree ah)
________	a condition of involuntary emission of urine; bed-wetting	**enuresis** (en yoo **REE** sis)
________	presence of glucose in the urine	**glycosuria** (glye kohs **YOO** ree ah)
________	presence of blood in the urine	**hematuria** (hee mah **TOO** ree ah)
________	the inability to hold urine	**incontinence** (in **KON** tih nens)
________	presence of ketone in the urine	**ketonuria** (kee toh **NOO** ree ah)
________	excessive urination during the night	**nocturia** (nok **TOO** ree ah)
________	scanty urination	**oliguria** (ol ig **YOO** ree ah)
________	excessive urination	**polyuria** (pol ee **YOO** ree ah)
________	pus in the urine	**pyuria** (pye **YOO** ree ah)

EXPLANATION FRAME

Urinalysis is a laboratory procedure that may involve the physical, chemical, and microscopic examination of urine. It is a valuable diagnostic tool, as abnormal conditions or diseases may be quickly and easily detected because the physical and chemical constituents of normal urine are constant. A freshly voided specimen will provide for more accurate test results as certain changes may occur if urine is left standing.

13.17 **True or False.** Because the physical and chemical constituents of normal urine are constant, urinalysis is a valuable diagnostic tool.

true

EXPLANATION FRAME

Some abnormal constituents that may be found in urine during a chemical examination are:

- Protein. An important sign of renal disease, acute glomerulonephritis, pyelonephritis.

(*continued*)

continued

Answer Column

- Glucose. Diabetes mellitus, pain, excitement, acromegaly, liver damage.
- Ketone and acetone. Uncontrolled diabetes mellitus.
- Bilibrubin. Liver disease, biliary obstruction, congestive heart failure.
- Blood. Renal disease, trauma.
- Nitrites. Bacteriuria.
- Urobilinogen. Absent—biliary obstruction.
  Reduced—antibiotic therapy.
  Increased—early warning of hepatic or hemolytic disease.

13.18 A fruity sweet odor from urine is indicative of the presence of __________, which is associated with diabetes mellitus.

acetone
(**ASS** eh tone)

13.19 A __________ is an instrument used to measure the specific gravity of urine.

The word elements used to build this term are:

__________ combining form that means urine

__________ suffix that means instrument to measure

urinometer
(yoo rih **NOM** eh ter)

urin / o

-meter

13.20 __________ is the crushing of a kidney stone.

The word elements used to build this term are:

__________ combining form that means stone

__________ suffix that means crushing

lithotripsy
(**LITH** oh trip see)

lith / o

-tripsy

13.21 A __________ is a hollow, flexible tube that can be inserted into a body cavity, organ, or vessel to withdraw fluids, to introduce fluids into a body cavity, to monitor pressure, and/or to visualize the body part. An example of a catheter is the Foley, an indwelling catheter, that is retained in the bladder by a balloon inflated with air or liquid. It is used for the purpose of draining urine from the bladder.

catheter
(**KATH** eh ter)

13.22 __________ is the excessive amounts of urea and other nitrogenous waste products in the blood that occurs with renal failure.

uremia
(yoo **REE** mee ah)

ANSWER COLUMN

EXPLANATION FRAME

Drugs that are generally used for diseases and disorders of the urinary system include diuretics, urinary tract antibacterials, urinary tract antiseptics, and other drugs, such as Pyridium.

13.23 A __________ decreases reabsorption of sodium chloride by the kidneys, thereby increasing the amount of salt and water excreted in the urine. This action reduces the amount of fluid retained in the body and prevents/relieves edema.

diuretic
(dye yoor **RET** ik)

13.24 Urinary tract __________, especially sulfonamides, are used for treating acute, uncomplicated urinary tract infections.

antibacterials
(an tih bak **TEE** ree als)

13.25 Urinary tract __________ may inhibit the growth of microorganisms by bacteri**cidal**, bacterio**static**, **anti**-infective, and/or **anti**bacterial action.

Note: **-cidal** means to kill; **-static** means to control; and the prefix **anti** means against.

antiseptics
(an ti **SEP** tiks)

13.26 __________ (phenazopyridine HCl) has an analgesic, anesthetic action on the urinary tract mucosa. The patient should be advised that this medication causes the urine to turn a reddish-orange color and may stain clothing.

Pyridium
(pye **RID** ee um)

13.27 A blood urea nitrogen __________ test is used to determine the amount of urea that is excreted by the kidneys. Abnormal results indicate renal disease.

BUN

13.28 A __________ (**cyst / o**) examination is a visual exam of the bladder and urethra via a lighted cystoscope. Abnormal results may indicate the presence of renal calculi, a tumor, prostatic hyperplasia, and/or bleeding.

cystoscopic
(sis toh **SKOP** ik)

Answer Column

13.29 An __________ (intravenous pyelogram) is an x-ray record of the kidneys, ureters, and bladder. A radiopaque substance is intravenously injected and abnormal results may indicate renal calculi, kidney or bladder tumors, and kidney disease.

IVP

13.30 ABBREVIATIONS

Write in the correct abbreviation for the following:

		Answer
__________	albumin/globulin ratio	**A/G**
__________	acute glomerulonephritis	**AGN**
__________	blood urea nitrogen	**BUN**
__________	clean catch	**CC**
__________	chronic glomerulonephritis	**CGN**
__________	chronic renal failure	**CRF**
__________	cystoscopic examination	**cysto**
__________	end-stage renal disease	**ESRD**
__________	genitourinary	**GU**
__________	interstitial cystitis	**IC**
__________	intake and output	**I & O**
__________	intravenous pyelogram	**IVP**
__________	kidney, ureter, and bladder	**KUB**
__________	sodium	**Na**
__________	peritoneal dialysis	**PD**
__________	urinalysis	**UA**
__________	urinary tract infection	**UTI**

IN THE SPOTLIGHT

CYSTITIS

Cystitis is an inflammation of the urinary bladder. Each year, in the United States, approximately 10 million people seek treatment for urinary tract infections, with cystitis being the most common. Cystitis is most often caused by an ascending infection from the urethra. It is more common in the female, because of the short length of the urethra, which promotes the transmission of bacteria from the skin and genitals to the internal bladder. The most common type of bacteria that causes cystitis in the female is *Escherichia coli* (*E. coli*), the colon bacillus. This bacillus is constantly present in the alimentary canal and is normally nonpathogenic, but when it enters the urinary tract and is transmitted to the bladder, it can cause infection. Cystitis in men is usually secondary to some other type of infection such as epididymitis, prostatitis, gonorrhea, syphilis, and/or kidney stone.

Diagnosis is determined by the history of the symptoms, microscopic urinalysis, urine culture, dipstick, or gram stain. The symptoms of cystitis include:

- Frequency
- Hematuria
- Pain or spasm in the region of the bladder and pelvic area
- Urgency
- Pyuria
- Chills and fever
- Burning sensation and pain during urination

Treatment of cystitis usually consists of taking an antibiotic or antibacterial agent for a specified number of times and days, depending on the type of infection and its severity. The sulfonamides and antibiotics such as penicillins, cephalosporins, tetracyclines, and aminoglycosides are generally the drugs of first choice. Always ask the patient if he or she is allergic to any medication before the initiation of drug therapy. Note: If there is any question about a person's hypersensitivity to an antibiotic and/or sulfa drugs, an appropriate skin test should be performed before the initiation of drug therapy.

CASE STUDY

Please read the following case study and then work frames 13.31–13.34 . Write in your answer in the answer column. Check your responses with the answers provided at the end of frame 13.34.

A 21-year-old female was seen by a physician and the following is a synopsis of the visit.

PRESENT HISTORY: The patient states that she goes to the bathroom a lot and that it "burns" and "hurts." She also has chills and fever.

SIGNS AND SYMPTOMS: Chief Complaints: Frequency, burning sensation and pain during urination, chills, and fever.

DIAGNOSIS: Acute cystitis. The diagnosis was determined by a history of the symptoms, and a complete urinalysis (physical, chemical, and microscopic) that revealed red blood cells, white blood cells, and bacteria.

TREATMENT: The physician ordered a sulfonamide and Pyridium and provided her with written Guidelines to Help Avoid Cystitis (Female).

(*continued*)

PREVENTION: In the United States, approximately 10 million people seek treatment for urinary tract infections each year, with cystitis being the most common. Cystitis is most often caused by an ascending infection from the urethra and it is more common in the female, because of the short length of the urethra, which promotes the transmission of bacteria from the skin and genitals to the internal bladder. The most common type of bacterium that causes cystitis in females is *Escherichia coli (E. coli),* the colon bacillius.

Guidelines to Help Avoid Cystitis (Female)

- Drink 8 glasses or more of water/day.
- Females should wipe themselves from front to back to avoid contaminating the urinary meatus.
- Have sexual partner wear a condom.
- Do not use vaginal deodorants, bubble baths, colored toilet paper, and other substances that could cause irritation to the urinary meatus.
- Wear cotton underclothes and keep the genital area dry.

13.31 Signs and symptoms of cystitis include frequency, burning ____________ and pain during urination, chills, and fever.

13.32 The most common type of bacterium that causes cystitis in the female is ____________.

13.33 The diagnosis was determined by a history of the symptoms and a complete ____________ that revealed red blood cells, white blood cells, and bacteria.

13.34 Treatment included a ____________, Pyridium, and written Guidelines to Help Avoid Cystitis (Female).

CASE STUDY ANSWERS

13.31 sensation

13.32 *Escherichia coli (E. coli)*

13.33 urinalysis

13.34 sulfonamide

REVIEW A: WORD ELEMENTS

This review allows you to check your knowledge of some of the word elements presented in this unit. In the spaces provided, write the meaning of the word elements that are identified as **Prefix (P), Word Root (R), Combining Form (CF),** and/or **Suffix (S).**

MEDICAL WORD	*WORD ELEMENT*	*MEANING*
1. nephritis	nephr (R)	____________
	-itis (S)	____________
2. nephroma	nephr / o (CF)	____________
	-oma (S)	____________
3. ureteroplasty	ureter / o (CF)	____________
	-plasty (S)	____________
4. pyelocystitis	pyel / o (CF)	____________
	cyst (R)	____________
	-itis (S)	____________
5. glomerular	glomerul (R)	____________
	-ar (S)	____________
6. cystectomy	cyst (R)	____________
	-ectomy (S)	____________
7. cystoscope	cyst / o (CF)	____________
	-scope (S)	____________
8. urethralgia	urethr (R)	____________
	-algia (S)	____________
9. urethropexy	urethr / o (CF)	____________
	-pexy (S)	____________
10. dysuria	dys (P)	____________
	-uria (S)	____________
11. polyuria	poly (P)	____________
	-uria (S)	____________
12. urinometer	urin / o (CF)	____________
	-meter (S)	____________

REVIEW B: MEDICAL TERMS

Please place the correct letter from column II on the appropriate line of column I.

COLUMN I		COLUMN II
______	1. renal	A. the process of emptying the bladder
______	2. ureters	B. inflammation of the renal glomeruli
______	3. urethropraxis	C. an x-ray record of the bladder
______	4. nephrons	D. a condition of increased flow of urine
______	5. glomerulitis	E. scanty urination
______	6. cystogram	F. pertaining to the kidney
______	7. micturition	G. tubes that transport urine from the kidney to the bladder
______	8. diuresis	H. crushing of a kidney stone
______	9. oliguria	I. structural and functional units of the kidney
______	10. lithotripsy	J. obstruction of the urethra

REVIEW C: DISEASES AND DISORDERS

Please provide the correct disease or disorder for each of the following descriptions.

1. ______ ______ is an acute pain that occurs in the kidney area and is caused by blockage during the passage of a stone.
2. ______ ______ is cessation of proper functioning of the kidney.
3. ______ is inflammation of the kidney and renal pelvis.
4. ______ is inflammation of the kidney involving primarily the glomeruli.
5. ______ is a hernia of the bladder that protrudes into the vagina.

REVIEW D: UNSCRAMBLE THE WORDS

Unscramble the following medical terms and place the correct term on the line directly across from the scrambled word.

1. paythorhpen ______
2. redalbd ______
3. ratheur ______
4. diov ______
5. iauryp ______
6. oneteca ______
7. ontekiaur ______
8. iaurtameh ______

REVIEW E: DRUGS USED FOR THE URINARY SYSTEM

Please provide the correct answer for each of the following descriptions.

1. ____________ decrease reabsorption of sodium chloride by the kidneys.
2. ____________ are used for treating acute, uncomplicated urinary tract infections.
3. ____________ may inhibit the growth of microorganisms by bactericidal and/or bacteriostatic action.
4. ____________ has an analgesic, anesthetic action on the urinary tract mucosa.

REVIEW F: ABBREVIATIONS

Please provide the correct abbreviation and/or meaning for the abbreviation.

1. __________ acute glomerulonephritis
2. CRF __________
3. __________ genitourinary
4. IVP __________
5. __________ sodium
6. UA __________

14 THE FEMALE REPRODUCTIVE SYSTEM: GYNECOLOGY AND OBSTETRICS

LEARNING CONCEPTS

- the female reproductive system
- essential terminology
- pronunciation guide
- word elements
- explanation frames
- terminology that describes a malpositioned uterus
- breast cancer: signs and symptoms, risk factors
- breast self-examination
- selected diseases and disorders
- drugs used for the female reproductive system
- abbreviations
- in the spotlight: stem cells
- case study: annual pap smear and breast exam
- review exercises

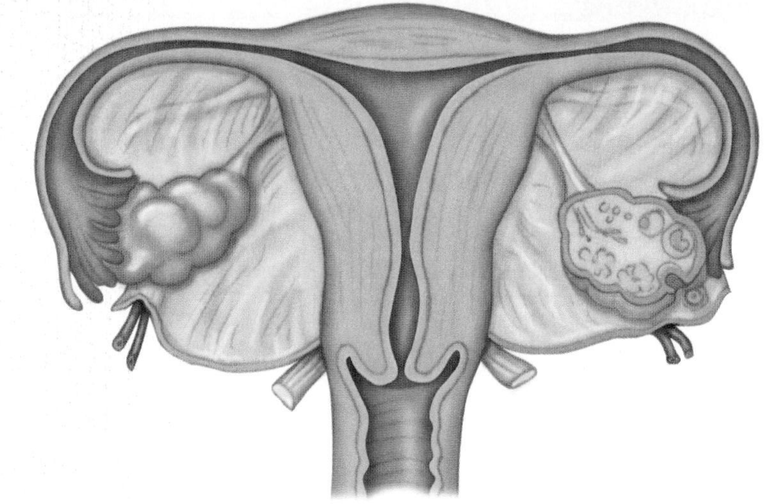

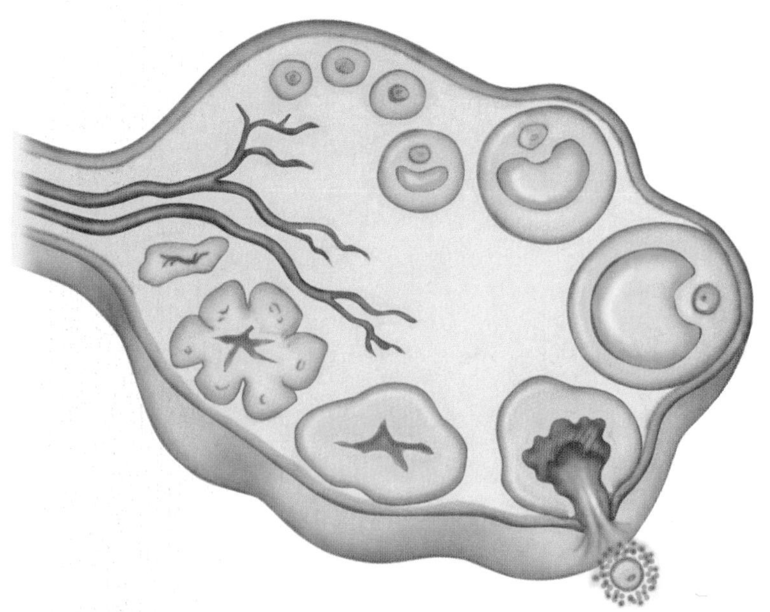

OBJECTIVES

ON COMPLETION OF THIS UNIT, YOU SHOULD BE ABLE TO:

- Briefly describe the female reproductive system.
- Describe the primary functions of the various organs or structures of the female reproductive system.
- Identify and give the meaning of the primary word elements for this unit.
- Analyze, build, spell, and pronounce selected medical words.
- Describe selected diseases/disorders of the female reproductive system.
- Define selected terms that describe a malpositioned uterus.
- Explain why mammography and breast self-exam are valuable detection and screening methods for breast cancer.
- List eight possible signs and symptoms of breast cancer.
- List seven risk factors for breast cancer in order of their importance.
- Describe selected drugs that are used for the female reproductive system diseases or disorders.
- Define selected abbreviations that pertain to the female reproductive system.
- Define stem cells.
- Describe embryonic stem cells and state from where they may be obtained.
- Describe adult stem cells and state where they are found in the body.
- Describe a stem-cell line.
- List several medical uses for stem cells.
- Complete the Case Study on Pap Smear Routine Annual with Gyn Exam and Mammogram Routine Exam.
- Successfully complete the review section.

TECH LINK

CD-ROM Use the CD-ROM enclosed with your textbook to gain additional reinforcement through interactive word building exercises, spelling games, labeling activities, and additional quizzes.

www.prenhall.com/rice Use the above address to access the free, interactive Companion Website created specifically for this textbook. Get hints, instant feedback, and textbook references to chapter-related multiple choice and true/false questions, fill-in-the-blank, and labeling exercises. In addition, you will find an audio glossary, and essay questions.

The female reproductive system consists of the ovaries, fallopian tubes, uterus, vagina, vulva, and breasts. See Table 14–1. The ovaries are the primary sex organs of the female and their activity is primarily controlled by the anterior lobe of the pituitary gland. The ovaries produce ova (the female reproductive cells) and hormones. In an average normal woman more than 400 ova may be produced during her reproductive years.

The ovary is also an endocrine gland, producing estrogen and progesterone. Estrogen is the female sex hormone and progesterone is a steroid hormone. These hormones are essential in promoting growth, development, and maintenance of the secondary sex organs and characteristics. They also prepare the uterus for pregnancy, promote development of the mammary glands, and play a vital role in a woman's emotional well-being and sexual drive.

TABLE 14–1 THE FEMALE REPRODUCTIVE SYSTEM

Organ/Structure	Primary Functions
The Uterus	Organ of the cyclic discharge of menses; provides place for the nourishment and development of the fetus; contracts during labor to help expel the fetus
The Fallopian Tubes (Uterine Tubes Oviducts)	Serve as a duct for the conveyance of the ovum from the ovary to the uterus; serve as ducts for the conveyance of spermatozoa from the uterus toward the ovary
The Ovaries	Production of ova and hormones
The Vagina	Female organ of copulation; serves as a passageway for the discharge of menstruation; serves as a passageway for the birth of the fetus
The Vulva	External female genitalia
Mons pubis	Provides pad of fatty tissue
Labia majora	Provides two folds of adipose tissue
Labia minora	Lies within the labia majora and encloses the vestibule
Vestibule	Opening for the urethra, the vagina, and two excretory ducts of Bartholin's glands
Clitoris	Erectile tissue that is homologous to the penis of the male; produces pleasurable sensations during the sexual act
The Breast	Following childbirth, mammary glands produce milk

ANSWER COLUMN

14.1 ____________ is the study of the female reproductive system.
The word elements used to build this term are:
____________ combining form that means female
____________ suffix that means study of

gynecology
(gigh neh **KOL** oh jee)
gynec / o
-logy

14.2 A ____________ is a physician who specializes in the study of the female reproductive system.

gynecologist
(gigh neh **KOL** oh jist)

EXPLANATION FRAME

The female reproductive system consists of the ovaries, fallopian tubes, uterus, vagina, vulva, and breasts. See Figure 14–1. The uterus is a muscular, hollow, pear-shaped organ having three identifiable areas: the body or upper portion, the isthmus or central area, and the cervix, which is the lower cylindrical portion or neck. The fundus is the bulging surface of the body of the uterus extending from the internal os (mouth) of the cervix upward above the fallopian tubes. See Figure 14–2.

The three primary functions of the uterus are as follows: (1) It is the organ of the cyclic discharge of a bloody fluid called menses; (2) it is a place for the protection and nourishment of the fetus during pregnancy; (3) during labor, the muscular uterine wall contracts rhythmically and powerfully to expel the fetus from the uterus.

PRIMARY WORD ELEMENTS

The following word elements (prefixes, roots, combining forms, and suffixes) will be used to build medical terms that relate to this unit. Please commit these to memory.

PREFIX

PREFIX	MEANING	PREFIX	MEANING
a	without, lack of	**nulli**	none
ante	before	**post**	after, behind
dys	bad, difficult, painful	**pre**	before, in front of
intra	within	**primi**	first
multi	many, much	**retro**	backward
neo	new		

COMBINING FORM

COMBINING FORM / ROOT	MEANING	COMBINING FORM / ROOT	MEANING
amni / o	lamb	**nat**	birth
bartholin	Bartholin's glands	**o / o**	ovum, egg
cervic	cervix, neck	**oophor**	ovary
cervic / o	cervix, neck	**oophor / o**	ovary
colp	vagina	**ovar**	ovary
colp / o	vagina	**ovari / o, ovar/ i**	ovary
flex	to bend	**para**	to bear
genital	belonging to birth	**partum**	labor
gravida	pregnant	**pause**	cessation
gynec / o	female	**salping**	tube, fallopian tube
hyster	uterus, womb	**salping / o**	tube, fallopian tube
hyster / o	uterus, womb	**uter**	uterus, womb
mamm, mast	breast	**uter / o**	uterus, womb
mamm / o, mast / o	breast	**vagin**	vagina
men / o	month	**vers**	turning
metr	uterus, womb	**vesic**	bladder
metr / i, metr / o	uterus, womb		

SUFFIX

SUFFIX	MEANING	SUFFIX	MEANING
-al	pertaining to	**-itis**	inflammation
-algia, -dynia	pain	**-logy**	study of
-cele	hernia, tumor, swelling	**-malacia**	softening
-centesis	surgical puncture	**-oma**	tumor
-ectomy	surgical excision	**-pathy**	disease
-genesis	formation, produce	**-pexy**	surgical fixation
-gram	mark, record	**-plasty**	surgical repair
-graphy	recording	**-rrhagia**	bursting forth
-ia, -osis	condition of	**-rrhaphy**	suture
-ist	one who specializes	**-rrhea**	flow

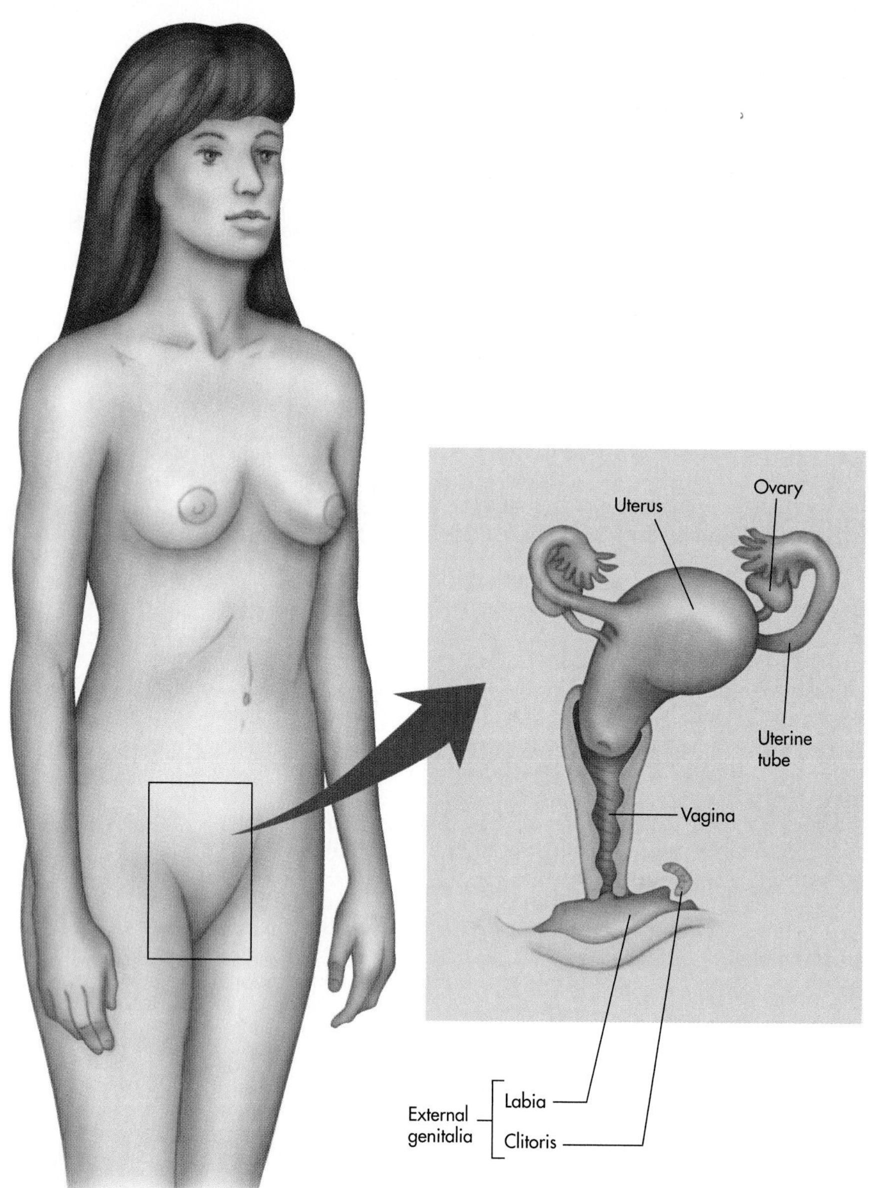

FIGURE 14–1
The female reproductive system: vagina, uterine (fallopian) tube, ovary, uterus, and external genitalia.

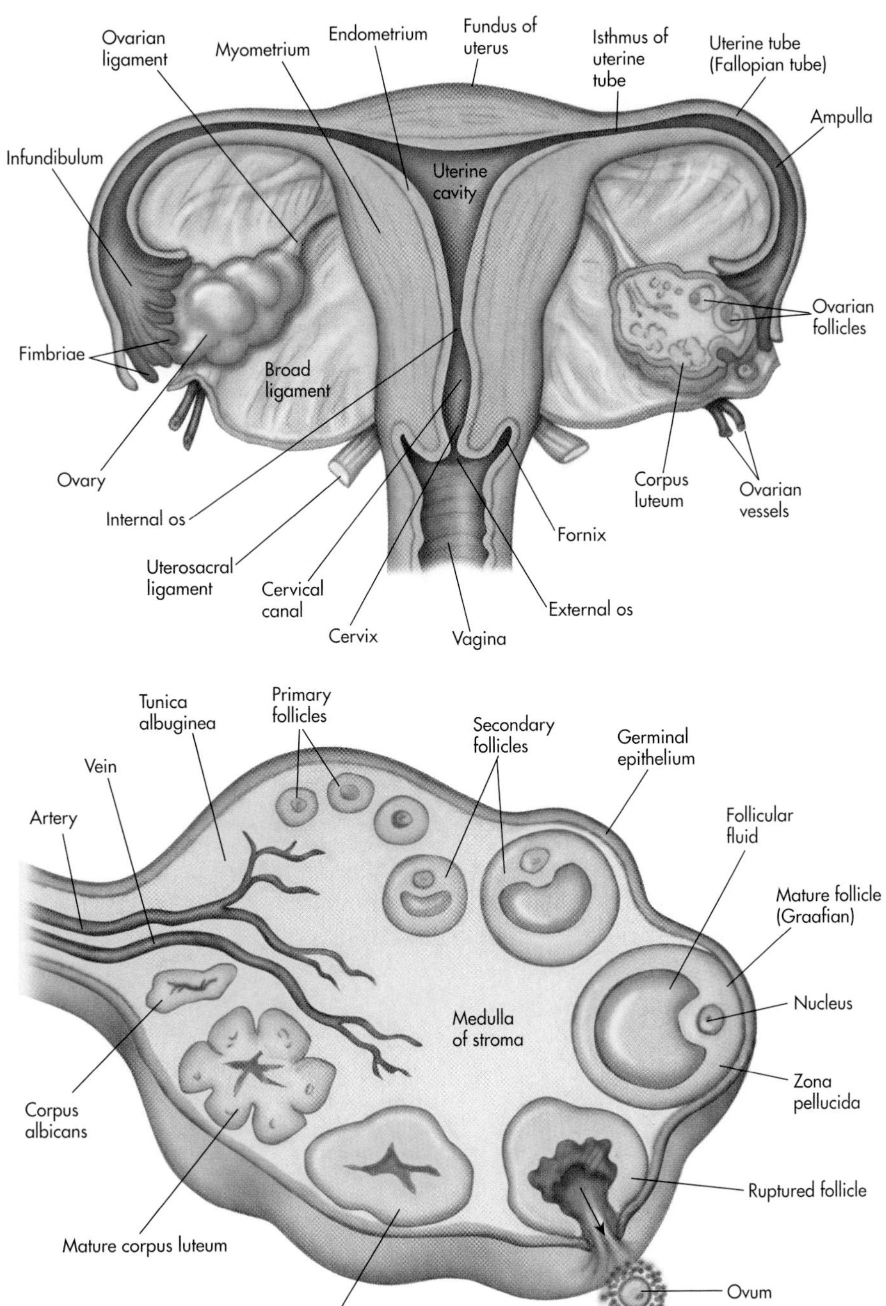

■ **FIGURE 14–2**

The uterus, ovaries, and associated structures with an expanded view of a mammalian ovary showing stages of graafian follicle and ovum development.

Answer Column

14.3 There are several word elements that mean uterus. In this frame the medical terms that are built by using the combining form **hyster / o** and the root **hyster** will be presented.

		Answer
___________	uterine pain; SYN: hysterodynia	**hysteralgia** (hiss ter **AL** jee ah)
___________	surgical excision of the uterus	**hysterectomy** (hiss ter **EK** toh mee)
___________	inflammation of the uterus	**hysteritis** (hiss ter **EYE** tis)
___________	incision into the uterus; also called a cesarean section	**hysterotomy** (hiss ter **OT** oh mee)
___________	an instrument used in the biopsy of uterine tissue	**hysteroscope** (**HISS** ter oh scope)
___________	surgical excision of the entire uterus	**panhysterectomy** (pan hiss ter **EK** toh mee)
___________	surgical excision of the uterus and one or both ovaries	**hystero-oophorectomy** (hiss ter oh off oh **REK** toh mee)
___________	surgical excision of the uterus and fallopian tube	**hysterosalpingectomy** (hiss ter oh sal pin **JEK** toh mee)

14.4 The combining forms **metr / i** and **metr / o** and the root **metr** mean uterus. Medical terms that are built using these word elements are:

		Answer
___________	inflammation of the uterus	**metritis** (meh **TRY** tis)
___________	uterine carcinoma	**metrocarcinoma** (meh troh kar sin **NOH** mah)
___________	uterine pain	**metrodynia** (meh troh **DIN** ee ah)
___________	softening of the uterus	**metromalacia** (meh troh mah **LAY** she ah)
___________	muscular wall of the uterus	**myometrium** (my oh **MEE** tree um)
___________	inflammation of the muscular wall of the uterus	**myometritis** (my oh meh **TRY** tis)
___________	a condition in which endometrial tissue occurs in various sites in the abdominal or pelvic cavity	**endometriosis** (en doh mee tree **OH** sis)

ANSWER COLUMN

14.5 The combining form **uter / o** and the root **uter** mean uterus. Medical terms that are built using these word elements are:

		Answer
___________	pertaining to the uterus	**uterine** (**YOO** ter in)
___________	hernia containing the uterus	**uterocele** (**YOO** ter oh seel)
___________	surgical repair of the uterus	**uteroplasty** (**YOO** ter oh plas tee)
___________	an instrument for viewing the uterine cavity	**uteroscope** (**YOO** ter oh scope)
___________	incision of the uterus	**uterotomy** (yoo ter **OT** oh mee)
___________	pertaining to within the uterus	**intrauterine** (in trah **YOO** ter in)
___________	refers to the ovaries and the fallopian tubes	**uterine adnexa** (**YOO** ter in add **NEK** sah)
___________	is a benign tumor of the uterus that contains fiber-like tissue	**uterine fibroid tumor** (**YOO** ter in **FIGH** broid **TOO** mor)

EXPLANATION FRAME

The normal position of the uterus is with the cervix pointing toward the lower end of the sacrum and the fundus toward the suprapubic regions. The uterus may become malpositioned due to weakness of its supporting ligaments. Trauma, disease processes of the uterus, or multiple pregnancies may contribute to the weakening of the supporting ligaments. Anteflexion, retroflexion, anteversion, and retroversion are some of the terms that are used to describe a malpositioned uterus.

14.6 ___________ is the process of bending forward of the uterus at its body and neck.

anteflexion (an tee **FLEK** shun)

14.7 ___________ is the process of bending the body of the uterus backward at an angle with the cervix usually unchanged from its normal position.

retroflexion (ret roh **FLEK** shun)

14.8 ___________ is the process of turning the fundus forward toward the pubis, with the cervix tilted up toward the sacrum.

anteversion (an tee **VER** zhun)

14.9 ___________ is the process of turning the uterus backward, with the cervix pointing forward toward the symphysis pubis.

retroversion (ret roh **VER** zhun)

Answer Column

14.10 The combining form **cervic / o** and the root **cervic** mean cervix, neck. In this unit, **cervic / o** pertains to the **cervix uteri**.

Medical terms that are built using these word elements are:

		Answer
__________	pertaining to the cervix of an organ, as the cervix uteri	**cervical** (**SER** vih kal)
__________	inflammation of the cervix uteri	**cervicitis** (ser vih **SIGH** tis)
__________	inflammation of the cervix and vagina	**cervicocolpitis** (ser vih kol **PYE** tis)
__________	inflammation of the cervix of the uterus and vagina	**cervicovaginitis** (ser vih koh vaj ih **NYE** tis)
__________	pertaining to the cervix uteri and bladder	**cervicovesical** (ser vih koh **VES** ih kal)

14.11 A __________ (Pap smear) is a screening technique to aid in the detection of cervical/uterine cancer and cancer precursors. Pap smears are graded on a five-point scale, with No. 1 being normal and No. 5 being carcinoma in situ., cancer that has not spread. Abnormal squamous cells of undetermined significance is No. 2; doctors refer to it as Ascus. It means that some cervical cells on the Pap smear look abnormal, but not abnormal enough to be considered precancerous.

Both false-positive and false-negative results have been experienced with Pap smears. Accordingly, any lesion should be biopsied unless not indicated clinically. The Pap smear should not be used as a sole means to diagnose or exclude malignant and premalignant lesions. It is a screening procedure only.

Answer: **Papanicolaou** (pap ah **NIK** oh low)

14.12 __________ and curettage (D&C) is a surgical procedure that expands the cervical canal of the uterus (dilation) so that the surface lining of the uterine wall can be scraped (curettage). It is often used after a spontaneous abortion and as a diagnostic tool for analysis of the endometrium.

Answer: **dilation** (dye **LAY** shun)

EXPLANATION FRAME

The menstrual cycle is a periodic recurrent series of changes occurring in the uterus, ovaries, vagina, and breasts. The human cycle averages 28 days in length, measured from the beginning of menstruation. Ovulation usually occurs around the 14th day before the next menstrual period begins.

14.13 __________ is the process of discharging the menses.

Answer: **menstruation** (men stroo **AY** shun)

		Answer Column
14.14	___________ ___________ syndrome (TSS) is a rare and sometimes fatal disease caused by a toxin or toxins produced by certain strains of the bacterium *Staphylococcus aureus*. It has occurred in young menstruating women, most of whom were using vaginal tampons for menstrual protection.	**toxic shock** (**TOKS** ik shok)
14.15	___________ is the medical term that describes the initial menstrual period. The average age of menarche in the United States is 12.8 years.	**menarche** (men **AR** kee)
14.16	___________ is the process in which an ovum is discharged from the cortex of the ovary.	**ovulation** (ov yoo **LAY** shun)
14.17	___________ is abdominal pain that occurs midway between the menstrual periods at ovulation. This dull pain has a duration of a few minutes to a few hours.	**mittelschmerz** (**MIT** el shmertz)
14.18	___________ is the permanent cessation of menstrual activity. It is also called the climacteric and/or the change of life. Natural menopause will occur in 25% of women by age 47, in 50% by age 50, in 75% by age 52, and in 95% by age 55.	**menopause** (**MEN** oh pawz)
	The word elements used to build this term are:	
	___________ combining form that means month	**men / o**
	___________ root that means cessation (process of stopping)	**pause**
14.19	___________ is excessive bleeding at the time of a menstrual period, either in number of days or amount of blood or both.	**menorrhagia** (men oh **RAY** jee ah)
	The word elements used to build this term are:	
	___________ combining form that means month	**men / o**
	___________ suffix that means to burst forth	**-rrhagia**
14.20	___________ is a lack of the monthly flow or menstruation.	**amenorrhea** (ah men oh **REE** ah)
	The word elements used to build this term are:	
	___________ prefix that means lack of	**a**
	___________ combining form that means month	**men / o**
	___________ suffix that means flow	**-rrhea**

Answer Column

14.21 __________ is a difficult or painful monthly flow. The prefix **dys** means difficult, painful.

dysmenorrhea
(dis men oh **REE** ah)

EXPLANATION FRAME

The fallopian tubes extend laterally from either side of the uterus and end near each ovary. A fallopian tube consists of an isthmus, ampulla, infundibulum, and its opening, the ostium. Surrounding each ostium are fimbriae or finger-like processes. These processes work to propel the discharged ovum into the tube, where ciliary action aids in moving it toward the uterus. Fallopian tubes are also called uterine tubes or oviducts. See Figure 14–2.

The primary functions of the fallopian tubes are:

- Each tube serves as a duct for the conveyance of the ovum from the ovary to the uterus.
- The tubes serve as ducts for the conveyance of spermatozoa from the uterus toward the ovary.

14.22 The finger-like processes that work to propel a discharged ovum from the ovary into a fallopian tube are called __________.

fimbriae
(**FIM** bree ay)

14.23 The combining form **salping / o** and the root **salping** mean fallopian tube. Medical terms that are built with these word elements are:

__________ surgical excision of a fallopian tube

__________ inflammation of a fallopian tube

__________ surgical excision of an ovary and a fallopian tube

salpingectomy
(sal pin **JEK** toh mee)
salpingitis
(sal pin **JIGH** tis)
salpingo-oophorectomy
(sal ping goh oh off oh **REK** toh mee)

EXPLANATION FRAME

The ovaries are almond-shaped organs attached to the uterus by the ovarian ligament and lie close to the fimbriae of the fallopian tubes. See Figure 14–2. The functional activity of the ovary is primarily controlled by the anterior lobe of the pituitary gland. Two functions have been identified for the ovary:

- The production of ova—the female reproductive cells, and
- The production of hormones—estrogen and progesterone

ANSWER COLUMN

14.24 ___________ means concerning or resembling the ovary.
An **ovarian cyst** is a sac that develops in the ovary. It consists of one or more chambers containing fluid. It may have to be removed surgically or it could rupture on its own.

ovarian
(oh **VAY** ree an)

14.25 The combining forms **ovari / o** and **ovar / i** and the root **ovar** mean ovary. Medical terms that begin with these word elements are:

___________	surgical excision of an ovary	**ovariectomy** (oh var ee **EK** toh mee)
___________	ovarian hernia	**ovariocele** (oh **VAR** ee oh seel)
___________	surgical puncture and drainage of an ovarian cyst	**ovariocentesis** (oh var ee oh sen **TEE** sis)
___________	surgical excision of the ovaries and uterus	**ovariohysterectomy** (oh vay ree oh hiss ter **EK** toh mee)
___________	disease of the ovary	**ovariopathy** (oh var ee **OP** ah thee)
___________	inflammation of an ovary	**ovaritis** (oh vah **RYE** tis)

14.26 The combining form **oophor / o** and the root **oophor** also mean ovary. Medical terms that begin with these word elements are:

___________	surgical excision of an ovary	**oophorectomy** (oh off oh **REK** toh mee)
___________	inflammation of an ovary	**oophoritis** (oh off oh **RIGH** tis)
___________	surgical excision of the uterus and ovaries	**oophorohysterectomy** (oh off oh roh hiss ter **EK** toh mee)
___________	malignant tumor of an ovary	**oophoroma** (oh off oh **ROH** mah)
___________	surgical fixation of a displaced ovary	**oophoropexy** (oh off oh roh **PEK** see)
___________	surgical excision of an ovary and fallopian tube	**oophorosalpingectomy** (oh off oh roh sal pin **JEK** toh mee)

ANSWER COLUMN

14.27 A __________ is an instrument used to examine the ovaries and fallopian tubes. It may also be used during a female sterilization procedure. A small incision is made in the umbilicus and the laparoscope is inserted through this opening. The fallopian tubes are identified and then either tied off, clamped, or cauterized or portions of them destroyed by a laser. This procedure is called a tubal ligation.

laparoscope (**LAP** ah roh scope)

14.28 The combining form **o / o** means ovum, egg.

__________ means formation of the ovum

__________ means ovum, egg

__________ suffix that means formation, produce

oogenesis (oh oh **JEN** eh sis)
o / o
-genesis

14.29 __________ is the process in which an ovum becomes impregnated by a spermatozoon. This normally occurs in the fallopian tube.

fertilization (fer til ih **ZAY** shun)

14.30 __________ is the process of the union of the male's sperm and the female's ovum; fertilization.

conception (kon **SEP** shun)

14.31 A __________ is the mature male sex or germ cell. Spermatozoa is the plural of spermatozoon.

spermatozoon (sper mat oh **ZOH** on)

EXPLANATION FRAME

A zygote is the fertilized ovum. The zygote is produced by the union of two gametes (spermatozoon and ovum). A blastocyst is an embryonic cell mass that attaches to the uterus wall and is a stage in the development of a mammalian embryo. An embryo is a stage of prenatal development between the 2nd and 8th week. The fetus is the developing young in the uterus from the 3rd month to birth. See Figure 14–3.

14.32 A __________ is also an **o / o / sperm**. An oosperm is a cell formed by the union of the spermatozoon with the ovum; the fertilized ovum.

zygote (**ZY** gote)

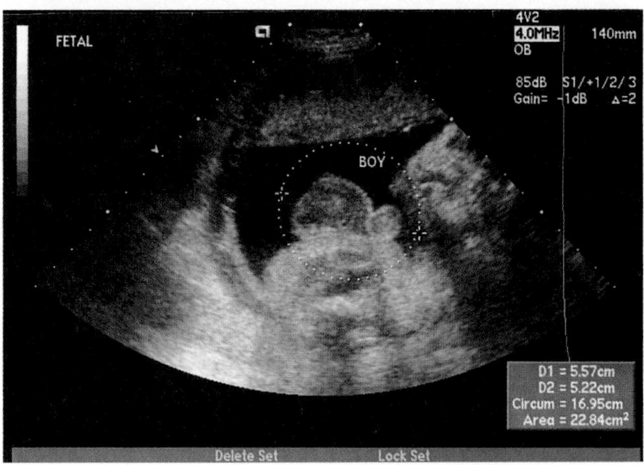

FIGURE 14–3
Ultrasonogram showing a male fetus. *(Courtesy of Nancy West.)*

	ANSWER COLUMN
14.33 ____________ is a temporary condition that occurs within a woman's body from the time of conception through the embryonic and fetal periods to birth. It lasts approximately 280 days (40 weeks; 10 lunar months; 9⅓ calendar months).	**pregnancy** (**PREG** nan see)
14.34 ____________ is the surgical puncture of the amniotic sac to obtain a sample of amniotic fluid.	**amniocentesis** (am nee oh sen **TEE** sis)
14.35 ____________ pertaining to before childbirth.	**prenatal** (pre **NAY** tl)
14.36 ____________ pertaining to the first 4 weeks after birth.	**neonatal** (nee oh **NAY** tal)
14.37 ____________ pertaining to after childbirth.	**postpartum** (post **PAR** tum)
14.38 ____________ refers to a woman during her first pregnancy.	**primigravida** (prigh mih **GRAV** ih dah)
14.39 ____________ refers to a woman who has borne one infant.	**primipara** (prigh **MIP** eh rah)
14.40 ____________ refers to a woman who has borne no offspring.	**nullipara** (null **IP** ah rah)

Answer Column

14.41 __________ refers to a woman who has borne more than one infant.

multipara (mull **TIP** ah rah)

EXPLANATION FRAME

The vagina is a musculomembranous tube extending from the vestibule to the uterus. See Figure 14–4. It is 10 to 15 cm in length and is situated between the bladder and the rectum. A fold of mucous membrane, the hymen, partially covers the external opening of the vagina.

The vagina has three basic functions:

- It is the female organ of **copulation** (sexual intercourse).
- It serves as a passageway for the discharge of menstruation.
- It serves as a passageway for the birth of the fetus.

14.42 __________ is inflammation of the vagina. Vaginitis may be caused by microorganisms such as gonococci, chlamydia, staphylococci, streptococci, spirochetes; viruses; irritation from use of strong chemicals in douching; fungus infection (candidiasis); protozoal infection (*Trichomonas vaginalis*); neoplasms of cervix or vagina; and/or irritation from foreign bodies such as pessaries and/or tampons.

vaginitis (vaj in **EYE** tis)

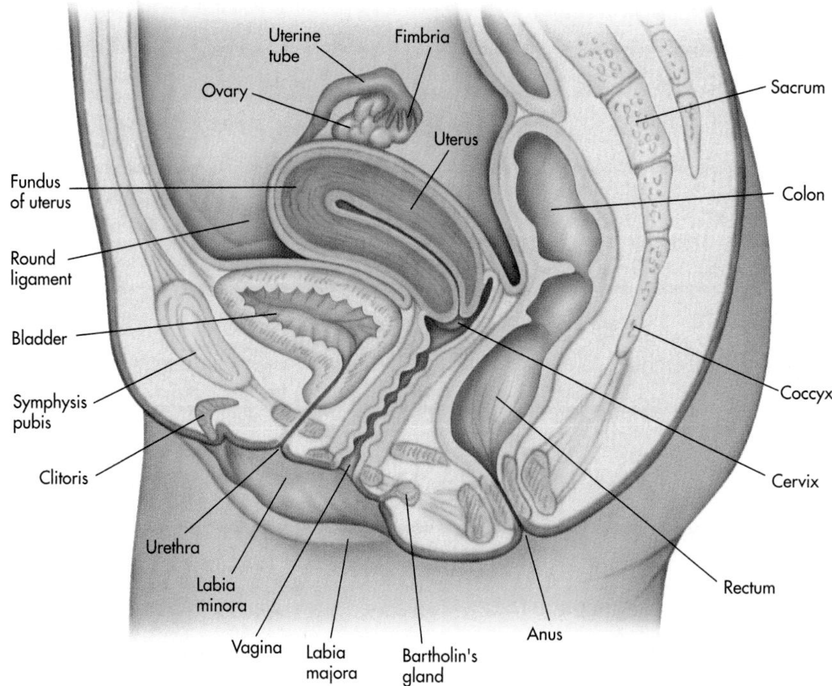

FIGURE 14–4
Sagittal section of the female pelvis, showing organs of the reproductive system.

Answer Column

14.43 The combining form **colp / o** and the root **colp** mean vagina. Medical terms that begin with these word elements are:

		Answer
__________	inflammation of the vagina	**colpitis** (kol **PYE** tis)
__________	hernia into the vagina	**colpocele** (**KOL** poh seel)
__________	inflammation of the vagina and bladder	**colpocystitis** (kol poh sis **TYE** tis)
__________	pain in the vagina; SYN: colpalgia	**colpodynia** (kol poh **DIN** ee ah)
__________	surgical repair of the vagina and perineum	**colpoperineoplasty** (kol poh per ih **NEE** oh plas tee)
__________	suture of the vagina	**colporrhaphy** (kol **POR** ah fee)
__________	an instrument used for examination of the tissues of the vagina and cervix by means of a magnifying lens	**colposcope** (**KOL** poh scope)
__________	examination of vaginal and cervical tissues by using a colposcope	**colposcopy** (kol **POSS** koh pee)

EXPLANATION FRAME

The vulva or the pudendum consists of five organs that comprise the external female genitalia: The **mons pubis** is a pad of fatty tissue of triangular shape and is the rounded area over the symphysis pubis; the **labia majora** are the two folds of adipose tissue, which are large lip-like structures, lying on either side of the vaginal opening; the **labia minora** are two thin folds of skin that lie within the labia majora and enclose the vestibule; the **vestibule** is the cleft between the labia minora and four structures open into it: the urethra, the vagina, and two excretory ducts of Bartholin's glands. See Figure 14–4. These glands produce a mucous secretion that lubricates the vagina; the **clitoris** is a small organ consisting of sensitive erectile tissue that is homologous to the penis of the male. Between the vulva and the anus is an external region known as the perineum. It is composed of muscle covered with skin.

14.44 The __________ are male or female reproductive organs. — **genitalia** (jen ih **TAY** lee ah)

The word elements used to build this term are:

		Answer
__________	root that means belonging to birth	**genital**
__________	suffix that means condition	**-ia**

ANSWER COLUMN

14.45 A __________ is a wart-like growth of the skin, usually seen on the external genitalia or near the anus.

condyloma (kon dih **LOH** mah)

14.46 Condyloma __________ is an ordinary wart in the genital and perianal areas. It is caused by various types of human papilloma virus. It may be spread from one area containing a wart inoculating an area that it contacts. The virus that causes the wart is usually sexually transmitted. It is also called a genital wart.

acuminatum (ah kyoo mih **NAY** tum)

14.47 The external region between the vulva and the anus is called the __________.

perineum (pair ih **NEE** um)

14.48 An __________ is an incision of the perineum. During the second stage of labor it may be used to prevent tearing of the perineum and to facilitate delivery of the fetus.

episiotomy (eh peez ee **OT** oh mee)

14.49 __________ is inflammation of Bartholin's glands.

bartholinitis (bar toh lin **EYE** tis)

14.50 A __________ abscess is a localized collection of pus that develops when Bartholin's glands become occluded in an acute inflammatory process.

Bartholin's (**BAR** toh linz)

14.51 A Bartholin's __________ is commonly formed in chronic inflammation of Bartholin's glands. A cyst is a closed sac or pouch that contains fluid, semifluid, or solid material.

cyst (**SIST**)

EXPLANATION FRAME

The breast or mammary glands are compound alveolar structures consisting of 15 to 20 glandular tissue lobes separated by septa of connective tissue. See Figure 14–5. The areola is the dark, pigmented area found in the skin over each breast, and the nipple is the elevated area in the center of the areola. During pregnancy, the areola changes from its pinkish color to a dark brown or reddish color.

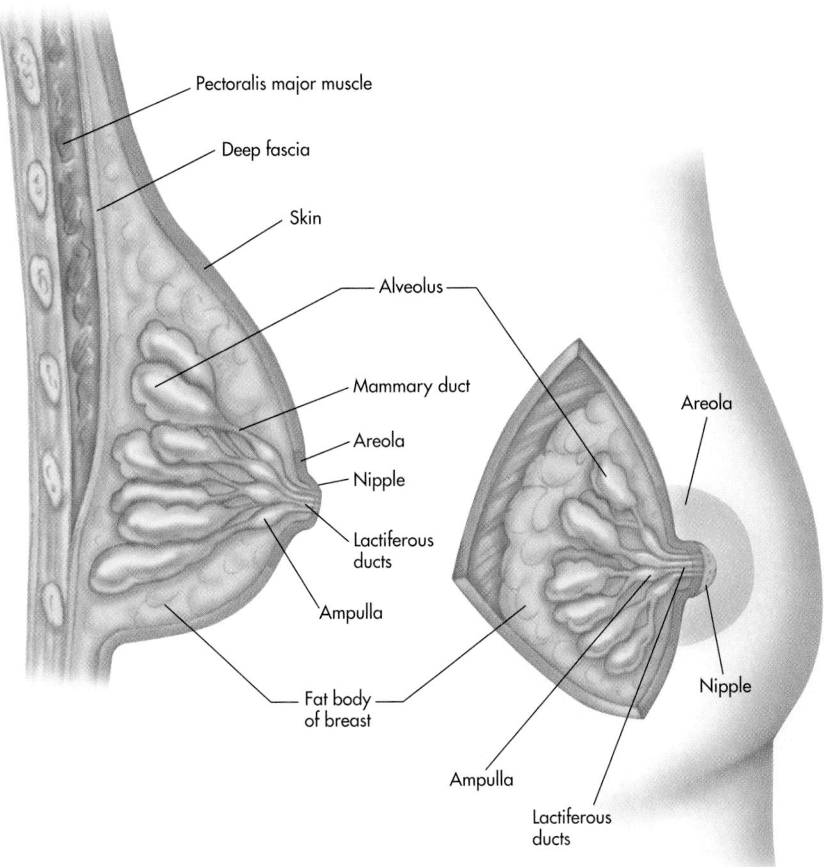

FIGURE 14–5
The breast and its structures.

ANSWER COLUMN

14.52 The combining form **mamm / o** and the roots **mamm** and **mast** mean breast.

Medical terms that begin with these word elements are:

		Answer
___________	is the process of obtaining x-ray pictures of the breast. It is used as a screening tool for breast cancer and as a means to diagnose early breast cancer.	**mammography** (mam **OG** rah fee)
___________	x-ray record (film) of the breast (See Figure 14–6 and Figure 14–7.)	**mammogram** (**MAM** oh gram)
___________	surgical repair of the breast	**mammoplasty** (**MAM** moh plas tee)
___________	surgical excision of the breast; SYN: mammectomy	**mastectomy** (mass **TEK** toh mee)
___________	inflammation of the breast	**mastitis** (mas **TYE** tis)

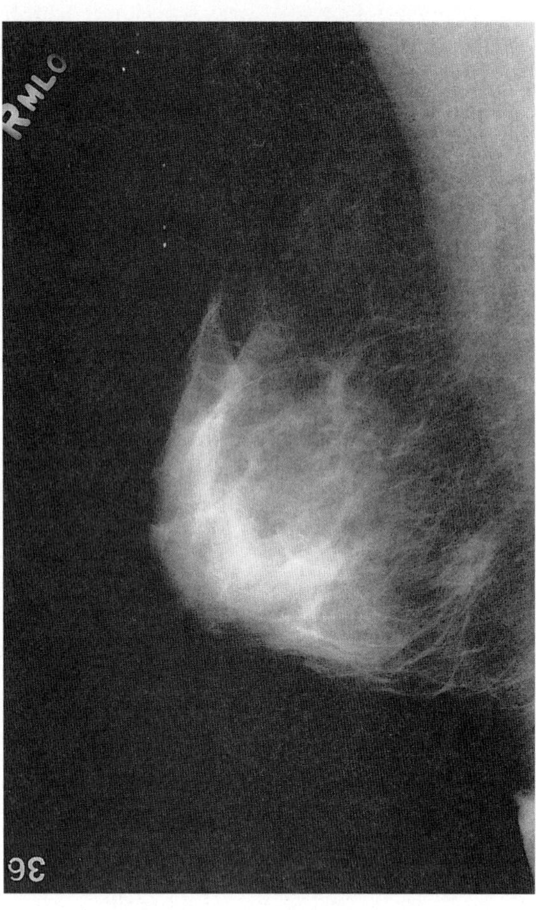

■ **FIGURE 14–6**
Normal mammogram. *(Courtesy of Teresa Resch.)*

ANSWER COLUMN

14.53 Diseases of the breast may range from mild to fatal. ___________ disease of the breast is a condition in which there are palpable lumps in the breast, usually associated with pain and tenderness, that fluctuate with the menstrual cycle and become progressively worse until menopause. *This condition is also referred to as mammary dysplasia or cystic disease of the breast.*

fibrocystic
(figh broh **SIS** tik)

14.54 There are an estimated 200 different kinds of cancer. The exact cause is unknown, but with ___________ there is an abnormal process wherein a cell or group of cells undergoes changes and no longer carries on normal cell functions. Malignant cells usually multiply rapidly, forming a mass of abnormal cells that enlarges, ulcerates, and sheds malignant cells to surrounding tissues. This process destroys the normal cells, with malignant cells taking their places, and often results in the formation of a tumor.

cancer
(**KAN** ser)

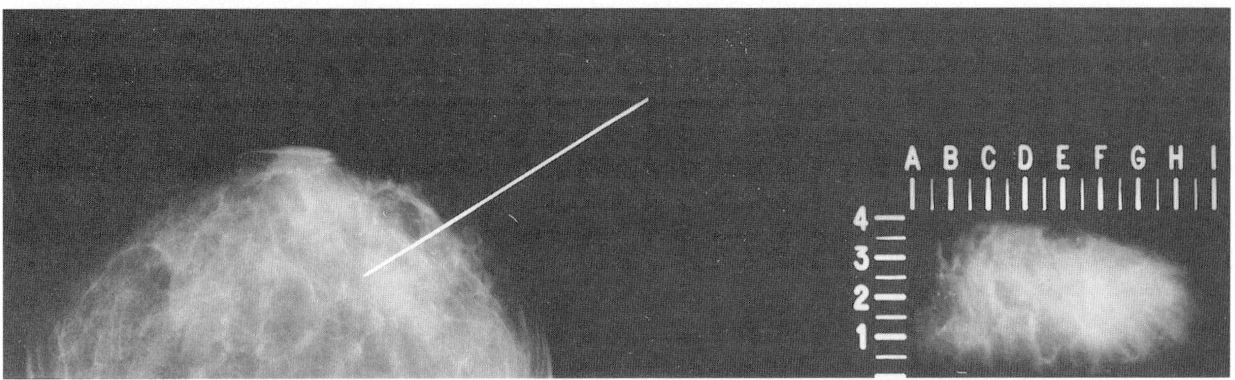

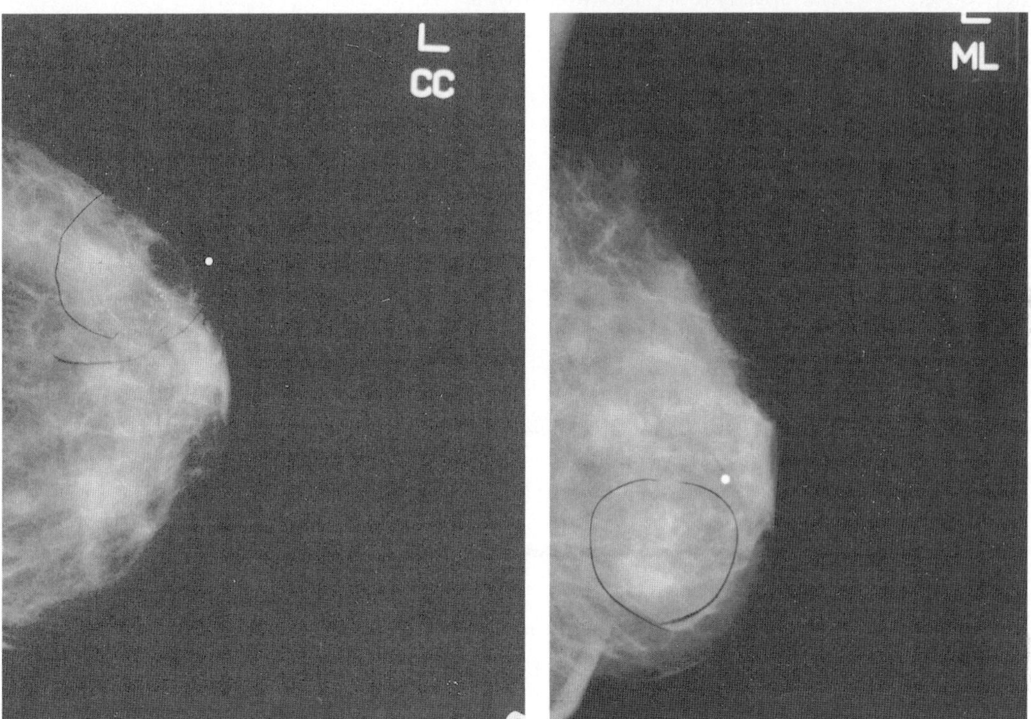

FIGURE 14–7
Mammogram showing cancer with microcalcifications. *(Courtesy of Teresa Resch.)*

EXPLANATION FRAME

This year approximately 182,000 women and approximately 1000 men will be diagnosed with breast cancer. It kills about 46,000 women a year and is the leading cause of death in women between the ages of 32 and 52. More than 90% of all breast lumps are discovered by women themselves. The majority of these lumps are benign (noncancerous) but of those that are not, early detection and treatment are essential. When performed properly, mammography and breast self-exam are valuable detection and screening methods for breast cancer.

Answer Column

14.55 ___________ ___________ ___________ (BSE) is the visual inspection and manual examination of the breast. Women should perform the Breast Self-Exam once a month and should look for changes in contour, symmetry, "dimpling" of the skin, retraction of the nipple(s), discharge, and the presence of lumps. See Figure 14–8.

breast self-examination

EXPLANATION FRAME

Approximately 50% of malignant tumors of the breast appear in the upper, outer quadrant and extend into the armpit. Eighteen percent of breast cancers occur in the nipple area, 11% in the lower outer quadrant, and 6% in the inner quadrant. Signs and symptoms of breast cancer are generally insidious and may include:

- Unusual secretions from the nipple
- Changes in the nipple's appearance
- Nontender, movable lump in early stage; as cancer advances, lump often becomes fixed in one place
- Well-localized discomfort that may be described as a burning, stinging, or aching sensation
- Dimpling or peau d'orange (orange-peel appearance) over the area of cancer of the breast
- Asymmetry and an elevation of the affected breast
- Nipple retraction
- Pain in the later stages

14.56 ___________ is a term that is used to indicate a disease that comes on in such a manner as to make the patient unaware of its onset.

insidious
(in **SID** ee us)

14.57 ___________ means lack of symmetry (same in size, shape, and relative position of parts on opposite sides of the body).

asymmetry
(ay **SIM** eh tree)

14.58 ___________ means of bad kind; growing worse. It is a term that is used to indicate a cancerous growth.

malignant
(mah **LIG** nant)

14.59 ___________ means a shortening; the act of drawing backward or the state of being drawn back.

retraction
(ree **TRAK** shun)

WHY DO THE BREAST SELF-EXAM?

There are many good reasons for doing a breast self-exam each month. One reason is that it is easy to do and the more you do it, the better you will get at it. When you get to know how your breasts normally feel, you will quickly be able to feel any change, and early detection is the key to successful treatment and cure.

REMEMBER: A breast self-exam could save your breast – and save your life. Most breast lumps are found by women themselves, but in fact, most lumps in the breast are not cancer. Be safe, be sure.

WHEN TO DO BREAST SELF-EXAM

The best time to do breast self-exam is right after your period, when breasts are not tender or swollen. If you do not have regular periods or sometimes skip a month, do it on the same day every month.

NOW, HOW TO DO BREAST SELF-EXAM

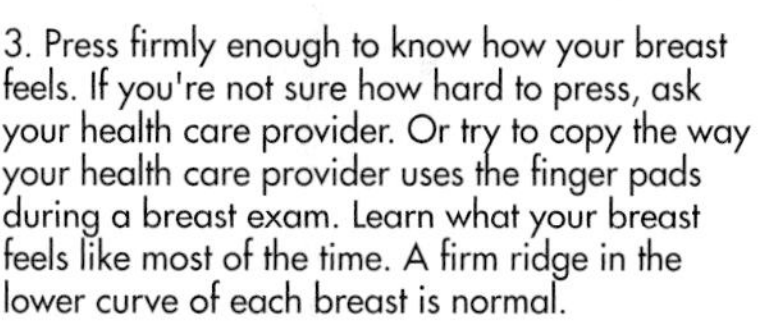

1. Lie down and put a pillow under your right shoulder. Place your right arm behind your head.

2. Use the finger pads of your three middle fingers on your left hand to feel for lumps or thickening. Your finger pads are the top third of each finger.

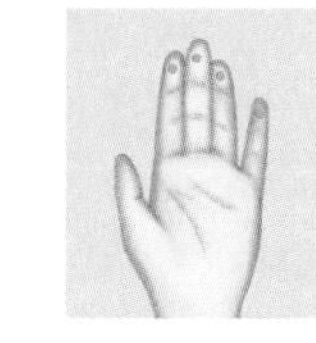

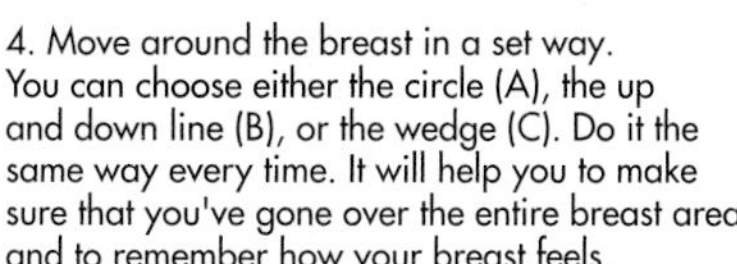

3. Press firmly enough to know how your breast feels. If you're not sure how hard to press, ask your health care provider. Or try to copy the way your health care provider uses the finger pads during a breast exam. Learn what your breast feels like most of the time. A firm ridge in the lower curve of each breast is normal.

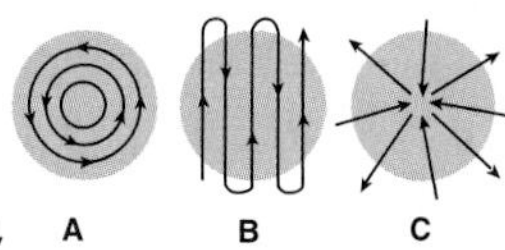

4. Move around the breast in a set way. You can choose either the circle (A), the up and down line (B), or the wedge (C). Do it the same way every time. It will help you to make sure that you've gone over the entire breast area, and to remember how your breast feels.

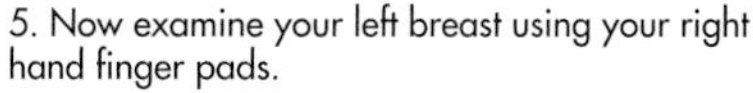

5. Now examine your left breast using your right hand finger pads.

6. If you find any changes, see your doctor right away.

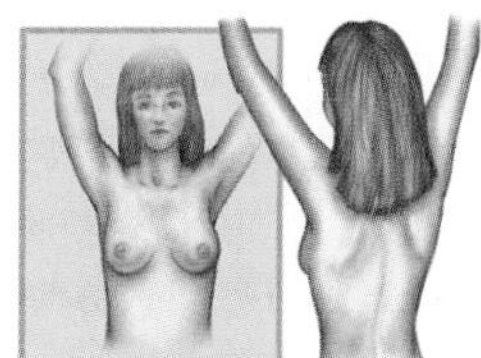

FOR ADDED SAFETY:

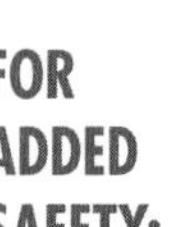

You should also check your breasts while standing in front of a mirror right after you do your breast self-exam each month. See if there are any changes in the way your breasts look: dimpling of the skin, changes in the nipple, or redness or swelling.

You might also want to do a breast self-exam while you're in the shower. Your soapy hands will glide over the wet skin, making it easy to check how your breasts feel.

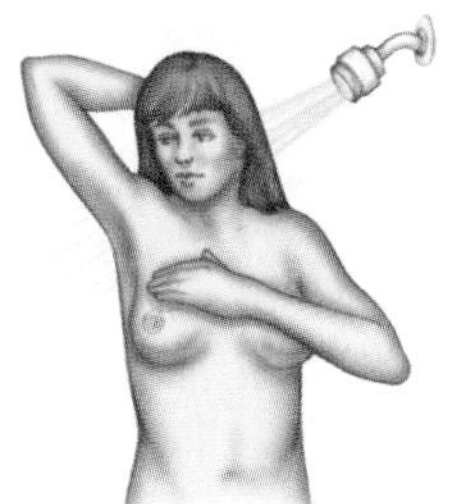

FIGURE 14–8
Breast self-examination.

EXPLANATION FRAME

Following are the risk factors for breast cancer in order of importance.

- Family history—increased risk when breast cancer occurs before menopause in mother, sister, or daughter, especially if cancer occurs in both breasts
- Over age 50 and nullipara (borne no offspring)
- Having a first baby after age 30
- History of chronic breast disease, especially epithelial hyperplasia
- Exposure to ionizing radiation of more than 50 rad during adolescence
- Obesity
- Early menarche, late menopause

Drugs that are generally used for diseases and disorders of the female reproductive system include various combinations of estrogens and progesterone.

14.60 __________ are used for a variety of conditions. They may be used in the treatment of amenorrhea, dysfunctional bleeding, and hirsutism and in palliative therapy for breast cancer in women and prostatic cancer in men.

estrogens
(**ESS** troh jens)

14.61 Estrogens are also used as __________ therapy in the treatment of uncomfortable symptoms that are related to menopause. It is believed that estrogen replacement therapy is useful in preventing osteoporosis, Alzheimer's disease, and heart disease in women.

replacement

14.62 __________ are synthetic preparations of progesterone. They are used to prevent uterine bleeding and are combined with estrogen for treatment of amenorrhea. They may be used in cases of infertility and threatened or habitual miscarriage.

progestins
(proh **JES** tins)

14.63 Oral __________ contain mixtures of estrogen and progestin in various levels of strength. The estrogen in the pill inhibits ovulation and the progestin inhibits pituitary secretion of luteinizing hormone (LH), causing changes in the cervical mucus that renders it unfavorable to penetration by sperm.

contraceptives
(kon trah **SEP** tivs)

ANSWER COLUMN

14.64 ____________ is an ascending infection from the vagina or cervix to the uterus, fallopian tubes, and broad ligaments. It may be caused by almost any bacterium and early treatment with appropriate antibiotics is important to prevent occlusion of the fallopian tubes that could lead to infertility.

pelvic inflammatory disease (PID)
(**PELL** vik in **FLAM** mah toh ree dih **ZEEZ**)

14.65 ABBREVIATIONS

Write in the correct abbreviation for the following:

		Answer
____________	abdominal hysterectomy	**AH**
____________	breast self-examination	**BSE**
____________	dilation (dilatation) and curettage	**D&C**
____________	dysfunctional uterine bleeding	**DUB**
____________	gynecology	**GYN**
____________	hormone replacement therapy	**HRT**
____________	hysterosalpingography	**HSG**
____________	in vitro fertilization	**IVF**
____________	luteinizing hormone	**LH**
____________	last menstrual period	**LMP**
____________	marital history	**MH**
____________	Papanicolaou (smear)	**Pap**
____________	pelvic inflammatory disease	**PID**
____________	previous menstrual period	**PMP**
____________	premenstrual syndrome	**PMS**
____________	toxic shock syndrome	**TSS**

IN THE SPOTLIGHT

STEM CELLS

In August of 2001 President George W. Bush announced support for limited stem cell research. Stem cells are master cells that have the ability to transform themselves into other cell types, including those in the brain, heart, bones, muscles, and skin.

Embryonic stem cells are cells contained in embryos that have the ability to transform themselves into virtually any other type of cell in the body. About five days after fertilization, the human embryo becomes a blastocyst, which is a hollow sphere of about 100 cells. Cells in its outer layer go on to form the placenta and other organs needed to support fetal development in the uterus. The inner cells go on to form nearly all of the tissues of the body. These are the embryonic stem cells used in research.

Embryonic stem cells may be obtained:

- From surplus frozen embryos left in storage at clinics for in vitro fertilization (IVF) and destined to be destroyed
- From clinics that gain consent from donors to fuse egg and sperm to create embryos specifically to obtain stem cells

Adult stem cells have already differentiated into specific cell or tissue types but have a limited ability to transform into specialized cell types. They have been found in the brain and blood and certain other organs. Adult stem cells are more specialized than embryonic stem cells and give rise to specific cell types. Although named adult stem cells, they can be harbored in mature tissue in the bodies of children, as well as adults.

A stem-cell line consists of stem cells from an embryo that continue to divide indefinitely in the laboratory. This is a lineage of cells that can be sold to laboratories for use in research. Fewer than a dozen stem-cell lines have been created under specific criteria that would allow them to be used in federally funded research. The criteria specify that they come from surplus embryos donated from fertility clinics where they would otherwise have been destroyed.

Scientists hope to harness the transformational qualities of stem cells to provide treatments for a variety of diseases affecting millions of people worldwide. It may be possible to replace tissues and organs damaged by disease or injury to restore healthy functioning. For example, in people with Parkinson's disease, injecting stem cells into the area of the brain that controls muscle movement, where the disease kills nerve cells, might regenerate the neurons and reverse the illnesses. This procedure would be a stem-cell transplantation.

Therapeutic applications of stem cells also could treat diabetes; Alzheimer's disease; stroke; heart attack; multiple sclerosis; blood, bone and bone marrow ailments; severe burns by providing skin grafts; spinal cord injuries; and cancer patients who have lost cells and tissue because of radiation and chemotherapy.

Other possible medical uses for stem cells are using them to test a drug's therapeutic effects and toxic side effects in human tissue without using a laboratory animal as a proxy. In addition, they may be harnessed and packaged to deliver gene therapy to specific targets in the body to treat genetic problems.

CASE STUDY

Please read the following case study and then work frames 14.66–14.69. Write in your answer in the answer column. Check your responses with the answers provided at the end of frame 14.69.

A 54-year-old female was seen by a physician and the following is a synopsis of the visit.

PRESENT HISTORY: The patient states that she is feeling fine and is seeing the doctor for her annual Pap smear and breast exam. She is on estrogen replacement therapy and Atenolol for hypertension. A mammogram was scheduled at a local hospital.

SIGNS AND SYMPTOMS: Chief Complaint: none.

DIAGNOSIS: Pap Smear Routine Annual with Gyn Exam and Mammogram Routine Exam. The routine mammogram was abnormal. She was informed by her physician that she would need to have another mammogram and it was scheduled for the following day. The patient was most concerned about the possibility of having breast cancer, but the results of her second mammogram were within normal limits.

TREATMENT: Continue estrogen replacement therapy and medication regimen for hypertension. Return for her annual Pap smear, breast exam, and mammogram next August.

14.66 Give the meaning for the abbreviation Pap __________.

14.67 Give the meaning for the abbreviation Gyn __________.

14.68 Atenolol is a medication prescribed for __________.

14.69 Treatment included continuing __________ replacement therapy and medication for hypertension.

CASE STUDY ANSWERS

14.66 Papanicolaou (smear)
14.67 gynecology
14.68 hypertension
14.69 estrogen

REVIEW A: WORD ELEMENTS

This review allows you to check your knowledge of some of the word elements presented in this unit. In the spaces provided, write the meaning of the word elements that are identified as **Prefix (P), Word Root (R), Combining Form (CF),** and/or **Suffix (S)**.

MEDICAL WORD	*WORD ELEMENT*	*MEANING*
1. gynecology	gynec / o (CF)	________
	-logy (S)	________
2. hysteralgia	hyster (R)	________
	-algia (S)	________
3. hysterectomy	hyster (R)	________
	-ectomy (S)	________
4. metritis	metr (R)	________
	-itis (S)	________
5. uteroplasty	uter / o (CF)	________
	-plasty (S)	________
6. cervicitis	cervic (R)	________
	-itis (S)	________
7. menopause	men / o (CF)	________
	pause (R)	________
8. menorrhagia	men / o (CF)	________
	-rrhagia (S)	________
9. dysmenorrhea	dys (P)	________
	men / o (CF)	________
	-rrhea (S)	________
10. salpingectomy	salping (R)	________
	-ectomy (S)	________
11. ovariocentesis	ovari / o (CF)	________
	-centesis (S)	________
12. oophoropexy	oophor / o (CF)	________
	-pexy (S)	________

REVIEW B: MEDICAL TERMS

Please place the correct letter from column II on the appropriate line of column I.

COLUMN I		COLUMN II
______	1. myometrium	A. the process of turning the uterus backward
______	2. intrauterine	B. the process of discharging the menses
______	3 uterine adnexa	C. the initial menstrual period
______	4. retroversion	D. the ovaries and the fallopian tubes
______	5. anteversion	E. process in which the ovum is discharged from the ovary
______	6. menstruation	F. muscular wall of the uterus
______	7. menarche	G. abdominal pain that occurs at ovulation
______	8. ovulation	H. the process of turning the fundus forward toward the pubis
______	9. mittelschmerz	I. lack of the monthly flow or menstruation
______	10. amenorrhea	J. pertaining to within the uterus

REVIEW C: DISEASES AND DISORDERS

Please provide the correct disease or disorder for each of the following descriptions.

1. ______ ______ is a sac that develops in the ovary.
2. ______ is inflammation of the vagina.
3. ______ is a wart-like growth of the skin, usually seen on the external genitalia or near the anus.
4. ______ is inflammation of Bartholin's glands.
5. ______ disease of the breast is a condition in which there are palpable lumps in the breast. This condition is also referred to as mammary dysplasia or cystic disease of the breast.

REVIEW D: UNSCRAMBLE THE WORDS

Unscramble the following medical terms and place the correct term on the line directly across from the scrambled word.

1. inereut ____________
2. taliondi ____________
3. aeirbmif ____________
4. paroslapeoc ____________
5. zatilioniterf ____________
6. necpocniot ____________
7. yteogz ____________
8. talinegia ____________

REVIEW E: DRUGS USED FOR THE FEMALE REPRODUCTIVE SYSTEM

Please provide the correct answer for each of the following descriptions.

1. ____________ may be used in the treatment of amenorrhea, dysfunctional bleeding, and a variety of other conditions.
2. ____________ replacement therapy is used in the treatment of uncomfortable symptoms of menopause.
3. ____________ are synthetic preparations of progesterone.
4. ____________ contraceptives contain mixtures of estrogen and progestin in various strengths.

REVIEW F: ABBREVIATIONS

Please provide the correct abbreviation and/or meaning for the abbreviation.

1. ____________ abdominal hysterectomy
2. D&C ____________
3. ____________ gynecology
4. Pap ____________
5. ____________ premenstrual syndrome
6. toxic shock syndrome ____________

15 THE MALE REPRODUCTIVE SYSTEM: UROLOGY

LEARNING CONCEPTS

- the male reproductive system
- essential terminology
- pronunciation guide
- word elements
- explanation frames
- prostatism: signs and symptoms
- sexually transmited diseases: symptoms and treatment
- drugs used for the male reproductive system
- abbreviations
- in the spotlight: erectile dysfunction
- case study: benign prostatic hyperplasia
- review exercises

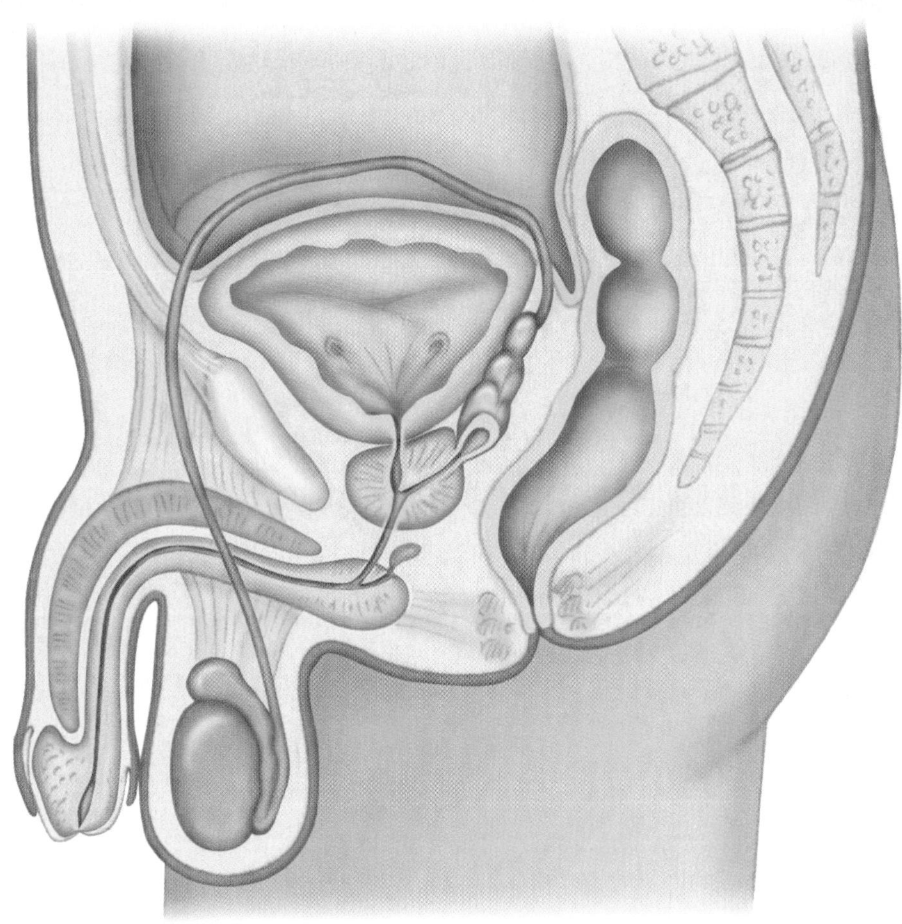

OBJECTIVES

ON COMPLETION OF THIS UNIT, YOU SHOULD BE ABLE TO:

- Briefly describe the male reproductive system.
- Describe the primary functions of the various organs or structures of the male reproductive system.
- Identify and give the meaning of the primary word elements for this unit.
- Analyze, build, spell, and pronounce selected medical words.
- Describe selected diseases/disorders of the male reproductive system.
- List five symptoms usually associated with benign prostatic hyperplasia (BPH).
- Describe selected sexually transmitted diseases (STDs).
- Give the symptoms of and treatment for selected sexually transmitted diseases for the male, female, and newborn.
- Describe selected drugs that are used for the male reproductive system diseases or disorders.
- List five signs of possible anabolic steroid abuse.
- Define selected abbreviations that pertain to the male reproductive system.
- List the causes of erectile dysfunction.
- Describe the treatment for erectile dysfunction.
- Complete the Case Study on Benign Prostatic Hyperplasia.
- Successfully complete the review section.

TECH LINK

CD-ROM Use the CD-ROM enclosed with your textbook to gain additional reinforcement through interactive word building exercises, spelling games, labeling activities, and additional quizzes.

www.prenhall.com/rice Use the above address to access the free, interactive Companion Website created specifically for this textbook. Get hints, instant feedback, and textbook references to chapter-related multiple choice and true/false questions, fill-in-the-blank, and labeling exercises. In addition, you will find an audio glossary, and essay questions.

The male reproductive system consists of the testes, various ducts and tubes, the urethra, and the accessory glands: bulbourethral, prostate, and the seminal vesicles. The supporting structures and accessory sex organs are the scrotum and the penis. See Table 15–1.

The testes are two ovoid-shaped organs located in the scrotum. Within the testes are small tubes called the seminiferous tubules. It is within these tubes that spermatozoa are formed. An average normal male produces approximately 200 million sperm each day.

Cells within the testes also produce the male sex hormone, testosterone, which is responsible for the development of secondary male characteristics during puberty. Testosterone is essential for normal growth and development of the male accessory sex organs. It plays a vital role in the erection process of the penis and thus is necessary for the reproductive act. Additionally, it affects the growth of hair on the face, muscular development, and vocal timbre.

TABLE 15–1 THE MALE REPRODUCTIVE SYSTEM

Organ/Structure	Primary Functions
The Scrotum	Contains testes and connecting tubes; contractile action brings the testes closer to the perineum, where they can absorb sufficient body heat to maintain the viability of the spermatozoa
The Penis	Male organ of copulation; site of the orifice for the elimination of urine and semen from the body
The Testes	Contains seminiferous tubules that are the site of the development of spermatozoa; cells within the testes also produce the male sex hormone, testosterone
The Epididymis	Storage site for the maturation of sperm
The Ductus Deferens or Vas Deferens	Excretory duct of the testis
The Seminal Vesicles	Produce a slightly alkaline fluid that becomes a part of the seminal fluid or semen
The Prostate Gland	Secretes an alkaline fluid that aids in maintaining the viability of spermatozoa
The Bulbourethral or Cowper's Glands	Produce a mucous secretion before ejaculation, which becomes a part of the semen
The Urethra	Transmits urine and semen out of the body

Answer Column

15.1 ____________ is the study of the urinary system. Because the male reproductive organs also function as urinary organs, it is this specialty area that is concerned with diseases and disorders of the male reproductive system.

urology
(yoo **RALL** oh jee)

EXPLANATION FRAME

In the male, the scrotum and the penis are the external organs of reproduction. The scrotum is a pouch-like structure located behind the penis. It is suspended from the perineal region and is divided by a septum into two sacs, each containing one of the testes along with its connecting tube called the epididymis. The penis is the male organ of copulation and the site of the orifice for the elimination of urine and semen from the body. The penis has three longitudinal columns of erectile tissue that are capable of enlargement when engorged with blood, as is the case during sexual stimulation. See Figure 15–1 and Figure 15–2.

15.2 The ____________ is composed of erectile tissue covered with skin. The glans penis is the cone-shaped head of the penis and is the site of the urethral orifice.

penis
(**PEE** nis)

PRIMARY WORD ELEMENTS

The following word elements (prefixes, roots, combining forms, and suffixes) will be used to build medical terms that relate to this unit. Please commit these to memory.

PREFIX

PREFIX	MEANING	PREFIX	MEANING
a	without, lack of	**hydro**	water
circum	around	**hypo**	below, deficient
epi	upon	**oligo**	little, scanty

COMBINING FORM

COMBINING FORM / ROOT	MEANING	COMBINING FORM / ROOT	MEANING
balan	glans penis	**spadias**	a rent, an opening
balan / o	glans penis	**sperm, spermat**	seed (sperm)
cis	to cut	**sperm / i, spermat / o**	seed (sperm)
crypt	hidden	**testicul**	testicle
cyst	bladder	**ureth**	urethra
didym	testis	**urethr / o**	urethra
orch, orch / i, orchi / o	testicle	**varic / o**	twisted vein
orchid, orchid / o	testicle	**vas**	vessel
pen	penis	**vesicul**	vesicle
phim	a muzzle	**zo / o**	animal
prostat	prostate	**zoon**	life
prostat / o	prostate		

SUFFIXES

SUFFIX	MEANING	SUFFIX	MEANING
-al	pertaining to	**-ion**	process
-algia	pain	**-itis**	inflammation
-blast	immature cell, germ cell	**-megaly**	enlargement, large
-cele	hernia, tumor, swelling	**-pexy**	surgical fixation
-cide	to kill	**-phraxis**	to obstruct
-cyst	bladder	**-plasty**	surgical repair
-ectomy	surgical excision	**-tomy**	incision
-genesis	formation, produce	**-uria**	urine
-ia, -ism, -osis	condition of		

ANSWER COLUMN

15.3 The foreskin or __________ is the loose skin fold that covers the glans penis. The foreskin contains glands that secrete a lubricating fluid called __________. The foreskin may be removed by a surgical procedure known as __________.

prepuce (PRE pyoos)

smegma (SMEG mah)

circumcision
(ser kum **SIH** zhun)

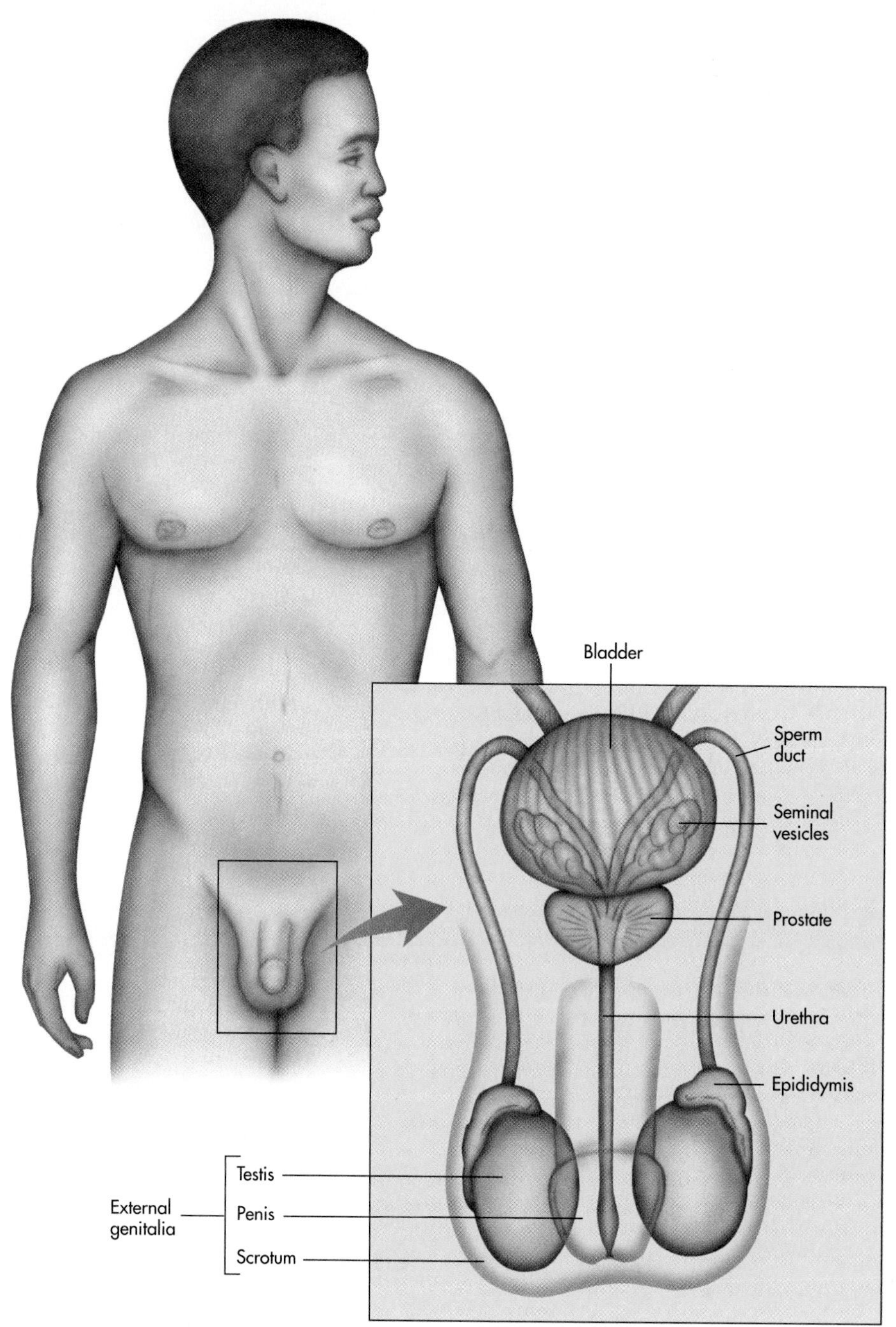

FIGURE 15–1

The male reproductive system: seminal vesicles, prostate, urethra, sperm duct, epididymis, and external genitalia.

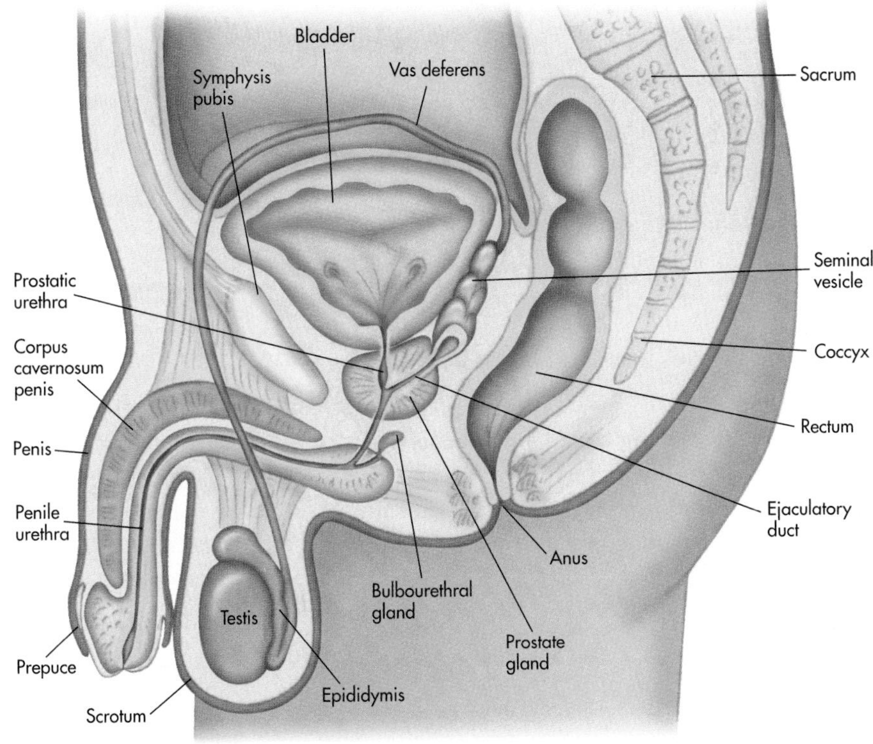

FIGURE 15–2
Sagittal section of the male pelvis, showing the organs of the reproductive system.

		ANSWER COLUMN
15.4	The word elements used to build the term **circum / cis / ion** are:	
	__________ prefix that means around	**circum**
	__________ root that means to cut	**cis**
	__________ suffix that means process	**-ion**
15.5	The combining form **balan / o** and the root **balan** mean glans penis. Medical terms that are built using these word elements are:	
	__________ inflammation of the glans penis	**balanitis** (bal ah **NYE** tis)
	__________ herniation of the glans penis through a rupture of the prepuce	**balanocele** (**BAL** ah noh seel)
	__________ surgical repair of the glans penis	**balanoplasty** (**BAL** an noh plas tee)

ANSWER COLUMN

FOR REVIEW: SUFFIXES

-itis inflammation
-cele hernia, tumor, swelling
-plasty surgical repair

15.6 The root **pen** means penis. Medical terms that use this word element are:

__________ pertaining to the penis

__________ __________ is a device implanted in the penis that makes it become erect. The device is usually in the form of inflatable plastic cylinders implanted in each corpus cavernosum of the penis. In most patients, this device permits the attaining of a nearly physiologic erection

__________ inflammation of the penis

penile (**PEE** nile)
penile prosthesis (**PEE** nile pross **THEE** sis)
penitis (pee **NYE** tis)

15.7 __________ is a condition of narrowing of the opening of the prepuce wherein the foreskin cannot be drawn back over the glans penis.

phimosis (fih **MOH** sis)

15.8 A __________ is a thin, flexible protective sheath, usually latex, worn over the penis during copulation to help prevent impregnation or venereal disease.

condom (**KON** dum)

EXPLANATION FRAME

The testes (testicles), male gonads, are located in the scrotum. See Figure 15–1 and Figure 15–2. The interior of each testis is divided into about 250 wedge-shaped lobes by fibrous tissues. Coiled within each lobe are one to three small tubes called the seminiferous tubules. These tubules are the site of the development of spermatozoa. Cells within the testes also produce the male sex hormone, testosterone, which is responsible for the development of secondary male characteristics during puberty.

15.9 The combining forms **orchi / o** and **orchid / o** and the roots **orch** and **orchid** mean testis; testicle. Medical terms that are built using these word elements are:

__________ a congenital condition in which there is a lack of one or both testes; SYN: anorchidism

__________ surgical excision of a testicle; SYN: orchidectomy

anorchism (an **OR** kiszm)
orchiectomy (or kee **EK** toh mee)

continued

		ANSWER COLUMN
____________	surgical fixation of a testicle; SYN: orchidopexy	**orchiopexy** (or kee oh **PEK** see)
____________	surgical repair of a testicle; SYN: orchidoplasty	**orchioplasty** (**OR** kee oh plas tee)
____________	incision into a testicle; SYN: orchidotomy	**orchiototmy** (or kee **OT** oh mee)
____________	inflammation of a testicle (testis)	**orchitis** (or **KIGH** tis)
____________	a condition in which the testes fail to descend into the scrotum; SYN: cryptorchidism	**cryptorchism** (krip **TOR** kizm)

15.10 A ____________ is a collection of serous fluid in a sac-like cavity, especially the tunica vaginalis testis. It may also refer to a serous tumor of the testes or associated structures.

hydrocele (**HIGH** droh seel)

The word elements used to build this term are:

____________	prefix that means water	**hydro**
____________	suffix that means hernia, tumor, swelling	**-cele**

15.11 The root **testicul** also means testicle. The medical term ____________ means pertaining to the testicle. The suffix **-ar** means pertaining to.

testicular (tes **TIK** yoo lar)

EXPLANATION FRAME

Testicular cancer usually occurs in men younger than 40 years of age. It is the most common type of cancer in men between the ages of 20 and 35 years. The cause is unknown and if not treated in the early stages, the cancer can spread through the lymphatic system to the lymph nodes in the abdomen, chest, and neck, and eventually to the lungs. The first sign is often a painless lump discovered in the testicle. Treatment includes an orchiectomy, followed by radiation therapy and chemotherapy.

15.12 The medical term ____________ means to remove the testicles or ovaries; to geld, to spay. A male who has been castrated is called an eunuch.

castrate (**KASS** trayt)

EXPLANATION FRAME

Each testis is connected by efferent ductules to an epididymis, which is a coiled tube lying on the posterior aspect of the testis. The epididymis is between 13 and 20 feet in length but is coiled into a space less than 2 inches (5 cm) long and ends in the ductus deferens. Each epididymis functions as a storage site for the maturation of sperm. See Figure 15–2.

Answer Column

15.13 __________ is the surgical excision of the epididymis.
The word elements used to build this term are:
__________ prefix that means upon
__________ root that means testis
__________ suffix that means surgical excision

epididymectomy
(ep ih did ih **MEK** toh mee)
epi
didym
-ectomy

15.14 __________ is inflammation of the epididymis.
The prefix **epi** means upon, the root **didym** means testis, and the suffix __________ means inflammation.

epididymitis
(ep ih did ih **MYE** tis)
-itis

EXPLANATION FRAME

The ductus deferens or vas deferens is a slim muscular tube, about 45 cm in length, and is a continuation of the epididymis. See Figure 15–2. It is described as the excretory duct of the testis and extends from a point adjacent to the testis to enter the abdomen through the inguinal canal. It is later joined by the duct from the seminal vesicle. Between the testis and the part of the abdomen known as the internal inguinal ring, the ductus deferens is contained within a structure known as the spermatic cord.

15.15 A __________ is an enlargement and twisting of the veins of the spermatic cord. *This condition commonly occurs on the left side and is seen in adolescent males. Surgery is usually required for persistent symptomatic varicocele.*

varicocele
(**VAIR** ih koh seel)

15.16 The root **vas** means a vessel or duct. __________ is inflammation of the vas deferens.

vastitis
(vah **SIGH** tis)

15.17 __________ is the surgical excision of the vas deferens. It is usually performed bilaterally to produce sterility in the male. *To be sure of sterility the male should have about two dozen ejaculations to help ensure that sterility has been accomplished. At least two ejaculates should be free of sperm before one considers this a safe method of birth control.*

vasectomy
(vas **EK** toh mee)

EXPLANATION FRAME

There are two seminal vesicles, each connected by a narrow duct to a ductus deferens, which then forms a short tube, the ejaculatory duct, that penetrates the base of the prostate gland and opens into the prostatic portion of the urethra. The seminal vesicles produce a slightly alkaline fluid that becomes a part of the seminal fluid or semen. See Figure 15–1.

ANSWER COLUMN

15.18 __________ is the fluid transporting medium for spermatozoa discharged during ejaculation.

semen
(SEE men)

15.19 __________ is the expulsion of seminal fluid from the male urethra. *Ejaculation is a reflex phenomenon. It occurs normally during copulation, masturbation, or as a nocturnal emission. The volume of an ejaculation is from 2 to 5 mL and may contain 60 to 150 million sperm/mL.*

ejaculation
(ee jak yoo **LAY** shun)

EXPLANATION FRAME

A typical sperm has a head, neck, middle, and tail. Not all sperm are normal. Some may have two heads, an aplastic head, an irregular head, an elongated head, two or more tails, or no tail. See Figure 15–3.

15.20 The combining forms **sperm / i** and **spermat / o** and the roots **sperm** and **spermat** mean seed, sperm. Medical terms that are built using these word elements are:

__________ the sperm germ cell

spermatoblast
(SPER mah toh blast)

__________ a cyst of the epididymis that contains spermatozoa; SYN: spermatocele

spermatocyst
(SPER mah toh sist)

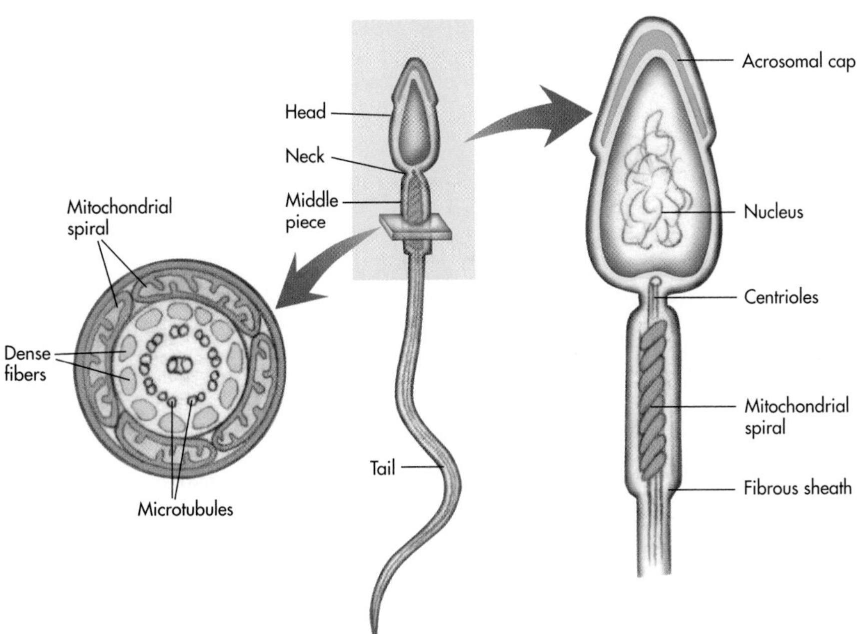

■ **FIGURE 15–3**
The basic structure of a spermatozoon (sperm).

ANSWER COLUMN

continued

		Answer
____________	the formation of spermatozoa	**spermatogenesis** (sper mat oh **JEN** eh sis)
____________	the male sex cell. The plural form is spermatozoa	**spermatozoon** (sper mat oh **ZOH** on)
____________	discharge of semen with the urine	**spermaturia** (sper mah **TOO** ree ah)
____________	an agent that kills sperm	**spermicide (SPER** mih side)

15.21 ____________ is a condition in which there is a lack of spermatozoa in the semen. The word elements used to build this term are:

		Answer
____________	prefix that means lack of	**a**
____________	combining form that means animal	**zo / o**
____________	root that means seed	**sperm**
____________	suffix that means condition of	**-ia**

Answer: **azoospermia** (ah zoh oh **SPER** mee ah)

15.22 ____________ is a condition in which there is a scanty amount of spermatozoa in the semen. The word elements used to build this term are:

		Answer
____________	prefix that means scanty	**oligo**
____________	root that means seed	**sperm**
____________	suffix that means condition of	**-ia**

Answer: **oligospermia** (ol ih goh **SPER** mee ah)

15.23 ____________ is a condition in which there is a lack of secretion of the male seed; sperm. The word elements used to build this term are:

		Answer
____________	prefix that means lack of	**a**
____________	root that means seed	**spermat**
____________	suffix that means condition of	**-ism**

Answer: **aspermatism** (ah **SPER** mah tizm)

EXPLANATION FRAME

The prostate gland is about 4 cm wide and weighs about 20 grams. It is composed of glandular, connective, and muscular tissue and lies behind the urinary bladder. It surrounds the first 2.5 cm of the urethra and secretes an alkaline fluid that aids in maintaining the viability of spermatozoa. See Figure 15–4.

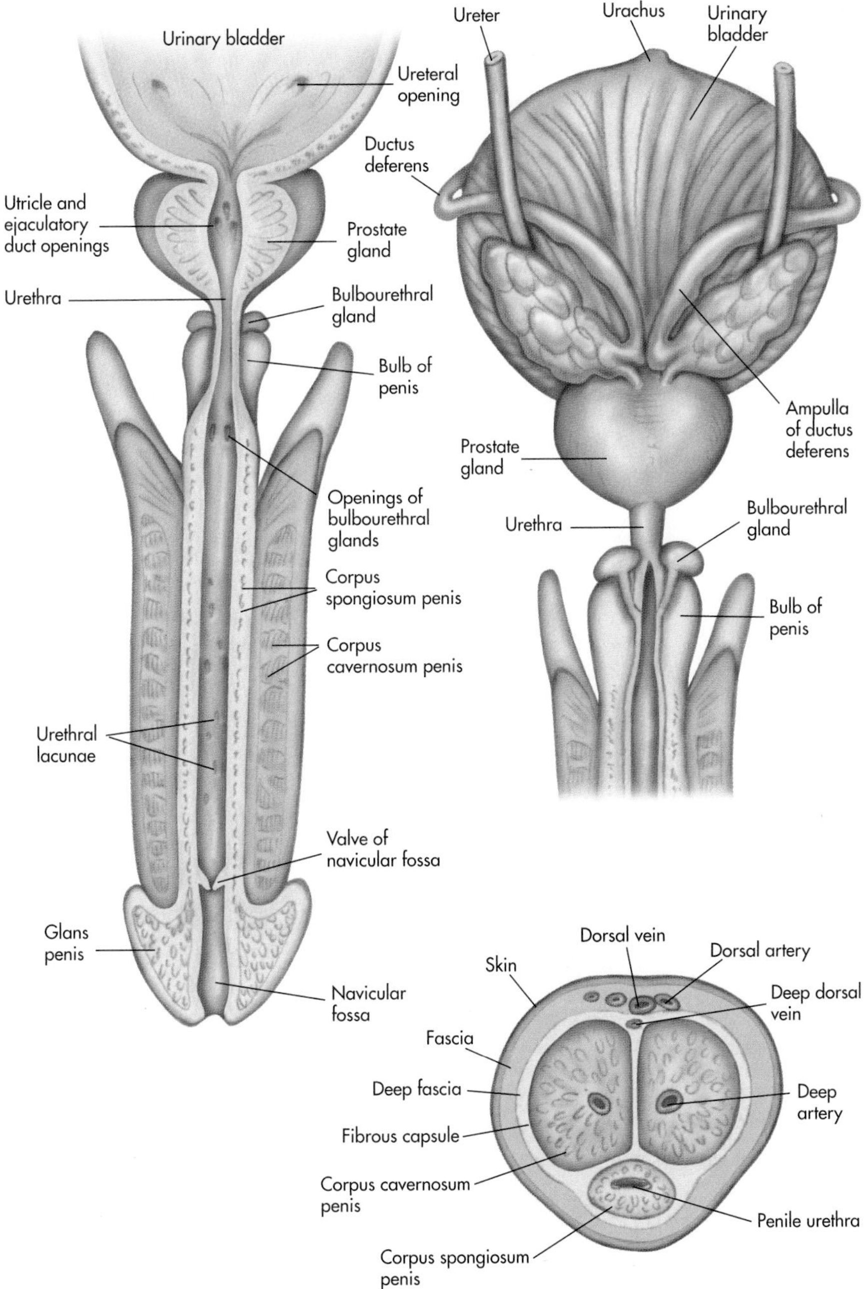

FIGURE 15-4
The structures of the bladder, prostate gland, and penis.

	ANSWER COLUMN
15.24 Enlargement of the prostate that can occur in older men is called benign __________ hyperplasia (hypertrophy).	**prostatic** (pross **TAT** ik)

Answer Column

EXPLANATION FRAME

Benign prostatic hyperplasia (BPH) is enlargement of the prostate gland; it may occur in men who are 50 years of age and older. As the prostate enlarges, it compresses the urethra, thereby restricting the normal flow of urine. This restriction generally causes a number of symptoms and can be referred to as prostatism. Symptoms usually include:

- A weak or hard-to-start urine stream
- A need to urinate often, especially at night
- A feeling of urgency
- Acute urinary retention
- Recurrent urinary infections

15.25 __________ is any condition of the prostate that interferes with the flow of urine from the bladder.

prostatism
(PROSS tah tixm)

EXPLANATION FRAME

By age 60, four out of five men may have an enlarged prostate and suffer urinary difficulties. By age 75, one in eleven men may develop prostate cancer. Approximately 165,000 new cases of prostate cancer occur each year with a death toll of 34,000 lives. It is recommended that men age 40 and up should have a digital rectal exam each year and that men age 50 and over should have a prostate-specific antigen (PSA) blood test each year. Those men who are at high risk should have the exam and blood test at an earlier age.

15.26 **True or False.** *Prostate-specific antigen (PSA) is a urine test that is used to screen for prostate cancer. Prostate-specific antigen is a blood test that measures concentrations of a special type of protein known as prostate-specific antigen. Increased level indicates prostate disease or possibly prostate cancer.*

false

15.27 The combining form **prostat / o** and the root **prostat** mean prostate. Medical terms that are built using these word elements are:

__________ pain in the prostate

__________ surgical excision of the prostate

__________ inflammation of the prostate

prostatalgia
(pross tah **TAL** jee ah)
prostatectomy
(pross tah **TEK** toh mee)
prostatitis
(pross tah **TYE** tis)

ANSWER COLUMN

continued

_______ inflammation of the prostate and bladder — **prostatocystitis** (pross tah toh sis **TYE** tis)

_______ enlargement of the prostate — **prostatomegaly** (pross tah toh **MEG** ah lee)

EXPLANATION FRAME

The bulbourethral or Cowper's glands are two small pea-sized glands located below the prostate and on either side of the urethra. A duct about 2.5 cm long connects them with the wall of the urethra. The bulbourethral glands produce a mucus secretion before ejaculation, which becomes a part of the semen. The male urethra is approximately 20 cm long and extends from the urinary bladder to the external urethral orifice at the head of the penis. It serves to transmit urine and semen out of the body. See Figure 15–4.

15.28 _______ is a congenital defect in which the urethra opens on the dorsum (back) of the penis.
The prefix _______ means upon and the root _______ means a rent, an opening.

Answer: **epispadias** (ep ih **SPAY** dee as); **epi** **spadias**

15.29 _______ is a congenital defect in which the urethra opens on the underside of the penis. The prefix _______ means under and the root **spadias** means a rent, an opening.

Answer: **hypospadias** (high poh **SPAY** dee as); **hypo**

15.30 The combining form **urethr / o** and the root **urethr** mean urethra. Medical terms that are built using these word elements are:

_______ pertaining to the urethra — **urethral** (yoo **REE** thral)

_______ pain in the urethra; SYN: urethrodynia — **urethralgia** (yoo ree **THRAL** jee ah)

_______ surgical excision of the urethra or part of it — **urethrectomy** (yoo ree **THREK** toh mee)

_______ obstruction of the urethra; SYN: urethremphraxis — **urethrophraxis** (yoo ree throh **FRAK** sis)

_______ spasm of the urethra; SYN: urethrismus — **urethrism** (**YOO** ree thrizm)

_______ inflammation of the urethra — **urethritis** (yoo ree **THRYE** tis)

ANSWER COLUMN

15.31 ___________ means pertaining to or resulting from intercourse. Venereal diseases are the most common causes of urethritis in the male and vaginitis in the female.

venereal (veh **NEER** ee al)

EXPLANATION FRAME

Syphilis is a sexually transmitted disease (STD) that may be passed from person to person through sexual contact or from mother to child. It is caused by a bacterium, *Treponema pallidum.* Treatment of syphilis is with antibiotics such as penicillin, tetracycline, or erythromycin.

Venereal disease research laboratory (VDRL) is an antigen serologic test that is used to determine the presence of *Treponema pallidum.*

15.32 ___________ is a venereal disease caused by a bacterium, *Treponema pallidum.*

syphilis (**SIF** ih lis)

EXPLANATION FRAME

Genital warts are caused by the human papilloma virus (HPV). In the male these warts appear as cauliflower-like growths on the penis and perianal area. In the female they appear as cauliflower-like growths around the vagina and perianal area. Treatment choices are: laser surgery, chemotherapy, cryosurgery, and/or cauterization.

15.33 The human papilloma virus (HPV) causes ___________ warts.

genital (**JEN** ih tal)

EXPLANATION FRAME

Trichomonas is a parasitic protozoa that causes trichomoniasis, a sexually transmitted disease (STD).

SYMPTOMS

Male	Usually asymptomatic. Can lead to cystitis, urethritis, prostatitis
Female	White frothy vaginal discharge, burning and itching of vulva. Can lead to cystitis, urethritis, vaginitis
Treatment	Flagyl (metronidazole)

15.34 **True or False**. Trichomoniasis is caused by a protozoon.

true

ANSWER COLUMN

EXPLANATION FRAME

Herpes genitalis is a sexually transmitted disease caused by the herpes simplex virus-2 (HSV-2).

SYMPTOMS OF HERPES GENITALIS DURING THE ACTIVE PHASE ARE

Male	Fluid-filled vesicles (blisters) on penis. Rupture causes acute pain and itching
Female	Blisters in and around vagina
Newborn	Can be infected during vaginal delivery. Severe infection, physical and mental damage
Treatment	Valtrex (valacyclovir) is an antiviral drug that may be used to relieve symptoms of herpes genitalis during the acute phase. There is no cure for this disease

15.35 Valtrex may be used to relieve symptoms of __________ genitalis.

herpes (**HER** peez)

EXPLANATION FRAME

Gonorrhea is a sexually transmitted disease that is caused by a bacterium, *Neisseria gonorrhoeae.* **Symptoms include:**

Male	Purulent urethral discharge, dysuria, urinary frequency
Female	Purulent vaginal discharge, dysuria, urinary frequency, abnormal menstrual bleeding, abdominal tenderness. Can lead to PID and sterility
Treatment	Antibiotics

15.36 Symptoms of gonorrhea in the male include a purulent urethral discharge, __________, and urinary frequency.

dysuria
(dis **YOO** ree ah)

EXPLANATION FRAME

Chlamydia is a sexually transmitted disease caused by the bacterium *Chlamydia trachomatis*. It may be asymptomatic or cause the following **symptoms:**

Male	Mucopurulent discharge from penis, burning, itching in genital area, dysuria, swollen testes. Can lead to sterility
Female	Mucopurulent discharge from vagina, cystitis, pelvic pain, cervicitis. Can lead to pelvic inflammatory disease (PID) and sterility
Treatment	Antibiotics

Answer Column

15.37 __________ is a sexually transmitted disease caused by the bacterium *Chlamydia trachomatis*.

chlamydia (klah **MID** ee ah)

EXPLANATION FRAME

Drugs that are generally used for diseases and disorders of the male reproductive system include androgenic hormones and androgen hormone inhibitors.

Testosterone is the most important androgen, and adequate secretions of this hormone are necessary to maintain normal male sex characteristics, the male libido, and sexual potency.

Proscar (finasteride) is an androgen hormone inhibitor that may be used to help relieve the symptoms of benign prostatic hyperplasia.

15.38 __________ is an androgenic hormone. Its therapeutic use includes primary hypogonadism; to stimulate puberty in carefully selected males, relieve male menopause, and stimulate sperm production in oligospermia; and in cases of impotence due to androgen deficiency.

testosterone (tes **TOSS** ter ohn)

15.39 Side effects of testosterone therapy may include nausea, __________, jaundice, and edema. Another side effect that may occur in the male is frequent or persistent erection of the penis. In the adolescent male a sign of premature epiphyseal closure would be a side effect. The adolescent male who is on testosterone therapy should have bone development checked every 6 months.

vomiting (**VOM** it ing)

15.40 Testosterone therapy may be used in the female when there is advanced inoperable metastatic __________ cancer.

breast (BREST)

15.41 Side effects of testosterone therapy in the female may include hoarseness, acne, changes in __________ periods, and growth of hair on face and/or body.

menstrual (**MEN** stroo al)

ANSWER COLUMN

EXPLANATION FRAME

Anabolic steroids may be abused by individuals who seek to increase muscle mass, strength, and overall athletic ability. This form of use of anabolic (testosterone) is illegal. **Some of the signs of possible abuse include:**

- Flu-like symptoms (sneezing, coughing, rhinorrhea, malaise)
- Headaches
- Muscle aches
- Dizziness
- Bruises

15.42 Signs of possible anabolic steroid abuse include flu-like symptoms, headaches, muscle aches, dizziness, and ___________.

bruises (BROOZES)

15.43 ABBREVIATIONS

Write in the correct abbreviation for the following:

		Answer
___________	benign prostatic hyperplasia (hypertrophy)	**BPH**
___________	gonorrhea	**GC**
___________	dihydrotestosterone	**DHT**
___________	human papilloma virus	**HPV**
___________	herpes simplex virus-2	**HSV-2**
___________	nocturnal penile tumescence	**NPT**
___________	prostate-specific antigen	**PSA**
___________	suprapubic prostatectomy	**SPP**
___________	sexually transmitted diseases	**STDS**
___________	serologic test for syphilis	**STS**
___________	*Treponema pallidum* agglutination (test)	**TPA**
___________	transurethral resection	**TUR**
___________	transurethral resection of the prostate	**TURP**
___________	urogenital	**UG**
___________	venereal disease	**VD**
___________	venereal disease research laboratory (test)	**VDRL**
___________	Wassermann reaction	**WR**

IN THE SPOTLIGHT

ERECTILE DYSFUNCTION

According to the National Institute of Health (NIH), erectile dysfunction (impotence) affects as many as 20 million men in the United States. It was once thought to be an unavoidable result of aging but now is understood to be caused by a variety of factors.

Erectile dysfunction (ED) is the inability to achieve or maintain an erection sufficient for sexual intercourse. It occurs when not enough blood is supplied to the penis, when the smooth muscle in the penis fails to relax, or when the penis does not retain the blood that flows into it. According to studies by NIH, 5% of men have some degree of erecitle dysfunction at age 40 and approximately 15% to 25% at age 65 or older. Although the likelihood of erectile dysfunction increases with age, it is not an inevitable part of aging. About 80 percent of erectile dysfunction has a physical cause.

Some physical causes of erectile dysfunction are:

- *Vascular diseases.* Arteriosclerosis, hypertension, high cholesterol, and other medical conditions can obstruct blood flow.
- *Diabetes.* Can alter nerve function and blood flow to the penis.
- *Prescription drugs.* Certain antihypertensive medications, cardiac medications, antihistamines, psychiatric medications, and other prescription drugs can cause erectile dysfunction.
- *Substance abuse.* Excessive use of tobacco, alcohol, and illegal drugs constrict blood vessels and can cause erectile dysfunction.
- *Neurological diseases.* Multiple sclerosis, Parkinson's disease, Alzheimer's, and other diseases can interrupt nerve impulses to the penis.
- *Surgery.* Prostate, colon, bladder, and other types of pelvic surgery may damage nerves and blood vessels.
- *Spinal injury.* Interruption of nerve impulses from the spinal cord to the penis can cause erectile dysfunction.
- *Other.* Hormonal imbalance, kidney failure, dialysis, and reduced testosterone levels can cause erectile dysfunction. Psychological problems such as depression and stress may also cause erectile dysfunction, as well as social problems such as unhappy relationships.

Erectile dysfunction can affect relationships and men should discuss the issue with their partners and seek medical advice. A medical evaluation is done when a man expresses concerns about his condition with his physician. Any underlying condition causing the problem should be treated.

Treatment may include counseling or sex therapy for men whose erectile dysfunction stems from emotional problems. Treatments for physical causes are based upon the cause. Viagra (sildenafil citrate) is an oral medication that may be prescribed for erectile dysfunction. It increases the body's ability to achieve and maintain an erection during sexual stimulation. It does not protect one from getting sexually transmitted diseases, including HIV. There is a potential for cardiac risk during sexual activity in patients with preexisting cardiovascular disease. Therefore, treatments for erectile dysfunction, including Viagra, generally should not be used in men for whom sexual activity is inadvisable because of their underlying cardiovascular status. The drug is potentially hazardous in those with acute coronary ischemia who are not on nitrates, those who have congestive heart failure, and those with borderline low blood pressure.

CASE STUDY

Please read the following case study and then work frames 15.44–15.48. Write in your answer in the answer column. Check your responses with the answers provided at the end of frame 15.48.

A 58-year-old male was seen by a physician and the following is a synopsis of the visit.

PRESENT HISTORY: The patient states that he is having difficulty with urination. He has a need to urinate often, especially at night, a sense of urgency, and a decrease in size and force of his urinary stream.

SIGNS AND SYMPTOMS: Chief Complaints: frequency, urgency, and decrease in size and force of the urinary stream.

DIAGNOSIS: Benign prostatic hyperplasia.

TREATMENT: Proscar (finasteride) was ordered by the physician to help relieve the symptoms of benign prostatic hyperplasia. It lowers the levels of dihydrotestosterone (DHT), which is a major factor in enlargement of the prostate. Lowering of DHT leads to shrinkage of the enlarged prostate gland in most men. It may take 6 months or more to determine if it is working for an individual. The patient was scheduled for a follow-up visit in 6 months and informed that side effects of Proscar may include impotence and less desire for sex, and that this medication can alter the prostate-specific antigen test (PSA) that is used to screen for prostate cancer.

15.44 The abbreviation DHT means ____________.

15.45 Signs and symptoms of benign prostatic hyperplasia include frequency, ____________, and decrease in size and force of the urinary stream.

15.46 Treatment included ____________ (finasteride).

15.47 Side effects of this medication may include ____________ and less desire for sex.

15.48 This medication can alter the ____________ -specific antigen test that is used to screen for prostate cancer.

CASE STUDY ANSWERS

15.44 dihydrotestosterone
15.45 urgency
15.46 Proscar
15.47 impotence
15.48 prostate

REVIEW A: WORD ELEMENTS

This review allows you to check your knowledge of some of the word elements presented in this unit. In the spaces provided, write the meaning of the word elements that are identified as **Prefix (P), Word Root (R), Combining Form (CF),** and/or **Suffix (S).**

MEDICAL WORD	*WORD ELEMENT*	*MEANING*
1. circumcision	circum (P)	________
	cis (R)	________
	-ion (S)	________
2. balanitis	balan (R)	________
	-itis (S)	________
3. balanoplasty	balan / o (CF)	________
	-plasty (S)	________
4. orchiectomy	orch / i (CF)	________
	-ectomy (S)	________
5. testicular	testicul (R)	________
	-ar (S)	________
6. epididymectomy	epi (P)	________
	didym (R)	________
	-ectomy (S)	________
7. epididymitis	epi (P)	________
	didym (R)	________
	-itis (S)	________
8. vasectomy	vas (R)	________
	-ectomyt (S)	________
9. oligospermia	oligo (P)	________
	sperm (R)	________
	-ia (S)	________
10. prostatectomy	prostat (R)	________
	-ectomy (S)	________
11. epispadias	epi (P)	________
	spadias (R)	________
12. urethral	urethr (R)	________
	-al (S)	________

REVIEW B: MEDICAL TERMS

Please place the correct letter from column II on the appropriate line of column I.

COLUMN I		COLUMN II
___________	1. penis	A. condition of narrowing of the opening of the prepuce
___________	2. prepuce	B. testes fail to descend into the scrotum
___________	3. smegma	C. to remove the testicles or ovaries
___________	4. phimosis	D. enlargement and twisting of the veins of the spermatic cord
___________	5. condom	E. pertaining to or resulting from intercourse
___________	6. cryptorchism	F. the foreskin
___________	7. castrate	G. fluid transporting medium for spermatozoa
___________	8. varicocele	H. thin, flexible protective sheath
___________	9. semen	I. lubricating fluid secreted by glands of the foreskin
___________	10. venereal	J. erectile tissue covered with skin

REVIEW C: SEXUALLY TRANSMITTED DISEASES

Please provide the correct disease or disorder for each of the following descriptions.

1. ___________ is a venereal disease caused by a bacterium, *Treponema pallidum.*
2. ___________ warts are caused by the human papilloma virus (HPV).
3. ___________ is a sexually transmitted disease caused by a parasitic protozoon.
4. ___________ genitalis is a sexually transmitted disease caused by the herpes simplex virus-2 (HSV-2).
5. ___________ is a sexually transmitted disease caused by a bacterium, *Neisseria gonorrhoeae.*

REVIEW D: UNSCRAMBLE THE WORDS

Unscramble the following medical terms and place the correct term on the line directly across from the scrambled word.

1. sitihcor ____________
2. uchneu ____________
3. ulatejcaion ____________
4. mierspedic ____________
5. ismurerth ____________
6. myaidalch ____________
7. heagonrro ____________
8. phisilsy ____________

REVIEW E: DRUGS USED FOR THE MALE REPRODUCTIVE SYSTEM

Please provide the correct answer for each of the following descriptions.

1. Testosterone is an ____________ hormone.
2. Testosterone may be used in the treatment of primary ____________; to stimulate puberty in carefully selected males, relieve male menopause, and stimulate sperm production in oligospermia; and in impotence due to androgen deficiency.
3. ____________ is an androgen hormone inhibitor that may be used to help relieve the symptoms of benign prostatic hyperplasia

REVIEW F: ABBREVIATIONS

Please provide the correct abbreviation and/or meaning for the abbreviation.

1. __________ benign prostatic hyperplasia (hypertrophy)
2. HPV ____________
3. __________ prostate-specific antigen
4. STDs ____________
5. __________ transurethral resection
6. VD ____________

APPENDIX A ANSWER KEY FOR THE REVIEW EXERCISES

■ UNIT 1 INTRODUCTION TO MEDICAL TERMINOLOGY

Review A: Prefixes

	PREFIX	MEANING
1.	ab	away from
2.	ab	away from
3.	ad	toward
4.	anti	against
5.	anti	against
6.	auto	self
7.	cac	bad
8.	centi	one-hundredth
9.	dia	through
10.	micro	small
11.	milli	one-thousandth

Review B: Word Roots and Combining Forms

	ROOT / CF	MEANING
1.	norm	norm, rule
2.	pyret	fever
3.	tuss	cough
4.	nom	law (self-governed)
5.	gastr / o	stomach
	enter / o	intestine
6.	kil / o	a thousand
7.	onc / o	tumor
	log	study of

Review C: Suffixes

	SUFFIX	MEANING
1.	-al	pertaining to
2.	-ic	pertaining to
3.	-ive	nature of, quality of
4.	-y	condition of
5.	-hexia	condition of
6.	-meter	to measure
7.	-gnosis	knowledge
8.	-logy	study of
9.	-gram	weight, mark, record
10.	-gram	weight, mark, record
11.	-gram	weight, mark, record
12.	-ist	one who specializes

Review D: Word Elements that Pertain to Color

1. albin, leuk / o
2. chlor / o
3. cirrh / o
4. cyan / o
5. erythr / o, rube / o
6. melan / o
7. poli / o
8. purpura
9. xanth / o

Review E: Forming Plural Endings of Medical Words

1. ganglia
2. gingivae
3. diagnoses
4. sera
5. phalanges
6. vertebrae
7. thrombi
8. fungi
9. spermatozoa
10. ova

■ UNIT 2 ORGANIZATION OF THE BODY

Review A: Organization of the Body

1. anatomy
2. physiology
3. atom
4. electron
5. proton
6. molecule
7. cells
8. protoplasm
9. tissue
10. system

Review B: Terms Used to Describe Direction

1. E
2. J
3. F
4. B
5. A
6. H
7. I
8. D
9. G
10. C

Review C: Terms Used to Describe Planes of the Body and Body Cavities

1. sagittal
2. transverse
3. coronal
4. ventral
5. thoracic
6. abdominal
7. pelvic
8. dorsal
9. cranial
10. abdominopelvic

Review D: Terms Used to Describe the Nine Regions of the Abdomen

1. right hypochondriac
2. left hypochondriac
3. epigastric
4. right lumbar
5. left lumbar
6. umbilical
7. right iliac, inguinal
8. left iliac, inguinal
9. hypogastric

Review E: Word Elements

1. ana (P) — up
   -tomy (S) — incision
2. physi / o (CF) — nature
   -logy (S) — study of
3. proto (P) — first
   -plasm (S) — a thing formed, plasma
4. hist / o (CF) — tissue
   -logy (S) — study of
5. adip (R) — fat
   -ose (S) — like
6. homeo (P) — same, similar
   -stasis (S) — control, stopping

■ UNIT 3 THE INTEGUMENTARY SYSTEM

Review A: Word Elements

1. covering
   pertaining to
2. upon, above
   skin
3. skin
   inflammation
4. skin
   study of
   one who specializes
5. skin
   study of
6. skin
   instrument to cut
7. red
   skin
8. skin
   pertaining to
9. black
   cancer
   tumor
10. black
    tumor
11. nail
    to eat
12. upon
    nail
    tissue

Review B: Medical Terms

1. E
2. G
3. H
4. B
5. I
6. A
7. J
8. C
9. D
10. F

Review C: Skin Signs

1. macule
2. papule
3. vesicle
4. crust
5. scale

Review D: Unscramble the Words

1. petechiae
2. pruritus
3. dehiscence
4. comedo
5. nevus
6. boil
7. wheal
8. rubeola

Review E: Drugs Used for the Integumentary System

1. keratolytics
2. emollients
3. antipruritic
4. Zovirax

Review F: Abbreviations

1. CC
2. diagnosis
3. Tx
4. history
5. Sx
6. PH

■ UNIT 4 THE SKELETAL SYSTEM

Review A: Word Elements

1. bone
   immature cell, germ cell
2. cartilage
   cells
3. within
   cartilage
   pertaining to
4. cartilage
   pertaining to
5. cartilage
   pain
6. cartilage
   surgical excision
7. cartilage
   disease
   study of
8. bone
   passage
   condition of
9. bone
   cancer
   tumor
10. bone
    bone marrow
    inflammation
11. bone
    softening
12. bone
    instrument to cut

Review B: Medical Terms

1. D
2. G
3. J
4. H
5. A
6. E
7. B
8. F
9. I
10. C

Review C: Types of Body Movements

1. eversion
2. pronation
3. supination
4. extension

Review D: Unscramble the Words

1. foramen
2. meatus
3. tubercle
4. trochanter
5. sinus
6. hallux
7. calcaneal
8. femur

Review E: Drugs Used for the Skeletal System

1. corticosteroids
2. Rheumatrex
3. analgesics
4. antirheumatic

Review F: Abbreviations

1. Ca
2. degenerative joint disease
3. Fx
4. joint
5. LAC
6. LLC
7. osteoarthritis
8. RA
9. short arm cast
10. Tx

■ UNIT 5 THE MUSCULAR SYSTEM

Review A: Word Elements

1. discharge
study of
one who specializes
2. fiber
muscle
inflammation
3. fiber
muscle
pain
4. tendon
pain
5. rod
muscle
tumor
6. difficult
nourishment, development
7. muscle
flesh
tumor
8. muscle
black
condition of
9. muscle
softening
10. muscle
weakness
11. a band
surgical repair

Review B: Medical Terms

1. E
2. G
3. J
4. A
5. C
6. B
7. I
8. D
9. F
10. H

Review C: Types of Exercise

1. active
2. isometric
3. passive
4. range of motion
5. relief of tension

Review D: Unscramble the Words

1. fibers
2. oxygen
3. tonicity
4. triceps
5. atrophy
6. flaccid
7. contracture
8. diaphragm

Review E: Drugs Used for the Muscular System

1. relaxants
2. antirheumatic
3. anti-inflammatory
4. analgesics

Review F: Abbreviations

1. BE
2. below knee
3. EMG
4. intramuscular
5. MD
6. physical therapy

■ UNIT 6 THE NERVOUS SYSTEM

Review A: Word Elements

1. nerve
   study of
2. cranium (skull)
   surgical excision
3. cranium (skull)
   hernia, herniation
4. cranium (skull)
   surgical repair
5. spinal cord
   inflammation
6. spinal cord
   disease
7. gray
   spinal cord
   inflammation
8. half
   paralysis, stroke
9. beside
   paralysis, stroke
10. four
    paralysis, stroke
11. half
    lack of
    eye, vision
12. lack of
    action

Review B: Medical Terms

1. H
2. E
3. F
4. I
5. G
6. B
7. J
8. C
9. D
10. A

Review C: Diseases and Disorders

1. coma
2. concussion
3. Alzheimer's
4. Reye's
5. sciatica

Review D: Unscramble the Words

1. central
2. cerebellar
3. temporal
4. aphasia
5. epilepsy
6. palsy
7. Parkinson's
8. sciatica

Review E: Drugs Used for the Nervous System

1. sedatives
2. hypnotics
3. anticonvulsants
4. anesthetics

Review F: Abbreviations

1. AD
2. amyotrophic lateral sclerosis
3. CNS
4. cerebrovascular accident
5. EEG
6. multiple sclerosis

■ UNIT 7 SPECIAL SENSES

Review A: Word Elements

1. ear
   nose
   larynx
   study of
2. hearing
   pertaining to
3. hearing
   pertaining to
4. to hear
   instrument to measure
5. ear
   inflammation
6. jingling
   pertaining to
7. eye
   study of
8. tear
   pertaining to
9. ciliary body
   stroke, paralysis
10. cornea
    inflammation
11. tone
    instrument to measure
12. eye
    disease

Review B: Medical Terms

1. G
2. D
3. F
4. A
5. B
6. J
7. C
8. I
9. H
10. E

Review C: Diseases and Disorders

1. Meniere's
2. deafness
3. cholesteatoma
4. glaucoma
5. cataract

Review D: Unscramble the Words

1. otodynia
2. endolymph
3. cerumen
4. vertigo
5. myopia
6. chalazion
7. accommodation
8. strabismus

Review E: Drugs Used for the Special Senses

1. antibiotics
2. antihistamines
3. mydriatics
4. antifungal

Review F: Answers

1. EENT
2. AU
3. AD
4. myopia
5. NVA
6. right eye

■ UNIT 8 THE ENDOCRINE SYSTEM

Review A: Word Elements

1. within
   to secrete
   study of
2. gland
   pain
3. gland
   softening
4. phlegm
   condition
5. gland
   deficient, below, under
   growth
6. extremity
   enlargement
7. nerve
   deficient, below, under
   growth
8. out, away from
   eye
   pertaining to
9. excessive, above
   calcium
   blood condition
10. excessive, many, much
    urine
11. excessive, many, much
    to eat

Review B: Medical Terms

1. E
2. J
3. F
4. A
5. B
6. C
7. I
8. D
9. H
10. G

Review C: Diseases and Disorders

1. acromegaly
2. diabetes insipidus
3. Addison's
4. Cushing's
5. diabetes mellitus

Review D: Unscramble the Words

1. adenosis
2. dwarfism
3. gigantism
4. thyrosis
5. tetany
6. insulin
7. cortisol
8. aldosterone

Review E: Drugs Used for the Endocrine System

1. thyroid
2. antithyroid
3. insulin
4. hypoglycemic

Review F: Abbeviations

1. ACTH
2. antidiuretic hormone
3. DI
4. diabetes mellitus
5. PTH
6. vasopressin

■ UNIT 9 THE CARDIOVASCULAR SYSTEM

Review A: Word Elements

1. heart
   study of
2. artery
   hardening
   condition of
3. fatty substance, porridge
   hardening
   condition of
4. heart
   pain
5. muscle
   heart
   pertaining to
6. a throwing in
   condition of
7. heart
   enlargement
8. electricity
   heart
   record
9. vein
   incision

Review B: Medical Terms

1. E
2. D
3. I
4. A
5. J
6. B
7. C
8. F
9. G
10. H

Review C: Diseases and Disorders

1. angina pectoris
2. myocardial infarction
3. cardiomyopathy
4. congestive
5. arrhythmia

Review D: Unscramble the Words

1. harvest
2. myocardium
3. septum
4. carotid
5. bradycardia

Review E: Drugs Used for the Cardiovascular System

1. digitalis
2. antiarrhythmic
3. vasopressors
4. nitrates
5. antihypertensive
6. anticoagulant
7. antilipemic

Review F: Abbreviations

1. BP
2. coronary artery disease
3. CMP
4. congestive heart failure
5. ECG, EKG
6. MI

■ UNIT 10 BLOOD, LYMPH, AND THE IMMUNE SYSTEM

Review A: Word Elements

1. blood
   study of
2. blood
   study
   one who specializes
3. red
   cell
4. many
   cell
   blood condition
5. clot
   surgical excision
6. clot
   destruction
7. white
   cell
8. eat, engulf
   cell
   condition of
9. immunity
   study of

Review B: Medical Terms

1. J
2. I
3. H
4. A
5. G
6. B
7. C
8. E
9. D
10. F

Review C: Diseases and Disorders

1. hemophilia
2. anemia
3. polycythemia
4. leukemia
5. lymphadenopathy

Review D: Unscramble the Words

1. antigen
2. hemoglobin
3. hemorrhage
4. perinicious
5. leukemia

Review E: Drugs Used for Blood, Lymph, and the Immune System

1. anticoagulants
2. antiplatelet
3. thrombolytic
4. hemostatic
5. hematinic
6. epoetin alfa
7. folic acid

Review F: Abbreviations

1. ABO
2. acquired immunodeficiency syndrome
3. RBC
4. Kaposi's sarcoma
5. Hb, Hgb, HGB
6. HIV

■ UNIT 11 THE DIGESTIVE SYSTEM

Review A: Word Elements

1. stomach
   intestine
   study of
2. gums
   inflammation
3. around
   contraction
4. intestine
   inflammation
5. appendix
   inflammation
6. anus, rectum
   study
   one who specializes
7. gall, bile
   bladder
   excision
8. pancreas
   inflammation
9. difficult
   to digest

Review B: Medical Terms

1. E
2. G
3. I
4. A
5. B
6. J
7. C
8. D
9. F
10. H

Review C: Diseases and Disorders

1. esophageal varices
2. esophageal reflux
3. Crohn's
4. cirrhosis
5. volvulus

Review D: Unscramble the Words

1. diarrhea
2. feces
3. enzyme
4. cirrhosis
5. liver

Review E: Drugs Used for the Digestive System

1. antacids
2. laxatives
3. antidiarrheal
4. antiemetics

Review F: Abbreviations

1. BM
2. gallbladder
3. GI
4. hepatitis A virus
5. pc
6. PP

■ UNIT 12 THE RESPIRATORY SYSTEM

Review A: Word Elements

1. nose
   pharynx
   inflammation
2. nose
   surgical repair
3. pharynx
   pain
4. larynx
   surgical excision
5. larynx
   new opening
6. trachea
   inflammation
7. bronchi
   instrument
8. lung
   inflammation
9. lung
   pertaining to
10. dark blue
    condition of
11. below, deficient
    oxygen
    condition of
12. difficult
    breathing

Review B: Medical Terms

1. G
2. E
3. J
4. A
5. I
6. B
7. C
8. D
9. F
10. H

Review C: Diseases and Disorders

1. asthma
2. coryza
3. emphysema
4. empyema
5. atelectasis

Review D: Unscramble the Words

1. pulmonary
2. pneumonia
3. hyaline
4. orthopnea
5. pleurisy
6. sputum
7. tuberculosis
8. artificial

Review E: Drugs Used for the Respiratory System

1. expectorants
2. mucolytics
3. decongestants
4. antitussives

Review F: Abbreviations

1. ARD
2. chronic obstructive pulmonary disease
3. PND
4. respiration
5. SOB
6. tuberculosis

■ UNIT 13 THE URINARY SYSTEM

Review A: Word Elements

1. kidney
   inflammation
2. kidney
   tumor
3. ureter
   surgical repair
4. renal pelvis
   bladder
   inflammation
5. glomeruli
   pertaining to
6. bladder
   surgical excision
7. bladder
   instrument
8. urethra
   pain
9. urethra
   surgical fixation
10. difficult, painful
    urine
11. excessive
    urine
12. urine
    instrument to measure

Review B: Medical Terms

1. F
2. G
3. J
4. I
5. B
6. C
7. A
8. D
9. E
10. H

Review C: Diseases and Disorders

1. renal colic
2. renal failure
3. pyelonephritis
4. glomerulonephritis
5. cystocele

Review D: Unscramble the Words

1. nephropathy
2. bladder
3. urethra
4. void
5. pyuria
6. acetone
7. ketonuria
8. hematuria

Review E: Drugs Used for the Urinary System

1. diuretics
2. antibacterials
3. antiseptics
4. Pyridium

Review F: Abbreviations

1. AGN
2. chronic renal failure
3. GU
4. intravenous pyelogram
5. Na
6. urinalysis

■ UNIT 14 THE FEMALE REPRODUCTIVE SYSTEM

Review A: Word Elements

1. female
study of
2. uterus
pain
3. uterus
surgical excision
4. uterus
inflammation
5. uterus
surgical repair
6. cervix
inflammation
7. month
cessation
8. month
to burst forth
9. difficult
monthly
flow
10. fallopian tube
surgical excision
11. ovary
surgical puncture
12. ovary
surgical fixation

Review B: Medical Terms

1. F
2. J
3. D
4. A
5. H
6. B
7. C
8. E
9. G
10. I

Review C: Diseases and Disorders

1. ovarian cyst
2. vaginitis
3. condyloma
4. bartholinitis
5. fibrocystic

Review D: Unscramble the Words

1. uterine
2. dilation
3. fimbriae
4. laparoscope
5. fertilization
6. conception
7. zygote
8. genitalia

Review E: Drugs Used for the Female Reproductive System

1. estrogen
2. estrogen
3. progestins
4. oral

Review F: Abbreviations

1. AH
2. dilatation and curettage
3. GYN
4. Papanicolaou (smear)
5. PMS
6. TSS

■ UNIT 15 THE MALE REPRODUCTIVE SYSTEM

Review A: Word Elements

1. around
   to cut
   process
2. glans penis
   inflammation
3. glans penis
   surgical repair
4. testicle
   surgical excision
5. testicle
   pertaining to
6. upon
   testis
   surgical excision
7. upon
   testis
   inflammation
8. vessel, duct
   surgical excision
9. scanty
   seed
   condition
10. prostate
    surgical excision
11. upon
    rent, an opening
12. urethra
    pertaining to

Review B: Medical Terms

1. J
2. F
3. I
4. A
5. H
6. B
7. C
8. D
9. G
10. E

Review C: Sexually Transmitted Diseases

1. syphilis
2. genital
3. trichomoniasis
4. herpes
5. gonorrhea

Review D: Unscramble the Words

1. orchitis
2. eunuch
3. ejaculation
4. spermicide
5. urethrism
6. chlamydia
7. gonorrhea
8. syphilis

Review E: Drugs Used for the Male Reproductive System

1. androgenic
2. hypogonadism
3. Proscar

Review F: Abbreviations

1. BPH
2. human papilloma virus
3. PSA
4. sexually transmitted diseases
5. TUR
6. venereal disease

APPENDIX B GLOSSARY OF WORD ELEMENTS

PREFIXES

A

a	no, not, without, lack of
ab	away from
ad	toward, near
ambi	both
an	no, not, without, lack of
ana	up
ant	against
ante	before
anti	against
apo	separation
auto	self

B

bi	two, double
brachy	short
brady	slow

C

cac	bad
cata	down
centi	a hundred
circum	around
con	with, together
contra	against

D

de	down, away from
deca	ten
di(a), dia	through, between
dif	apart, free from, separate
dipl	double
di(s)	two, apart
dys	bad, difficult, painful

E

ec	out, outside, outer
ecto	out, outside, outer
em	in
en	within
end	within, inner
endo	within, inner
ep	upon, over, above
epi	upon, over, above
eu	good, normal
ex	out, away from
exo	out, away from
extra	outside, beyond

H

hemi	half
hetero	different
homeo	similar, same, likeness
hydr	water
hydro	water
hyp	below, deficient
hyper	above, beyond, excessive
hypo	below, under, deficient

I

in	in, into, not
infer	below
infra	below
inter	between
intra	within

M

macro	large
mal	bad
mega	large, great
meso	middle
meta	beyond
micro	small
milli	one-thousandth
mono	one
multi	many, much

N

neo	new
nulli	none

O

olig	little, scanty
oligo	little, scanty

P

pan	all
par	around, beside
para	beside, alongside, abnormal
per	through
peri	around
poly	many, much, excessive
post	after, behind
pre	before
primi	first
pro	before
proto	first
pseudo	false

Q

quadri	four
quint	five

R

retro	backward

S

semi	half
sub	below, under, beneath
super	above, beyond
supra	above, beyond
sym	together
syn	together, with

T

tachy	fast
tetra	four
trans	across
tri	three

U

ultra	beyond
uni	one

■ WORD ROOTS/COMBINING FORMS

A

abdomin	abdomen
abdomin/o	abdomen
abort	to miscarry
absorpt	to suck in
acanth	a thorn
acetabul	vinegar cup
achill/o	Achilles' heel
acid	acid
acoust	hearing
acr	extremity, point
acr/o	extremity, point
aden	gland
aden/o	gland
adhes	stuck to
adip	fat
aer/o	air
agglutinat	clumping

albin	white
albumin	protein
alges	pain
alveol	small, hollow air sac
ambly	dull
ambul	to walk
amni/o	lamb
amputat	to cut through
amyl	starch
andr	man
ang/i	vessel
angin	to choke, quinsy
angi/o	vessel
anis/o	unequal
ankyl	stiffening, crooked, ankle
an/o	anus
anter	toward the front
anthrac	coal
aort	aorta
append	appendix, hang to
appendic	appendix, hang to
appendicul	to hang to
arachn	spider
arter	artery
arteri/o	artery
arthr	joint
arthr/o	joint
artific/i	not natural
atel	imperfect
ather/o	fatty substance, porridge
atri/o	atrium
aud/i	to hear
audi/o	to hear
auditor	hearing
aur	ear
auscultat	listen to
axi	axle
axill	armpit

B

bacter/i	bacteria
balan	glans penis
balan/o	glans penis
bartholin	Bartholin's glands
bil	bile
bil/i	bile, gall
bio	life
blephar	eyelid
blephar/o	eyelid
brach/i	arm
brachi/o	arm
bronch, bronch/i	bronchi
bronchiol	bronchiole
bronch/o	bronchi
bucc	cheek
burs	pouch

C

Calc	calcium
calc/i	calcium
calcane	heel
calciton	calcium
cancer	crab
capn	smoke
carcin	cancer
card	heart
card/i	heart
cardi/o	heart
carp	wrist
caud	tail
caus	heat
celi	abdomen, belly
centr	center
cephal	head
cephal/o	head
cept	receive
cerebell	little brain
cerebr/o	cerebrum
cervic	cervix, neck
cervic/o	cervix, neck
cheil	lip
chem/o	chemical
chlor/o	green
chol	gall, bile
chol/e	gall, bile
choledoch/o	common bile duct
chondr	cartilage
chondr/o	cartilage

chori/o	chorion
choroid/o	choroid
chromo	color
chym	juice
cirrh	orange-yellow
cirrh/o	orange-yellow
cis	to cut
clavicul	little key
cleid/o	clavicle
coagul	to clot
coccyg/o	tailbone
cochle/o	land snail
col	colon
col/i	colon
col/o	colon
coll/a	glue
collis	neck
col/o	colon
colon/o	colon
colp	vagina
colp/o	vagina
concuss	shaken violently
condyle	knuckle
congest	to heap together
con/i	dust
convuls	pulling together
corne	cornea
coron	crown
cortic	cortex
cost	rib
cox	hip
cran/i	skull
crani/o	skull
crine	to secrete
crin/o	to secrete
crur	leg
cry/o	cold
crypt	hidden
cubit	elbow
cubitus	to lie; a lying down
cutane	skin
cyan	dark blue
cycl/o	ciliary body
cyst	bladder, sac
cyst/i	bladder, sac
cyst/o	bladder, sac
cyt	cell
cyth	cell
cyt/o	cell

D

dacry	tear
dacry/o	tear
dactyl/o	finger or toe
dent	tooth
dent/i	tooth
derm	skin
dermat/o	skin
derm/o	skin
dextr/o	to the right
diastol	to expand
didym	testis
dilat	to widen
dist	away from the point of origin and/or attachment
dors	backward
dors/i	backward
duct	to lead
duoden	duodenum
duoden/o	duodenum
dur	dura, hard
dwarf	small

E

eg/o	I, self
electr/o	electricity
embol	to cast, to throw
emet	vomiting
encephal	brain
encephal/o	brain
enter	intestine
enter/o	intestine
eosin/o	rose-colored
episi/o	vulva, pudenda
erg	work
erget	work
erg/o	work

erysi	red
erythr/o	red
esophag	esophagus
esophag/e	esophagus
esophag/o	esophagus
esthet	feeling
eunia	a bed

F

fasc	a band (fascia)
fasc/i	a band (fascia)
fasci/o	a band (fascia)
femor	femur
fibr	fibrous tissue, fiber
fibrin	fibrous tissue, fiber
fibr/o	fibrous tissue, fiber
fibul	fibula
flex	to bend
format	a shaping
front	anterior; forehead
fung	fungus
fus	to pour

G

galact/o	milk
gastr	stomach
gastr/o	stomach
gen	formation, produce
genital	belonging to birth
ger	old age
gest	to carry
gigant	giant
gingiv	gums
gli	glue
glob	globe
globin	globule
glomerul	glomerulus, little ball
glomerul/o	glomerulus, little ball
gloss/o	tongue
glucag	sweet, sugar
gluc/o	sweet, sugar
glyc	glucose, sweet, sugar
glyc/os	sweet, sugar
gonad	seed
gravida	pregnant
gryp	curve
gynec/o	female

H

halat	breathe
halit	breathe
hallux	great (big) toe
hem	blood
hemat	blood
hemat/o	blood
hem/o	blood
hepar	liver
hepat	liver
hepat/o	liver
herni/o	hernia
hidr	sweat
hirsut	hairy
histam	histamine
hist/o	tissue
hol/o	whole
humer	humerus
hyal	glass
hydr	water
hypn	sleep
hypnot	sleep
hyster	womb, uterus
hyster/o	womb,uterus

I

icter	jaundice
ile	ileum
ili	ilium
illus	foot
immun	safe, immunity
immun/o	safe, immunity
infarct	infarct (necrosis of an area)
insul	insulin
insulin	insulin
integument	covering
irid	iris
ischi	ischium
is/o	equal

K

kal	potassium
kary/o	cell's nucleus
kel	tumor
keton	ketone
kerat	horn, cornea
kerat/o	horn, cornea
keton	ketone
kil/o	a thousand
kinet	motion
kyph	a hump

L

labi	lip
labyrinth	maze
labyrinth/o	maze
lacrim	tear
lamin	lamina, thin plate
lapar/o	flank, abdomen
laryng	larynx
laryng/e	larynx
laryng/o	larynx
later	side
laxat	to loosen
lei/o	smooth
lemma	sheath, rind, husk
letharg	drowsiness
leuk	white
leuk/a	white
leuk/o	white
levat	lifter
lingu	tongue
lip	fat
lipid	fat
lip/o	fat
lith	stone
lith/o	stone
lob	lobe
log	study
log/o	word
lord	bending
lumb	loin
lun	moon
lymph	lymph, clear fluid
lymph/o	lymph, clear fluid
lyt	destruction, to separate

M

mamm	breast
mamm/o	breast
mandibul	lower jawbone
man/o	thin
manus	hand
mast	breast
mast/o	breast
maxill	jawbone
meat	passage
medi	toward the middle
medull	marrow
melan	black
melan/o	black
men	month
men/o	month
mening	membrane (meninges)
mening/o	membrane (meninges)
menstruat	to discharge the menses
ment	chin
mes	middle
mester	month
metr	measure, womb, uterus
metr/i	womb, uterus
metr/o	womb, uterus
micturit	to urinate
mnes	memory
muc/o	mucus
mucus	mucus
muscul	muscle
muscul/o	muscle
my	muscle
myc	fungus
mydriat	dilation, widen
myel	bone marrow, spinal cord
myel/o	bone marrow, spinal cord
my/o	muscle
my/os	muscle
myring	drum membrane

myring/o	drum membrane
myx	mucus

N

nas/o	nose
nat	birth
necr	death
necr/o	death
nect	to bind, tie, connect
nephr	kidney
nephr/o	kidney
neur	nerve
neur/o	nerve
nid	nest
noct	night
nom	law
norm	rule
nucle	kernel, nucleus
nyctal	blind

O

occipit	back part of the skull
ocul	eye
olecran	elbow
onc/o	tumor
onych	nail
onych/i	nail
onych/o	nail
o/o	ovum, egg
oophor	ovary
oophor/o	ovary
ophthalm	eye
ophthalm/o	eye
opt	eye
opt/o	eye
or	mouth
orch	testicle
orch/i	testicle
orchid	testicle
orchid/o	testicle
orchi/o	testicle
orig	beginning
orth/o	straight
oscill	to swing
osm	smell
oste	bone
oste/o	bone
ot	ear
ot/o	ear
ovar	ovary
ovar/i	ovary
ovari/o	ovary
ovul	ovary
ox	oxygen
oxy	sour, sharp, acid

P

pachy	thick
pancreat	pancreas
paque	dark
para	to bear
pariet	a wall
partum	labor
patell	kneecap, patella
path	disease
pause	cessation
pect	chest
pector	chest
ped	foot, child
ped/i	foot, child
pedicul	louse
pelvi	pelvis
pen	penis
penile	penis
pept	to digest
perine	perineum
perine/o	perineum
pernic	destructive
phac	lens
phac/o	lens
phag	to eat, engulf
phag/o	to eat, engulf
phak	lentil, lens
phalange	closely knit row
pharyng	pharynx, throat
pharyng/o	pharynx, throat

phe/o	dusky
phim	a muzzle
phleb	vein
phleb/o	vein
phon	voice
phot/o	light
phragm	partition
phras	speech
physi/o	nature
pil/o	hair
pineal	pineal body
pin/o	to drink
pituitar	phlegm
plast	a developing
pleur	pleura
plicat	to fold
pneum/o	lung, air
pneumon	lung
poiet	formation
poli/o	gray
pollen	dust
pollex	thumb
por	passage
porphyr	purple
prand/i	meal
presby	old
press	to press
proct	anus, rectum
proct/o	anus, rectum
prostat	prostate
prostat/o	prostate
prosthesis	an addition
proxim	near the point of origin and/or attachment
prurit	itching
psor	an itching
psych	mind
psych/o	mind
pulm/o	lung
pulmon	lung
pulmon/o	lung
pulmonar	lung
pupill	pupil
purpura	purple
py	pus
pyel	renal pelvis
pyel/o	renal pelvis
pylor	pylorus, gate keeper
py/o	pus
pyret	fever
pyr/o	heat, fire

R

rach	spine
rachi	spine
rachi/o	spine
radi	radius
radic/o	spinal nerve root
radicul	spinal nerve root
radi/o	ray
ras	to scrape
rect/o	rectum
relaxat	to loosen
ren	kidney
ren/o	kidney
respirat	breathing
reticul/o	net
retin	retina
rhabd/o	rod
rheumat	discharge
rheumat/o	discharge
rhin	nose
rhin/o	nose
rhytid	wrinkle
rhytid/o	wrinkle
roent	roentgen
rotat	to turn
rrhyth	rhythm
rube/o	red

S

sacr	sacrum
sagitt	arrow-like
salping	tube, fallopian tube
salping/o	tube, fallopian tube
salpinx	tube, fallopian tube

sarc	flesh
sarc/o	flesh
scapul	shoulder blade
scler	hardening, sclera
scol/i	curvature
scop	to examine
sebace	sebum
seb/o	oil
semin	seed
senil	old
sept	putrefaction
ser/o	whey, serum
sert	to gain
sial	saliva
sider/o	iron
sigmoid	sigmoid colon
sigmoid/o	sigmoid colon
sin/o	a curve
sinus	a hollow curve
somat	body
somn	sleep
son	sound
spadias	a rent, an opening
spastic	convulsive
sperm	seed (sperm)
spermat	seed (sperm)
spermat/o	seed (sperm)
sperm/i	seed (sperm)
sphygm/o	pulse
spin	spine, a thorn
spir/o	breath
splen	spleen
splen/o	spleen
spondyl	vertebra
staped	stirrup
stat	standing still
steat	fat
sten	narrowing
ster	solid structure
stern	sternum
steth	chest
steth/o	chest
stigmat	point
stom	mouth
stomat	mouth
stomat/o	mouth
strict	to draw, to bind
sympath	sympathy
synov	joint fluid
systol	contraction

T

tele	distant
tempor	temples
tendin	tendon
tend/o	tendon
ten/o	tendon
tenon	tendon
tenos	tendon
tens	tension
tentori	tentorium, tent
terat	monster
testicul	testicle
tetan	stretched
thalass	sea
thel/i	nipple
therm	hot, heat
therm/o	hot, heat
thorac	chest
thorac/o	chest
thorax	chest
thromb	clot
thromb/o	clot
thym	thymus, mind, emotion
thym/o	thymus, mind, emotion
thyr	thyroid, shield
thyr/o	thyroid, shield
tibi	tibia
tinnit	a jingling
toc	birth
tom/o	to cut
ton	tone, tension
tonic	tone
ton/o	tone, tension
tonsill	tonsil, almond
top/o	place

torti	twisted
tox	poison
trache	trachea
trache/o	trachea
tract	to draw
trephinat	a bore
trich	hair
trich/o	hair
trigon	trigone
trism	grating
trop	turning
troph	a turning
tubercul	a little swelling
tuss	cough
tympan	eardrum

U

uln	ulna
umbilic	navel
ungu	nail
ur	urine
ure	urinate
urea	urea
uret	urine
ureter	ureter
ureter/o	ureter
urethr	urethra
urethr/o	urethra
urin	urine
urinat	urine
urin/o	urine
ur/o	urine
uter	uterus
uter/o	uterus
uve	uvea

V

vagin	vagina
vag/o	vagus, wandering
varic/o	twisted vein
vas	vessel
vascul	small vessel
vas/o	vessel
vector	a carrier
ven	vein
venere	sexual intercourse
ven/i	vein
ven/o	vein
ventr	near or on the belly side of the body
ventricul	ventricle
vermi	worm
vers	turning
vertebra	vertebra
vesic	bladder
vesicul	vesicle
vir	virus
viril	masculine
viscer	body organs
volunt	will
vuls	to pull

X

xanth/o	yellow
xen	foreign material
xer	dry
xer/o	dry
xiph	sword

Z

zo/o	animal
zoon	life

■ SUFFIXES

-ac	pertaining to
-ad	pertaining to
-age	related to
-al	pertaining to
-algesia	pain
-algia	pain
-ant	forming
-ar	pertaining to
-ary	pertaining to
-ase	enzyme
-asthenia	weakness
-ate	use, action

-betes	to go
-blast	immature cell, germ cell
-cele	hernia, tumor, swelling
-centesis	surgical puncture
-ceps	head
-cide	to kill
-clasia	a breaking
-clysis	injection
-cope	strike, cut
-crit	to separate
-cusis	hearing
-cuspid	point
-cyesis	pregnancy
-cyst	bladder, sac
-cyte	cell
-cytes	cells
-derma	skin
-dermis	skin
-desis	surgical binding
-dipsia	thirst
-drome	a course
-dynia	pain
-ectasis	dilation, dilatation, distention
-ectasy	dilation
-ectomy	surgical excision
-edema	swelling
-emesis	vomiting
-emia	blood condition
-emic	blood condition
-er	relating to, one who
-ergy	work
-esthesia	feeling
-form	shape
-fuge	to flee
-gen	formation, produce
-genes	produce
-genesis	formation, produce
-genic	formation, produce
-globin	protein
-gnosis	knowledge
-graft	pencil
-gram	weight, mark, record
-graph	to write, record
-graphy	recording
-hexia	condition of
-ia	condition of
-iasis	condition of
-ic	pertaining to
-in	chemical, pertaining to
-ine	pertaining to
-ion	process
-ism	condition of
-ist	one who specializes, agent
-itis	inflammation
-ity	condition of
-ive	nature of, quality of
-kinesis	motion
-lalia	to talk
-lemma	a sheath, rind
-lexia	diction
-liter	liter
-lith	stone
-logy	study of
-lymph	clear fluid
-lyse	destruction, to separate
-lysis	destruction, to separate
-malacia	softening
-mania	madness
-megaly	enlargement, large
-meter	instrument to measure, measure
-metry	measurement
-mnesia	memory
-morph	form, shape
-oid	resemble, form
-oma	tumor
-omion	shoulder
-opia	eye, vision
-opsia	eye, vision
-opsy	to view
-or	one who, a doer
-orexia	appetite
-ose	like
-osis	condition of
-ous	pertaining to
-paresis	weakness
-pathy	disease

-penia	lack of, deficiency
-pepsia	to digest
-pexy	surgical fixation
-phagia	to eat
-phasia	to speak
-pheresis	removal
-philia	attraction
-phobia	fear
-phoresis	to carry
-phragm	a fence
-phraxis	to obstruct
-physis	growth
-plasia	formation, produce
-plasm	a thing formed, plasma
-plasty	surgical repair
-plegia	stroke, paralysis
-pnea	breathing
-poiesis	formation
-praxia	action
-ptosis	prolapse, drooping
-ptysis	to spit, spitting
-puncture	to pierce
-rrhage	to burst forth, bursting forth
-rrhagia	to burst forth, bursting forth
-rrhaphy	suture
-rrhea	flow, discharge
-rrhexis	rupture
-scope	instrument
-scopy	to view, examine
-sepsis	decay
-sis	condition of
-some	body
-spasm	tension, spasm, contraction
-stalsis	contraction
-stasis	control, stopping
-staxis	dripping, trickling
-sthenia	strength
-stomy	new opening
-systole	contraction
-taxia	order
-therapy	treatment
-thermy	heat
-tic	pertaining to
-tome	instrument to cut
-tomy	incision
-tone	tension
-tripsy	crushing
-trophy	nourishment, development
-um	tissue
-ure	process
-uresis	to urinate
-uria	urine
-us	pertaining to
-verse	to turn
-y	condition of, pertaining to, process

APPENDIX C ABBREVIATIONS

A

A, Acc	accommodation
AB	abortion
Ab	antibody
ABC	aspiration biopsy cytology
ABGs	arterial blood gases
ABLB	alternate binaural loudness balance
ABO	blood group
ABR	auditory brainstem response
ac	before meals (ante cibum)
AC	air conditioning; anticoagulant
ACG	angiocardiography
ACS	American Cancer Society
ACTH	adrenocorticotropic hormone
AD	right ear (auris dexter); Alzheimer's disease; advance directive
ad lib	as desired; freely
adeno-CA	adenocarcinoma
ADH	antidiuretic hormone (vasopressin)
AE	above the elbow
AF	atrial fibrillation
AFB	acid-fast bacillus (TB organism)
AFP	alpha-fetoprotein
A/G	albumin/globulin ratio
Ag	antigen
AGN	acute glomerulonephritis
AH	abdominal hysterectomy
AHF	antihemophilic factor VIII
AHG	antihemophillic globulin factor VIII
AI	artificial insemination; aortic incompetence
AIDS	acquired immunodeficiency syndrome
AK	above knee
AKA	above-knee amputation
alk phos	alkaline phosphatase
ALL	acute lymphocytic leukemia
ALS	amyotrophic lateral sclerosis
AMA	American Medical Association
AMD	age-related macular degeneration
AMI	acute myocardial infarction
AML	acute myelogenous leukemia
ANS	autonomic nervous system
A&P	auscultation and percussion; anatomy and physiology
AP	anteroposterior
APTT	activated partial thromboplastin time
ARD	acute respiratory disease
ARDS	acute respiratory distress syndrome
ARF	acute renal failure
ARMD	age-related macular degeneration
AS	aortic stenosis; left ear (auris sinistra)
As, Ast, astigm	astigmatism
ASD	atrial septal defect
ASHD	arteriosclerotic heart disease
AST	aspartate aminotransferase
ATN	acute tubular necrosis
AU	both ears (auris unitas)

AV atrioventricular; arteriovenous
AVMs arteriovenous malformations
AVR aortic valve replacement

B

Ba barium
BAC blood alcohol concentration
BaE barium enema
baso basophil
BBB bundle branch block
BC bone conduction
BE below elbow
BG, bG blood sugar
bid twice a day
BIN, bin twice a night
BK below knee
BKA below-knee amputation
BM bowel movement
BMR basal metabolic rate
BNO bladder neck obstruction
BP blood pressure
BPH benign prostatic hyperplasia (hypertrophy)
BS bowel sounds
BSE breast self-examination
BT bleeding time
BUN blood urea nitrogen
Bx biopsy

C

c̄ with (cum)
C1, C2, etc. first cervical vertebra; second cervical vertebra
CA cancer
Ca calcium
CAD coronary artery disease
cap capsule
cath catheterization; catheter
CBC complete blood count
cc cubic centimeter
CC cardiac catheterization; chief complaint; clean catch
CCU coronary care unit
CDC Centers for Disease Control and Prevention
CDH congenital dislocation of the hip
CEA carcinoembryonic antigen
CGN chronic glomerulonephritis
CHD coronary heart disease
CHF congestive heart failure
Ci curie
Cib food (cibus)
CIS carcinoma in situ
CK creatine kinase
Cl chlorine
CLL chronic lymphocytic leukemia
cm centimeter
CML chronic myelogenous leukemia
CMP cardiomyopathy
CNS central nervous system
c/o complains of
CO_2 carbon dioxide
COLD chronic obstructive lung disease
COPD chronic obstructive pulmonary disease
CP cerebral palsy
CPD cephalopelvic disproportion
CPK creatine phosphokinase
CPR cardiopulmonary resuscitation
CR computerized radiography
CRF chronic renal failure
C&S culture and sensitivity
CS, C-section cesarean section
CSF cerebrospinal fluid
CTS carpal tunnel syndrome
CT computerized tomography
CUC chronic ulcerative colitis
CV cardiovascular
CVA cerebrovascular accident (stroke)
CVD cerebrovascular disease
CVS chorionic villus sampling
CWP childbirth without pain
CXR chest x-ray film; chest radiograph
cysto cystoscopic examination

D

/d per day
D diopter
dB decibel

D&C	dilation, dilatation and curettage
dc	discontinue
DC	discharge
DDS	Doctor of Dental Surgery
D&E	dilation and evacuation
decub	decubitus
derm	dermatology
DHT	dihydrotestosterone
DI	diabetes insipidus; diagnostic imaging
diff	differential count (white blood cells)
dil	dilute; diluted
DJD	degenerative joint disease
DM	diabetes mellitus
DNA	deoxyribonucleic acid
DNR	do not resuscitate
DO	doctor of osteopathy
DOA	dead on arrival
DOB	date of birth
DRE	digital rectal examination
DRGs	diagnostic related groups
DSA	digital subtraction angiography
DTaP	diphtheria, tetanus, and pertussis (vaccine)
DTRs	deep tendon reflexes
DUB	dysfunctional uterine bleeding
DVT	deep vein thrombosis
Dx	diagnosis

E

EBV	Epstein-Barr virus
ECF	extracellular fluid; extended care facility
ECG, EKG	electrocardiogram
ECHO	echocardiogram
ECT	electroconvulsive therapy
EDC	estimated date of confinement
EEG	electroencephalogram; electroencephalograph
EENT	eye, ear, nose, and throat
EGD	esophagogastroduodenoscopy
EM	emmetropia
EMG	electromyography
ENT	ear, nose, and throat
EOM	extraocular movement
eos, eosin	eosinophil
ERCP	endoscopic retrograde cholangiopancreatography
ERT	estrogen replacement therapy
ESL, ESWL	extracorporeal shock-wave lithotripsy
ESR, SR, sed rate	erythrocyte sedimentation rate; sedimentation rate
ESRD	end-stage renal disease
EST	electroshock therapy
ET	esotropia

F

F	Fahrenheit
FACP	Fellow, American College of Physicians
FACS	Fellow, American College of Surgeons
FBS	fasting blood sugar
FDA	Food and Drug Administration
FEF	forced expiratory flow
FEKG	fetal electrocardiogram
FEV	forced expiratory volume
FH	family history
FHR	fetal heart rate
FHT	fetal heart tone
FS	frozen section
FSH	follicle-stimulating hormone
FTND	full-term normal delivery
FUO	fever of undetermined origin
FVC	forced vital capacity
Fx	fracture

G

g	gram
GB	gallbladder
GC	gonorrhea
GCSF	granulocyte colony-stimulating factor
GERD	gastroesophageal reflux disease
GH	growth hormone
GI	gastrointestinal
GOT	glutamic oxaloacetic transaminase (AST)
GPT	glutamic pyruvic transaminase (ALT)
gr	grain
GTT	glucose tolerance test
gtt	drops (guttae)

GU	genitourinary
GYN	gynecology

H

h	hour
H	hypodermic; hydrogen
HAV	hepatitis A virus
HBV	hepatitis B virus
HCG	human chorionic gonadotropin
HCl	hydrochloric acid
HCO	bicarbonate
HCT, Hct	hematocrit
HD	hip disarticulation; hemodialysis; hearing distance
HDL	high-density lipoprotein
HDN	hemolytic disease of the newborn
HEENT	head, eyes, ears, nose, and throat
Hg	mercury
HGB, Hgb, Hb	hemoglobin
HIV	human immunodeficiency virus
HMD	hyaline membrane disease
HNP	herniated nucleus pulposus (herniated disk)
HPV	human papilloma virus
HRT	hormone replacement therapy
hs	at bedtime
HSG	hysterosalpingography
HSV-2	herpes simplex virus-2
HT	hypermetropia (hyperopia)
Hx	history
hypo	hypodermically

I

IAS	interatrial septum
IBS	irritable bowel syndrome
IC	interstitial cystitis
ICF	intracellular fluid
ICP	intracranial pressure
ICSH	interstitial cell-stimulating hormone
ICU	intensive care unit
I&D	incision and drainage
ID	intradermal
IDDM	insulin-dependent diabetes mellitus
Ig	immunoglobulin
IH	infectious hepatitis
IM	intramuscular
inj	injection
I&O	intake and output
IOP	intraocular pressure
IPPB	intermittent positive-pressure breathing
IQ	intelligence quotient
IRDS	infant respiratory distress syndrome
IS	intercostal space
ITP	idiopathic thrombocytopenia purpura
IU	international unit
IUD	intrauterine device
IUGR	intrauterine growth rate; intrauterine growth retardation
IV	intravenous
IVC	inferior vena cava; intravenous cholangiography
IVF	in vitro fertilization
IVP	intravenous pyelogram
IVS	interventricular septum

J

J	joule
jt	joint

K

K^+	potassium (an electrolyte)
KD	knee disarticulation
kg	kilogram
KS	Kaposi's sarcoma
KUB	kidney, ureter, and bladder

L

L, 1	liter
L1, L2, etc.	first lumbar vertebra, second lumbar vertebra, etc.
L, lt	left
L&A	light and accommodation
LA	left atrium
lab	laboratory
LAC	long arm cast
LAT, lat	lateral

LB	large bowel
lb	pound
LD	lactate dehydrogenase
LDL	low-density lipoprotein
LE	lupus erythematosus; lower extremity; left eye
LH	luteinizing hormone
liq	liquid; fluid
LLC	long leg cast
LLQ	lower left quadrant
LMP	last menstrual period
LP	lumbar puncture
LPN	licensed practical nurse
LRQ	lower right quadrant
LUQ	left upper quadrant
LV	left ventricle
lymphs	lymphocytes

M

M	molar; thousand; muscle
m	male; meter; minim
MCH	mean corpuscular hemoglobin
MCHC	mean corpuscular hemoglobin concentration
MCV	mean corpuscular volume
MD	medical doctor; muscular dystrophy
mEq	milliequivalent
mets	metastases
MG	myasthenia gravis
mg	milligram (0.001 gram)
MH	marital history
MI	myocardial infarction; mitral insufficiency
mix astig	mixed astigmatism
mL, ml	milliliter (0.001 liter)
mm	millimeter (0.001 meter; 0.039 inch)
mMol	millimole
MMR	measles, mumps, and rubella (vaccine)
mol wt	molecular weight
mono	monocyte
MRI	magnetic resonance imaging
MS	mitral stenosis; multiple sclerosis; musculoskeletal
MSH	melanocyte-stimulating hormone
mV	millivolt
MVP	mitral valve prolapse
MY	myopia

N

n	nerve
Na	sodium
NB	newborn
nCi	nanocurie
NIDDM	noninsulin-dependent diabetes mellitus
NMR	nuclear magnetic resonance
NPH	nonprotein nitrogen
NPO, npo	nothing by mouth (nulla per os)
NPT	nocturnal penile tumescence
NSAIDs	nonsteroidal anti-inflammatory drugs
NVA	near visual acuity

O

O	pint
O_2	oxygen
OA	osteoarthritis
OB	obstetrics
OB-GYN	obstetrics and gynecology
OCPs	oral contraceptive pills
OD	right eye (oculus dexter); overdose
od	once a day
OHS	open heart surgery
OM	otitis media
OR	operating room
ORTH, ortho	orthopedics; orthopaedics
OS	left eye (oculus sinister)
os	mouth opening; bone
OTC	over the counter
oto	otology
OU	both eyes (oculi unitas); each eye (oculus uterque)
OV	office visit
oz	ounce

P

P	pulse; phosphorus
PA	posteroanterior; pernicious anemia
PAC	premature arterial contraction

Pap	Papanicolaou (smear)
PAT	paroxysmal atrial tachycardia
Path	pathology
PBI	protein bound iodine
pc	after meals (post cibum)
PCP	*Pneumocystis carinii* pneumonia
PCV	packed cell volume
PD	peritoneal dialysis
PDR	*Physicians' Desk Reference*
PE	physical examination
PERRLA	pupils equal, regular, react to light, and accommodation
PET	positron emission tomography
PFT	pulmonary function test
PH	past history
pH	hydrogen ion concentration, degree of acidity
PID	pelvic inflammatory disease
PKU	phenylketonuria
PM, pm	afternoon, evening
PMH	past medical history
PMI	point of maximal impulse
PMP	previous menstrual period
PMS	premenstrual syndrome
PND	paroxysmal nocturnal dyspnea; postnasal drip
PNS	peripheral nervous system
PO, po	orally, by mouth (per os)
PP	postprandial (after meals)
PPD	purified protein derivative (TB test)
PPIs	proton pump inhibitors
pr	per rectum
prn	as necessary, as required, when necessary
PSA	prostate-specific antigen
PT	physical therapy; prothrombin time
pt	patient; pint
PTCA	percutaneous transluminal coronary angiography
PTH	parathormone
PTS	permanent threshold shift
PTT	partial thromboplastin time
PUD	peptic ulcer disease
PVC	premature ventricular contraction
PVD	peripheral vascular disease

Q

q	every
qam, qm	every morning
qd	every day (quaque die)
qh	every hour
q2h	every 2 hours
qid	four times a day
qns	quantity not sufficient
qpm, qn	every night
qs	quantity sufficient
qt	quart

R

R	respiration
R, rt	right
RA	right atrium; rheumatoid arthritis
rad	radiation absorbed dose
RAI	radioactive iodine
RAIU	radioactive iodine uptake
RBC	red blood cell; red blood cell (count)
RD	respiratory disease
RDS	respiratory distress syndrome
RE	right eye
REM	rapid eye movement
Rh	Rheseus blood (factor)
RLQ	right lower quadrant
RN	registered nurse
RNA	ribonucleic acid
R/O	rule out
ROM	range of motion
RP	retrograde pyelogram
RPM	revolutions per minute
RQ	respiratory quotient
RT	radiation therapy
RUQ	right upper quadrant
RV	right ventricle
Rx	take thou; prescribe; treatment; therapy

S

$\bar{s}$	without
SA, S-A	sinoatrial (node)
SAC	short arm cast

SAH	subarachnoid hemorrhage
SALT	serum alanine aminotransferase
SAST	serum aspartate aminotransferase
SC, sc, subq	subcutaneous
SD	shoulder disarticulation; standard deviation
seg, poly	polymorphonuclear neutrophil
SH	serum hepatitis
sh	shoulder
SIDS	sudden infant death syndrome
SK	streptokinase
SLE	systemic lupus erythematosus
SOB	shortness of breath
SOM	serous otitis media
sono	sonogram, sonography
SOP	standard operating procedure
sp gr, SG	specific gravity
SPP	suprapubic prostatectomy
SR	sedimentation rate
ss	one half
ST	esotropia
staph	staphylococcus
stat	immediately
STDs	sexually transmitted diseases
STH	somatotropin hormone
strep	streptococcus
STS	serologic test for syphilis
subcu, subq	subcutaneous
SVC	superior vena cava
SVD	spontaneous vaginal delivery
Sx	signs, symptoms
syr	syrup

T

T	temperature
T1, T2, etc.	thoracic vertebrae first, thoracic vertebrae second, etc.
T_3	triiodothyronine
T_4	thyroxine
T&A	tonsillectomy and adenoidectomy
tab	tablet
TAH	total abdominal hysterectomy
TB	tuberculosis
TENS	transcutaneous electrical nerve stimulation
THA	total hip arthroplasty
THR	total hip replacement
TIAs	transient ischemic attacks
tid	three times a day
TJ	triceps jerk
TKA	total knee arthroplasty
TKR	total knee replacement
TLC	tender loving care; total lung capacity
TMJ	temporomandibular joint
TNM	tumor, nodes, metastasis
top	topically
TPA	*Treponema pallidum* agglutination (test)
TPA, tPA	tissue plasminogen activator
TPN	total parenteral nutrition
TPR	temperature, pulse, respiration
tr, tinct	tincture
TSE	testicular self-exam
TSH	thyroid stimulating hormone
TSS	toxic shock syndrome
TTH	thyrotropic hormone
TTS	temporary threshold shift
TUR	transurethral resection
TURP	transurethral resection of the prostate
Tx	traction; treatment; transplant

U

U	units
UA	urinalysis
UC	uterine contractions
UG	urogenital
UGI	upper gastrointestinal
U&L, U/L	upper and lower
ULQ	upper left quadrant
ung	ointment
URI	upper respiratory infection
URQ	upper right quadrant
USP	United States Pharmacopeia
UTI	urinary tract infection
UV	ultraviolet

V

v	vein
VA	visual acuity
VC	vital capacity
VCG	vectorcardiogram
VCU, VCUG	voiding cystourethrogram
VD	venereal disease
VDRL	venereal disease research laboratory (syphilis test)
VF	visual field
VHD	ventricular heart disease
VLDL	very-low-density lipoprotein
vol	volume
vol %	volume percent
VP	vasopressin
VSD	ventricular septal defect
VT	ventricular tachycardia

W

WBC	white blood cell; white blood cell (count)
WDWN	well developed, well nourished
WR	Wassermann reaction
wt	weight
w/v	weight by volume

X

x	multiplied by
XM	cross match for blood (type and cross match)
XP	xeroderma pigmentosum
XR	x-ray
XT	exotropia
XX	female sex chromosomes
XY	male sex chromosomes

Y

YAG	yttrium-aluminum-garnet (laser)
YOB	year of birth
yr	year

Z

z	atomic number

■ CHARTING ABBREVIATIONS AND SYMBOLS

$\overline{aa}$	of each
ac	before meals (ante cibum)
AD	right ear (auris dextra)
ADL	activities of daily living
ad lib	as desired
adm	admission
AE	above the elbow
AJ	ankle jerk
AK	above knee
ALT	alanine aminotransferase
alt dieb	every other day
alt hor	every other hour
alt noc	every other night
AM, am	before noon (ante meridiem); morning
AMA	against medical advice
AMB	ambulate; ambulatory
ant	anterior
AP	anteroposterior
A-P	anterior-posterior
approx	approximately
AQ, aq	water
ASAP	as soon as possible
AS, LE	left ear (auris sinistra)
AV	atrioventricular
BE	below elbow
bid	twice a day
bin	twice a night
BK	below knee
BM	bowel movement
BMR	basal metabolic rate
BRP	bathroom privileges
C	Centigrade, Celsius, or calorie (kilocalorie)
caps	capsules
CBR	complete bed rest
CC	chief complaint; clean catch (urine)
CCU	cardiac (coronary) care unit
c/o	complains of

cont	continue
D	diopter
DC	discharge from hospital
dc	discontinue
DNA	does not apply
DNR	do not resuscitate
DNS	did not show
Dr	doctor
D/W	dextrose in water
Dx	diagnosis
EOM	extraocular movement
ER	emergency room
Ex	examination
F	Fahrenheit
FHS	fetal heart sounds
FHT	fetal heart tones
GB	gallbladder
GI	gastrointestinal
GU	genitourinary
h, hr	hour
hpf	high power field
hs	hour of sleep; bedtime (hora somni)
hypo	hypodermic injection
ICU	intensive care unit
IM	intramuscular
I&O	intake and output
IU	international unit
IV	intravenous
L	left
L&A	light and accommodation
LAT	lateral
LLQ	left lower quadrant
LMP	last menstrual period
LOA	left occipitoanterior
LPF	low power field (10x)
LUQ	left upper quadrant
L&W	living and well
MTD	right eardrum (membrana tympani dexter)
MTS	left eardrum (membrana tympani sinister)
neg	negative
NG	nasogastric
NPO	nothing by mouth
NS	normal saline
OD	right eye (oculus dexter)
OP	outpatient
OR	operating room
OS or OL	left eye (oculus sinister, oculus laevus)
OU	each eye (oculus uterque)
P	pulse
PA	posteroanterior
pc	after meals (post cibum)
PI	present illness
PO	postoperative
po	by mouth (per os)
PM, pm	afternoon or evening (post meridiem)
prn	as necessary, as required, when necessary
q	every (quaque)
qd	every day (quaque die)
qh	every hour (quaque hora)
q2h	every 2 hours
q4h	every 4 hours
qid	four times a day (quarter in die)
qm	every morning (quaque mane)
qn	every night (quaque nocte)
R	right; respiration
RBC	red blood cell (count)
Rh	Rhesus blood factor (Rh + or Rh -)
RLQ	right lower quadrant
R/O	rule out
ROM	range of motion; read only memory
RUQ	right upper quadrant
SC, sc, subq	subcutaneous
SOB	shortness of breath
SOS	if necessary (si opus sit)
stat	immediately
Sx	signs, symptoms
T, temp	temperature
tabs	tablets
TC&DB	turn, cough, deep breathe
tid	three times a day
tinct	tincture
TPN	total parenteral nutrition

trans	transverse
ULQ	upper left quadrant
ung	ointment
URQ	upper right quadrant
VS	vital signs
WBC	white blood cell (count)
WM, BM	white male, black male
WF, BF	white female, black female
x	times, power
–	negative
+	positive
F	female
M	male
+/–	positive or negative
*	birth
†	death
%	percent
#	number; pound
&	and
<	less than
=	equal
>	greater than
?	question
@	at
^	increase
™	trade mark
©	copyright
®	registered
¶	paragraph

APPENDIX D LIST OF TABLES AND FIGURES INCLUDED IN THE TEXT

TABLE 2–1	Elements Found in the Human Body
FIGURE 2–1.	The human body: levels of organization.
FIGURE 2–2.	Cells may be described as the basic building blocks of the human body. They have many different shapes and vary in size and function. These examples show the range of forms and sizes with the dimensions they would have if magnified approximately 500 times.
FIGURE 2–3.	Organ systems of the body with major functions.
FIGURE 2–4.	Planes of the body: coronal or frontal, transverse, and midsagittal.
FIGURE 2–5.	Body cavities.
FIGURE 2–6.	The nine regions of the abdominopelvic cavity.
FIGURE 2–7.	The four regions of the abdomen that are referred to as quadrants.
TABLE 3–1	The Integumentary System
FIGURE 3–1.	The integument: the epidermis, dermis, subcutaneous tissue, and its appendages.
FIGURE 3–2.	Melanoma. (Courtesy of Jason L. Smith, M.D.)
FIGURE 3–3.	Melanoma, forearm. (Courtesy of Jason L. Smith, M.D.)
FIGURE 3–4.	The fingernail, an appendage of the integument.
FIGURE 3–5.	Onychomycosis. (Courtesy of Jason L. Smith, M.D.)
FIGURE 3-6.	Hyperhidrosis. (Courtesy of Jason L. Smith, M.D.)
FIGURE 3–7.	Acne. (Courtesy of Jason L. Smith, M.D.)
FIGURE 3–8.	Skin signs are objective evidence of an illness or disorder. They can be seen, measured, or felt.
FIGURE 3–9.	Pediculosis capitis. (Courtesy of Jason L. Smith, M.D.)
FIGURE 3–10.	Psoriasis, back. (Courtesy of Jason L. Smith, M.D.)
FIGURE 3–11.	Varicella (chickenpox). (Courtesy of Jason L. Smith, M.D.)
FIGURE 3–12.	Keloid. (Courtesy of Jason L. Smith, M.D.)
FIGURE 3–13.	Wound dehiscence, back. (Courtesy of Jason L. Smith, M.D.)
FIGURE 3–14.	Nevus (mole). (Courtesy of Jason L. Smith, M.D.)
FIGURE 3–15.	Carbuncles. (Courtesy of Jason L. Smith, M.D.)
FIGURE 3–16.	Verrucae (warts). (Courtesy of Jason L. Smith, M.D.)
FIGURE 3–17.	Urticaria (hives). (Courtesy of Jason L. Smith, M.D.)
FIGURE 3–18.	Burn, second degree. (Courtesy of Jason L. Smith, M.D.)
FIGURE 3–19.	Male pattern alopecia. (Courtesy of Jason L. Smith, M.D.)

TABLE 4–1 The Skeletal System
FIGURE 4–1. Epiphyseal plate (arrows). (Courtesy of Teresa Resch.)
FIGURE 4–2. The skeleton can be divided into two main groups of bones: the axial and the appendicular skeleton.
FIGURE 4–3. The principal bones of the appendicular skeleton.
FIGURE 4–4. The parts of a long bone.
FIGURE 4–5. Types of body movements.
FIGURE 4–6. Abnormal curvatures of the spine: (A) kyphosis, (B) lordosis, (C) scoliosis.
FIGURE 4–7. Various types of fractures.
FIGURE 4–8. Vertebral regions, showing the four spinal curves.
FIGURE 4–9. The male pelvis is shaped like a funnel forming a narrower outlet than the female (A). The female pelvis is shaped like a basin (B).

TABLE 5–1 Selected Skeletal Muscles (Anterior View)
TABLE 5–2 Selected Skeletal Muscles (Posterior View)
TABLE 5–3 The Muscular System
FIGURE 5–1. Types of muscle tissue.
FIGURE 5–2. Selected skeletal muscles (anterior view).
FIGURE 5–3. Selected skeletal muscles and the Achilles tendon (posterior view).
FIGURE 5–4. A skeletal muscle consists of a group of fibers held together by connective tissue. It is enclosed in a fibrous sheath (fascia).

TABLE 6–1 The Nervous System
TABLE 6–2 Cranial Nerves and Functions
TABLE 6–3 Major Regions of the Brain and Their Functions
FIGURE 6–1. The nervous system is described as having two interconnected divisions: the central nervous system (CNS) consisting of the brain and spinal cord, and the peripheral nervous system (PNS) consisting of peripheral nerves.
FIGURE 6–2. The relationship of the 12 cranial nerves to specific regions of the brain.
FIGURE 6–3. The major regions of the brain.
FIGURE 6–4. The brain, its lobes, and principal sulci. The location of certain sensory and motor areas are shown.
FIGURE 6–5. The brain, spinal cord, and spinal nerves. An expanded view of a spinal nerve is shown.

TABLE 7–1 Special Senses: The Ear
TABLE 7–2 Special Senses: The Eye
FIGURE 7–1. The ear and its anatomic structures.
FIGURE 7–2. The cochlea.
FIGURE 7–3. The lacrimal apparatus and its anatomic structures.
FIGURE 7–4. The eyeball and its anatomic structures.
FIGURE 7–5. The Snellen eye chart. Individuals with normal vision can read line 8 of a full-sized chart at 20 feet (6.10 meters).

TABLE 8–1 The Endocrine System
TABLE 8–2 Summary of the Endocrine Glands, Hormones, and Hormone Functions

FIGURE 8–1. The primary glands of the endocrine system.
FIGURE 8–2. The thymus gland. Appearance and position (A), with anatomic structures (B).

TABLE 9–1 The Cardiovascular System
FIGURE 9–1. The conduction system of the heart. Action potentials for the SA and AV nodes, other parts of the conduction system, and the atrial and ventricular muscles are shown along with the correlation to recorded electrical activity (electrocardiogram-ECG/EKG).
FIGURE 9–2. The primary pulse points of the body.
FIGURE 9–3. Blood vessels: (A) normal artery, (B) constriction, (C) arteriosclerosis and atherosclerosis.
FIGURE 9–4. Coronary circulation. (A) Coronary vessels portraying the complexity and extent of the coronary circulation. (B) Coronary vessels that supply the anterior surface of the heart.
FIGURE 9–5. Sphygmomanometers: (A) aneroid type, (B) mercury type.
FIGURE 9–6. Uncontrolled hypertension can lead to kidney failure, stroke, heart attack, peripheral artery disease, and eye damage.
FIGURE 9–7. Hemangioma. (Courtesy of Jason L. Smith, M.D.)
FIGURE 9–8. Sclerosing hemangioma. (Courtesy of Jason L. Smith, M.D.)
FIGURE 9–9. A normal electrocardiogram (ECG/EKG).

TABLE 10–1 Blood and the Lymphatic System
TABLE 10–2 Types of Blood Cells and Functions
FIGURE 10–1. Traumatic hematoma. (Courtesy of Jason L. Smith, M.D.)
FIGURE 10–2. Hemorrhage, vein. (Courtesy of Jason L. Smith, M.D.)
FIGURE 10–3. The formed elements of blood: erythrocytes, leukocytes (neutrophils, eosinophils, basophils, lymphocytes, and monocytes), and thrombocytes (platelets).
FIGURE 10–4. The lymphatic system.
FIGURE 10–5. Lymphoma. (Courtesy of Jason L. Smith, M.D.)
FIGURE 10–6. Cutaneous T-cell lymphoma. (Courtesy of Jason L. Smith, M.D.)
FIGURE 10–7. The tonsils, lymph nodes, thymus, spleen, and lymphatic vessels with an expanded view of a lymph node.
FIGURE 10–8. Kaposi's sarcoma. (Courtesy of Jason L. Smith, M.D.)
FIGURE 10–9. Kaposi's sarcoma. (Courtesy of Jason L. Smith, M.D.)

TABLE 11–1 The Digestive System
FIGURE 11–1. The digestive system.
FIGURE 11–2. The oral cavity: (A) sagittal section, (B) anterior view as seen through the open mouth.
FIGURE 11–3. Gallbladder ultrasound. (Courtesy of Teresa Resch.)
FIGURE 11–4. Volvulus.
FIGURE 11–5. Peptic ulcer disease (PUD).
FIGURE 11–6. Upper GI series. (Courtesy of Teresa Resch.)

TABLE 12–1 The Respiratory System
FIGURE 12–1. The respiratory system: nasal cavity, pharynx, larynx, trachea, bronchus, and lung with expanded views of the trachea and alveolar structure.

FIGURE 12–2. The nose, nasal cavity, and pharynx: (A) nasal cartilages and external structures, (B) meatuses and positions of the entrance to the ethmoid and maxillary sinuses, (C) sagittal section of the nasal cavity and pharynx.

FIGURE 12–3. The larynx, trachea, bronchi, and lungs with an expanded view showing the structures of an alveolus and the pulmonary blood vessels.

TABLE 13–1 The Urinary System

FIGURE 13–1. The urinary system: kidneys, ureters, bladder, and urethra with expanded views of a nephron and the urine filled space within a bladder.

FIGURE 13–2. The kidney with an expanded view of a nephron.

FIGURE 13–3. Ultrasound liver and right kidney. (Courtesy of Teresa Resch.)

FIGURE 13–4. The organs of the urinary system with major functions.

TABLE 14–1 The Female Reproductive System

FIGURE 14–1. The female reproductive system: vagina, uterine (fallopian) tube, ovary, uterus, and external genitalia.

FIGURE 14–2. The uterus, ovaries, and associated structures with an expanded view of a mammalian ovary showing stages of graafian follicle and ovum development.

FIGURE 14–3. Ultrasonogram showing a male fetus. (Courtesy of Nancy West.)

FIGURE 14–4. Sagittal section of the female pelvis, showing organs of the reproductive system.

FIGURE 14–5. The breast and its structures.

FIGURE 14–6. Normal mammogram. (Courtesy of Teresa Resch.)

FIGURE 14–7. Mammogram showing cancer with microcalcifications. (Courtesy of Teresa Resch.)

FIGURE 14–8. Breast self-examination.

TABLE 15–1 The Male Reproductive System

FIGURE 15–1. The male reproductive system: seminal vesicles, prostate, urethra, sperm duct, epididymis, and external genitalia.

FIGURE 15–2. Sagittal section of the male pelvis, showing the organs of the reproductive system.

FIGURE 15–3. The basic structure of a spermatozoon (sperm).

FIGURE 15–4. The structures of the bladder, prostate gland, and penis.

INDEX

A

A/G, 308
AAFP, 245
AAP, 244
abbreviations pertaining to the,
  blood, lymph and the immune
    system, 244
  cardiovascular system, 220
  digestive system, 267–268
  endocrine system, 191
  female reproductive system, 337
  integumentary system, 63
  male reproductive system, 361
  muscular system, 116
  nervous system, 142
  respiratory system, 287–288
  skeletal system, 92
  special senses, 167
  urinary system, 308
abdomen, 23, 35
  regions of, 34*f*
abdominal cavity, 32
abdominal respiration, 284
abdominopelvic cavity, 33*f*, 34
  regions of, 34*f*
abducens nerve (VI), 129
abduct, 12, 16
abduction, 81
abnormal, 5, 10
ABO, 244
abrasion, 60
absorption, 251, 254, 259
accessory glands, 345
accessory nerve (XI), 129
accessory organs, 254
accommodation, 164
acetone, 306
Achilles tendinitis, 117
Achilles tendon, 103*f*, 117
ACIP, 244
acne, 52, 52*f*
acne vulgaris, 63
acoustic, 151
acoustic nerve (VIII), 129
acroarthritis, 87
acromegaly, 182
acromion, 87
ACTH, 191
Activase, 209
active exercise, 113
active immunization, 244
acyclovir, 62
AD, 142, 158
addisonian crisis, 192
Addison's disease, 188
adduct, 12, 16
adduction, 83
adenalgia, 180
adenectomy, 180
adenodynia, 180
adenohypophysis, 182
adenoma, 180
adenomalacia, 180
adenosclerosis, 180
adenosis, 180
ADH, 183, 191
adipose, 28
adrenal, 187, 188
adrenal glands, 187, 188
adrenal medulla, 189
adrenalectomy, 188
adrenocorticotropin hormone
    (ACTH), 177
adrenopathy, 188
adrenotropic, 188
adult stem cells, 338
aerobic exercise, 113
aeropleura, 283
aerothorax, 283
age-related osteoporosis, 93
aging-changes in the bones, joints,
    and muscles, 93
AGN, 308
AH, 337
AIDS, 242, 245, 246
air hunger, 284
albinism, 14, 15
albumin, 261, 297
albuminuria, 304
alcoholic cirrhosis, 262
aldosterone, 188
aldosteronism, 188
alimentary canal, 254
alopecia, 52, 63, 63*f*
ALS, 142
aluminum, 21, 267
alveolus, 282, 283
Alzheimer's disease, 139, 143
amblyopia, 159
amenorrhea, 323, 336
ametropia, 159
aminoglycosides, 309
amniocentesis, 327
amounts, prefixes pertaining to, 5
amoxicillin, 169
amphiarthrosis, 81
ampulla, 324
amputation, 112
amylase, 265
amyotrophic lateral sclerosis (ALS),
    139
anabolic steroids, 361
anal canal, 260
analgesic, 91, 116, 141, 158
anatomy, 24
androgen, 188
androgenic hormone, 360
androsterone, 178
anemia, 233
anencephaly, 130

anesthetic, 142
angina pectoris, 207, 222
angiography, 216
angioplasty, 216
angiospasm, 217
ankle, 23
anorchidism, 350
anorchism, 350
anorexia nervosa, 138
antacid, 266
antacid mixture, 266
antagonist, 108
anteflexion, 321
anterior, 30
anteversion, 321
anthracosis, 285
anti-inflammatory, 62, 91, 116
antiarrhythmic, 219
antibacterial, 307
antibiotic, 158, 166, 286
antibody, 241
anticholinergic, 157
anticoagulant, 219, 243, 261
anticonvulsant, 142
antidiarrheal, 267
antidiuretic hormone (ADH), 183, 191
antiemetic, 264, 267
antifungal, 62, 166
antigen, 241
antihistamine, 158, 286
antihypertensive, 219
antilipemic, 220
antiparkinsonian, 142
antiplatelet, 243
antipruritic, 62
antipyretic, 7, 10, 141, 158
antirheumatic, 92, 116
antiseptic, 63, 307
antithyroid, 191
antituberculosis, 287
antitussive, 7, 287
antiviral, 62, 166
anuria, 304
anus, 251
anvil, 154
apex, 30
aphagia, 138
aphasia, 137
aplastic anemia, 233
apnea, 284
aponeurosis, 110
apoplexy, 137
appendectomy, 260
appencices, 12
appendicitis, 260
appendicular skeleton, 72, 73*f*, 74*f*, 77
bones of, 74*f*
appendix, 12
apraxia, 138
arachnoid, 130
ARD, 287
ARDS, 287
areola, 330
arm, 23
armpit, 23
arrhythmia, 213
arteriosclerosis, 205
arteriovenous malformation, 143
arteritis, 202
artery, 13, 200, 202, 204, 214
artherectomy, 80
arthodesis, 81
arthralgia, 80
arthritis, 80
arthrocentesis, 80
arthropathy, 80
arthroplasty, 81
arthroscope, 81
articulation, 81
artificial pacemaker, 213
artificial respiration, 284
AS, 158
ascending colon, 260
ascites, 265
asepsis, 60
ASHD, 220
aspermatism, 354
assistive exercise, 113
asthma, 285
asymmetry, 334
ataxia, 138
atelectasis, 285
atelencephalia, 130
Atenolol, 339
athelete's foot, 53
atherosclerosis, 205
atom, 25
atria, 202
atrial fibrillation, 143
atrioventricular bundle, 202
atrioventricular node, 202
atrophy, 112
AU, 158
audible, 153
audiogram, 151
audiologist, 151
audiology, 151
audiometer, 151
audiometry, 153
auditory, 151
auditory canal, 151
aural, 153
aurical (pinna), 151
auscultation, 211
autoimmune, 241
autoimmune disease, 241
autoimmunity, 241
autologous, 241
autonomy, 7
avulsion, 60
axial skeleton, 72, 73*f*, 77
bones of, 72, 73*f*
axillary, 10
azoospermia, 354

B

B lymphocyte, 233
BAC, 244
bacteriuria, 305
bad breath, 266
balanitis, 349
balanocele, 349
balanoplasty, 349
baldness. *See* alopecia.
bartholinitis, 330
Bartholin's abcess, 330
Bartholin's cyst, 330
Bartholin's gland, 330
Basedow's disease, 184
basophil, 233
BC, 158
bedwetting, 305
belching, 264
benign, 8
benign prostatic hyperplasia (BPH), 356, 361
BG, 191
bG, 191
biceps brachii, 100
biceps femoris, 101
bile, 261
biliary cirrhosis, 262
bilirubin, 306
biology, 9
"black lung" disease, 285
bladder, 24, 295, 296*f*, 302
structure of, 355*f*
blastocyst, 338
blepharitis, 161
blepharoptosis, 161
blister, 53, 54*f*
blood, 28, 29*f*, 227, 228, 230, 231, 306
drugs for, 243
fluid part of, 236
formed elements of, 232*f*
blood clotting, 261
blood loss, 233
blood pressure, 210, 211
blood protein, 261
blood type, 236
blood urea nitrogen, 307
blood vessels, 206*f*
BM, 267
BMR, 191
body, 24
body cavity, 32, 33*f*
body levels of organization, 22*f*
body movement, types of, 81, 82*f*
body plane, 30
body planes of, 31*f*

boil, 60
bolus, 251, 254
bone, 24, 71
bone bruise, 115
bone spurs, 115
bones, 71
Bowman's capsule, 302
BP, 220
BPH, 356, 361, 363
brachial pulse point, 204, 205
brachialgia, 111
bradycardia, 213
brain, 32, 123, 130, 131*f*, 135*f*
lobes and sulci, 133*f*
major regions of, 131, 131*f*
"brain attack," 143
breast, 315, 316, 330, 331*f*
breast cancer, 333, 334, 360
risk factors for, 336
breast self-examination, 334, 335*f*
bronchi, 275, 277, 278*f*, 281, 282*f*
bronchiectasis, 281
bronchitis, 381
bronchodilator, 287
bronchomycosis, 281
bronchoplasty, 281
bronchoscope, 281
bronchoscopy, 288
bruise, 60, 425
BS, 267
BSE, 334, 335*f*
buccal, 255
bulbourethral gland, 345, 357–358
bulimia, 138
BUN, 307, 308
burn, 61, 61*f*
bursa, 83, 110
bursitis, 84, 114

C

Ca, 92
cachexia, 11
CAD, 220
calcaneal, 89
calcitonin, 184, 185
calcium, 21, 267
calciuria, 305
cancellous, 77
cancer, 48, 332, 333, 351, 356
Candida, 53
candidiasis, 53
capillary, 200, 214
Carafate, 267
carbon, 21, 23*f*
carbon dioxide, 275
carbuncle 60, 60*f*
cardiac catheterization, 217
cardiac muscle, 101
cardiodynia, 209
cardiogenic embolism, 143
cardiologist, 201
cardiology, 201
cardiomegaly, 209
cardiomyopathy, 214
cardiopulmonary, 10, 219
cardiopulmonary resuscitation (CPR), 219, 220
cardiovascular, 201
cardiovascular system, 28, 29*f*, 199
drugs for, 219–220
carotid dissection, 143
carotid point, 204, 205
carotid stenosis, 143
carpal, 89
cartilage, 71, 72, 79
castrate, 351
cataract, 164
catecholamine, 189
catheter, 306
caudal, 30
cavity, 32
CC, 63, 200, 308
CDC, 244
cecum, 260
cell, 25, 26*f*
cell membrane, 27
centimeter, 6
central nervous sytem (CNS), 123, 124*f*
cephalad, 30
cephalagia, 134
cephalohemometer, 134
cephalosporins, 309
cerebellar, 132
cerebellitis, 132
cerebellum, 131
cerebral aneurysm, 143
rupture of, 143
cerebral cortex, 133
cerebromalacia, 134
cerebrospinal, 134
cerebrovascular accident (CVA), 137, 142
cerebrum, 132
cerumen, 156
cervical, 87, 322
cervicitis, 322
cervicocolpitis, 322
cervicovaginitis, 322
cervicovesical, 322
cervix, 316, 321
cervix uteri, 322
CGN, 308
chalazion, 162
change of life, 323
cheek, 24
chest, 24, 210
chest pain, 207
chest x-ray, 288, 289
chewing, 266
Cheyne-Stokes respirations, 284
CHF, 220
chickenpox, 33, 56
chlamydia, 360
Chlamydia trachomatis, 360
chlorine, 21, 23*f*
chlorophyll, 14, 15
cholecystectomy, 262
cholecystitis, 263
cholecystogram, 263
cholecystokinin, 178
cholelithiasis, 264
cholesteatoma, 157
cholesterol, 207
cholinesterase inhibitor, 144
chondral, 80
chondralgia, 80
chondrectomy, 80
chondrocyte, 79
chondromalacia, 80
chondropathology, 80
choroid, 162
Christmas disease, 230
chromosome, 14
cib, 267
cicatrix, 57
ciliary body, 162, 164
circumcision, 349
circumduction, 83
cirrhosis, 262
clavicular, 10
climacteric, 323
clitoris, 329
closed fracture, 85
closed-angle glaucoma, 168
CMP, 220
CNS, 142
CO_2, 287
cobalt, 21, 23*f*
cochlea, 155*f*
COLD, 287
cold sore, 61
colipuncture, 260
colitis, 260
Colles' fracture, 86
colon, 260, 261
colon bacillus, 309
color, word elements pertaining to, 14
colostomy, 260
colpalgia, 329
colpitis, 329
colpocele, 329
colpocystitis, 329
colpodynia, 329
colpoperineoplasty, 329
colporrhaphy, 329
colposcope, 329
colposcopy, 329
coma, 139
combining form,4, 8, 13
comedo, 52, 59
comminuted fracture, 85

common cold, 285
compact bone, 77
compound fracture, 85
conception, 326
concussion, 139
condom, 350
condyle, 79
condyloma, 330
condyloma acuminatum, 330
cone, 164
congenital glaucoma, 168
congestive, 214
congestive heart failure, 143
conjunctiva, 159, 162
conjunctivitis, 162
connective, 27
constipation, 267
contraceptive, 336
contracture, 112
Cooley's anemia, 233
COPD, 287
copper, 21, 23*f*
cornea, 161, 163
coronal plane, 30
coronary circulation, 208*f*
corticosteroid, 91, 116, 287
cortisol, 188
coryza, 285
costal, 89
Cowper's gland, 357–358
CP, 142
CPR, 219, 220
cranial, 37
cranial cavity, 30
cranial nerve, 129
cranial nerves (12), specific regions of brain, 128*f*
craniectomy, 89, 134
craniocele, 89, 134
craniology, 89
cranioplasty, 87, 134
craniotomy, 89, 134
cranium, 134
crest, 79
cretinism, 184, 191
CRF, 308
crises, 12
crisis, 12
Crohn's disease, 259
crust, 53, 54*f*
cryotherapy, 115
cryptorchidism, 351
cryptorchism, 351
CT, 142
CUC, 267
Cushing's disease, 188
cutaneous, 46
CVA, 142
cyanosis, 284
cycloplegia, 162
cystectasy, 303
cystectomy, 303
cystic disease of the breast, 332
cystistaxis, 303
cystitis, 303, 309–310
cystocele, 303
cystogram, 303
cystoscope, 303
cytoscopic, 307
Cytotec, 267

D

D & C, 322, 337
dacryocystitis, 162
dacryoma, 162
dactylogram, 89
deafness, 157
debridement, 61
decongestant, 287
decubitus, 55
decubitus ulcer, 53
deep, 30
dehiscence, 59, 59*f*
deltoid, 100
dentalgia, 257
dentibuccal, 257
dentist, 257
dermatitis, 45
dermatologic disease, drugs for, 62
dermatologist, 45
dermatology, 9, 45
dermatome, 45
dermatomycosis, 47
dermis, 42
dermomycosis, 47
descending colon, 260
detoxify, 262
DHT, 361
DI, 191
diabetes, 186
diabetes insipidus, 183
diabetes mellitus, 186, 193
warning signs and symptoms of, 186
diagnosis, 5, 13
diagnostic procedures, suffixes used in, 9
diaphragm, 113
diaphysis, 77
diarrhea, 266
diarthrosis, 81
diastolic, 210
diencephalon, 132
digestion, 32, 251, 254, 259
digestive enzyme, 264
digestive system, 28, 29*f*, 250–273, 255*f*
  drugs for, 266–267
digitalis, 219
dihydro-testosterone, 363
dilation and curettage, 322, 337
diphtheria, 244
diplopia, 161
discharge, 51
distal, 30
diuresis, 305
diuretic, 166, 307
dizziness, 207
DJD, 92
DM, 191
dopamine, 189
dorsal, 30
dorsal cavity, 32
dorsiflexion, 81
drowsiness, 115
drugs for:
  blood, lymph, and immune system, 243
  cardiovascular system disease, 219–220
  dermatologic disease, 62–63
  digestive system disease, 266–267
  ear disease, 157–158
  endocrine system disease, 191
  eye disease, 166
  female reproductive system disease, 336
  male reproductive system disease, 360
  nervous system disease, 141
  respiratory system disease, 286–287
  skeletal system disease, 91–92
  urinary system disease, 307
dry, 46
DUB, 337
Duchenne's muscular dystrophy, 112, 118
ductus deferens, 351, 352
duodenum, 259
Dupuytren's contracture, 111
dura mater, 130
dwarfism, 182
Dx, 63
dysmenorrhea, 324
dyspepsia, 264
dysphasia, 137
dyspnea, 285
dystrophin, 111
dystrophy, 111
dysuria, 305

E

E. coli, 309
ear, 24, 149, 151
anatomical structures of, 152*f*
ear disease, drugs for, 154–158
earwax, 156
ECG, 220
echocardiography, 217
eclampsia, 143
eczema, 56

ED, 361
EEG, 142
EENT, 158
EGD, 267
ejaculation, 353
EKG, 220
elbow, 24
electrocardiogram, 217
  normal, 218*f*
electroencephalography, 130
electromyography, 109
electron, 25
elimination, 251, 254
EM, 167
embolism, 209
embolus, 137
embryonic stem cells, 338
emesis, 264
emmetropia, 161
emollient, 62
emphysema, 285
empyema, 285
encephalitis, 130
encephalocele, 130
encephalopathy, 130
endocardium, 202
endochondral, 79
endocrine system, 28, 29*f*, 174–196
  drugs for, 191
  primary glands of, 181*f*
endocrinologist, 180
endocrinology, 179
endolymph, 156
endometriosis, 320
endosteum, 877
ENT, 158
enteric, 259
enteritis, 259
enterocolitis, 259
enterogastrone, 178
enuresis, 305
enzyme, 265
eosinophil, 233
epidermis, 42, 43, 44*f*
epididymectomy, 352
epididymis, 346, 348*f*, 352
epididymitis, 309, 352
epigastric region, 34
epiglottis, 280
epilepsy, 140
epinephrine, 189
epiphyseal plate, 71, 72*f*
epiphysis, 78, 78*f*
episiotomy, 330
epispadias, 421
epistaxis, 285
epithelial, 27
epoetin alfa, 243
eponychium, 49
erectile dysfunction, 362
erection, 345
ergometer, 217
erosion, 53, 54*f*
eructation, 264
erythema, 46
erythroblast, 232
erythroclastic, 232
erythrocyte, 231, 232, 233
erythrocytosis, 232
erythroderma, 45
erythromycin, 358
erythropenia, 232
erythropoiesis, 232
Escherichia coli, 309
esophageal, 258
esophageal reflux, 258
esophageal varices, 258
esophagitis, 258
esophagogastroduodenoscopy, 259
esophagoscope, 258
esophagus, 251, 254, 257, 258
ESRD, 308
estradiol, 178
estriol, 178
estrogen, 315, 324, 336
estrone, 178
ethambutol, 288
eunuch, 351
eupnea, 285
eversion, 83
excretory system, 295
EXELON, 144
exercise, 113
exophthalmic, 184
exophthalmic goiter, 184
expectorant, 287
extension, 83
external respirarion, 275
extremity, 87
eye, 24, 148–172
  drugs for, 166
  external structure of, 159
eyeball, 163
  anatomic structures of, 163*f*
eyelid, 24, 159, 160, 161

F

facial nerve (VII), 129
fainting, 139
fallopian tube, 315, 316, 324
farsightedness, 161
fascia, 106
fasciectomy, 110
fasciodesis, 110
fascioplasty, 110
fascitis, 110
fat, 265
feces, 265
female pelvis, 328*f*
female reproductive system, 315–342, 318*f*
  drugs for, 336
  organs of, 328*f*
femora, 12
femoral point, 204
femoris, 12
femur, 74, 74*f*, 77
fertilization, 326
fetus, 316
fever blister, 61
fiber, 99
fiberoptics, 260
fibrinogen, 261
fibrocystic disease, 332
fibromyalgia, 105
fibromyositis, 105
fimbriae, 324
finasteride, 360, 363
finger, 24
fingernail. *See* nail.
fingerprint, 89
fissure, 53, 54*f*
flaccid, 111
Flagyl, 358
flatfoot, 89
flatus, 266
flexion, 81
flow, 51
fluorine, 21, 23*f*
folic acid, 243
follicle-stimulating hormone (FSH), 177
foot, 24
foramen, 78
foramina, 12
foreskin, 347
formed elements, 227, 230, 231, 232*f*
fracture, 85, 86
  types of, 86*f*
freckle, 53
frontal lobe, 133
frontal plane, 30
fundus, 316
fungus, 13, 50, 52
furuncle, 60
Fx, 92

G

gallbladder, 251, 252, 254, 262–264
gallbladder, ultrasonography of, 263
gallbladder, ultrasound of, 263*f*
gallstone, 263
gamma globulin, 261
ganglia, 13
gastric, 258
gastric juice, 258
gastric ulcer, 258, 269, 270
gastrin, 178
gastritis, 258

gastrocnemius, 100
gastroduodenitis, 258
gastrodynia, 258
gastroenteritis, 258
gastroenterologist, 252
gastroenterology, 14, 252
gastroesophageal reflux disease, 258
gastroesophagitis, 258
gastrointestinal tract, 254
gastroparesis, 258
gastrostomy, 258
GB, 268
GC, 361
gene therapy, 338
genital, 329
genital wart, 330, 422
genitalia, 329
genitourinary system, 295
genu valgum, 89
GERD, 268
GI, 268
gigantism, 182
gingivae, 13, 254
gingivitis, 254
gland, 180
endocrine, 181*f*
glans penis, 346
glaucoma, 165
glaucoma, closed-angle, 168
glaucoma, congenital, 168
glaucoma, normal-tension, 168
glaucoma, primary open-angle, 168
globin, 229
glomerular, 302
glomeruli, 297, 302
glomerulitis, 302
glomerulonephritis, 302
glossopharyngeal nerve (IX), 129
glossoplasty, 257
glossotomy, 257
glucagon, 185, 264
glucose, 306
gluteus maximus, 101
glycogen, 106
glycosuria, 305
goiter, 184
gonorrhea, 309, 359, 361
Graves' disease, 184
great toe, 24, 89
greenstick fracture, 86
growth hormone, 177–178, 182
GU, 308
gum, 24, 254
gynecologist, 316
gynecology, 316

H

H, 63
Haemophilus influenzae type b, 244
hair, 24, 41, 52
halitosis, 266
hallux, 89
hammer, 154
hand, 24
hardening, 205
harvest, 214
Hashimoto's disease, 184
HAV, 268
hay fever, 286
Hb, 244
HBV, 268
HD, 158
HDL, 207, 220
head, 24, 111, 134
head injuries, 143
hearing, 156
heart, 24, 199, 202
circulation in, 208*f*
conduction system of, 203*f*
heart attack, 209
heart disease, 207
heart transplant, 214
heartbeat, 202
heartburn, 266
heel, 24
heel bone, 89
Helicobacter pylori, 269
hemangioma, 214, 215*f*
hematinic, 243
hematocele, 230
hematocrit, 267
hematologist, 230
hematology, 9, 229
hematoma, 230, 231*f*
hematuria, 305
hemianopsia, 138
hemiparesis, 137
hemiplegia, 137
hemoglobin, 220
hemoglobinopathy, 230
hemolysis, 230
hemolyze, 230
hemophilia, 230
hemophobia, 230
hemopoiesis, 230
hemorrhage, 231, 231*f*
hemorrhagic fever, 231
hemorrhagic stroke, 143
hemostatic, 243
heparin, 261
hepatitis, 262, 268
hepatitis A (HAV), 268
hepatitis B (HBV), 242, 248, 268
hepatitis C (HCV), 268
hepatitis D (HDV), 268
hepatitis E (HEV), 268
hepatoma, 262
hepatomegaly, 262
hepatorrhexis, 262
hepatotoxin, 10
herpes genitalis, 423
herpes simplex, 61
herpes simplex virus-2, 359
herpes zoster, 57, 139
Herplex, 166
heterogeneous, 10
Hgb, 244
hidradenitis, 51
hilum, 301
hirsutism, 52
histamine H_2-receptor antagonist, 267
histologist, 28
histology, 27, 28
HIV, 242, 244
hives, 53
HMD, 287
homeostasis, 28
hordeolum, 162
hormonal imbalance, 362
hormone, 175, 177
HPV, 358, 361
HRT, 337
HSG, 337
HSV-2, 359, 361
HT, 167
human immunodeficiency virus (HIV), 242, 244
human papilloma virus (HPV), 358, 361
humerus, 77
humpback, 84
Hx, 63
hyaline membrane disease, 284
hydrocele, 351
hydrocephalus, 134
hydrochloric acid, 258
hydrocortisone, 188
hydrogen, 21, 23*f*
hypercalcemia, 185
hyperhidrosis, 51, 51*f*
hyperinsulinism, 187
hyperlipidemia, 210
hyperopia, 161
hyperparathyroidism, 185
hyperpnea, 28
hypertension, 211, 212*f*, 213
hypertension, uncontrolled, 212*f*
hyperthyroidism, 184, 191
hypnotic, 141
hypoadrenocorticism, 188
hypodermic, 46
hypodermoclysis, 47
hypogastric region, 34
hypoglossal nerve (XII), 129
hypoglycemia, 187
hypoglycemic, 191
hypoparathyroidism, 185
hyposecretion, 186
hypospadias, 357
hypotension, 213
hypothalamus, 132
hypothyroidism, 184

hypoxia, 284
hysteralgia, 320
hysterectomy, 320
hysteritis, 320
hystero-oophorectomy, 320
hysterodynia, 320
hysteropathy, 3
hysterosalpingectomy, 320
hysteroscope, 320
hysterotomy, 320

I

I & O, 308
IC, 361, 308
icteric, 58
IDDM, 186, 191
idoxuridine, 166
ileum, 259
iliac, 10
immune system, 227
drugs for, 243
immunity, 240–241, 244
immunization, 240–241, 244
immunologist, 241
immunology, 241
impetigo, 56
impotence, 362
incontinence, 305
incus, 154
indigestion, 264
infarct, 209
inferior, 30
infertility, 336
inflammation, 51
influenza, 245
infundibulum, 324
injection, 47
insertion, 106
insertional tendinitis, 117
insidious, 334
insulin, 178, 186, 187, 191, 264
insulin shock, 187
insulin-dependent diabetes mellitus (IDDM), 186, 191
integument, 43–44, 44*f*
integumentary system, 28, 28*f*, 40–68
  drugs for, 62–63
internal eye, 163
internal respiration, 275
interneuron, 125
interstitial cystitis, 309
intramuscular, 109
intraocular pressure, 166
intrauterine, 10, 321
intravenous pyelogram, 308
inversion, 83
involuntary muscle, 101
iodine, 29, 23*f*
IOP, 167
irides, 12
iris, 12, 164
iron deficiency anemia, 233
ischemic stroke, 143
islets of Langerhans, 185
isometric exercise, 113
isthmus, 324
IVF, 337
IVP, 308

J

jaundice, 58, 262
jejunum, 259
joint, 24, 81, 110
jt, 92

K

Kabikinase, 209
Kaposi's sarcoma, 242, 242*f*
keloid, 57, 58*f*
keratin, 49
keratitis, 161
keratolytic, 62
keratometer, 161
keratoplasty, 161
ketoacidosis, 191
ketone, 306
ketonuria, 305
kidney, 24, 295, 296*f*, 298, 299*f*
kidney stone, 298, 309
kilogram, 6
kneecap, 24
knock-knee, 89
Korotkoff's sound, 211
KUB, 308
Kussmaul's respiration, 284
kyphosis, 84, 84*f*, 85

L

labia majora, 329
labia minora, 329
labyrinthectomy, 155
labyrinthitis, 155
labyrinthotomy, 155
LAC, 92
laceration, 61
lacrimal, 162
lacrimal apparatus, 159, 160*f*
  anatomic structure of, 160
Laennec's portal cirrhosis, 262
laparoscope, 326
laparoscopic cholecystectomy, 263
large intestine, 251, 254, 260, 261
laryngeal, 280
laryngectomy, 280
laryngitis, 280
laryngoplasty, 280
laryngoscope, 280
laryngostomy, 280
larynx, 24, 275, 277, 278*f*, 280, 282*f*
laser angioplasty, 216
lateral, 30
latissimus dorsi, 101
laxative, 267
LDL, 207, 220
LE, 167
lecithin, 284
left hypochondriac region, 34
left iliac region, 34
left inguinal region, 34
left lower quadrant (LLQ), 35
left lumbar region, 34
left upper quadrant (LUQ), 35
leg, 24
lens, 164
lentigo, 55
lethargic, 190
lethargy, 190
leukapheresis, 235
leukemia, 235
leukocyte, 15, 231, 235
leukocytopenia, 235
leukocytosis, 235
leukopoiesis, 235
LH, 337
lice, 55
ligament, 110
lingual, 257
lip, 265
lipid, 210
lipoprotein, 207
lips, 24
lithotripsy, 306
liver, 24, 251, 254, 261, 262
LLC, 92
LMP, 337
long bone, 77
  features of, 78*f*
lordosis, 84, 84*f*
Lou Gehrig's disease, 139
low-grade fever, 288
lubb-dupp, 211
lumbar, 87
lung, 24, 275, 277, 278*f*, 282*f*, 283
lunula, 49
luteinizing hormone (LH), 177
lymph, 227, 228, 236, 237*f*
lymph node, 236, 239*f*
lymphadenitis, 238
lymphadenopathy, 238
lymphadenotomy, 238
lymphangiology, 238
lymphangioma, 238
lymphatic system, 28, 29*f*, 228, 237*f*, 236–239
drugs for, 243
lymphatic vessel, 236, 239*f*
lymphoid, 238
lymphoma, 38, 238*f*

lymphosarcoma, 238
lymphostasis, 238

M

macrocephalia, 134
macula lutea, 164
macule, 53, 54*f*
magnesium, 21, 267
male pelvis, 349*f*
male reproductive system, 345, 348*f*
  drugs for, 360
  organs of, 349*f*
malignant, 8, 334
malleus, 154
Malphigian corpuscle, 302
mammary dysplasia, 332
mammary gland. *See* breast
mammogram, 331, 332*f*
mammography, 331
mammoplasty, 331
manganese, 21, 23*f*
mastectomy, 331
mastication, 266
mastitis, 331
mastoid, 157
mastoidalgia, 157
mastoidectomy, 157
mastoiditis, 157
MDR TB, 288
meal, 264
measles, 61, 244, 245
meatus, 78
medial, 30
medical terminology, 4
medulla oblongata, 132, 283
medullary canal, 77
megacolon, 260
megaloblastic anemia, 233
meibomian gland, 162
melanin, 43, 47
melanocarcinoma, 47
melanocyte-stimulating hormone (MSH), 177
melanoma, 48, 48*f*
melatonin, 183
membrane, 27
menarche, 323
Meniere's disease, 157
meninges, 130
meningioma, 130
meningitis, 130
meningocele, 131
meningoencephalitis, 130
meningomyelocele, 131
meningopathy, 131
menopause, 323
menorrhagia, 323
menses, 316
menstrual cycle, 322–324
menstrual period, 360
menstruation, 322, 323
metacarpal, 89
metatarsal, 89
metritis, 320
metrocarcinoma, 320
metrodynia, 320
metromalacia, 320
metronidazole, 358
MH, 337
MI, 220
microcephalia, 134
microgram, 6
micturition, 304
midbrain, 132
middle ear, 154
migraine headaches, 143
miscarriage, 336
misoprostol, 267
mittelschmerz, 323
Mixoxidil, 63
molecule, 25
monilia, 53
monocyte, 233
mons pubis, 329
motor neuron, 123
mouth, 24, 251
movement, 108
MS, 142
mucolytic, 287
mucosal protective medications, 267
multidrug-resistant tuberculosis, 288
multipara, 328
multiple sclerosis, 140
mumps, 244, 245
muscle, 24. *See also specific type*
  classification of, 108
  types of, 100*f*
muscle fiber, 105
muscular dystrophy, 112
muscular system, 28, 29*f*, 99, 116
MY, 167
myalgia, 104
myasthenia, 109
myasthenia gravis, 140
Mycobacterium tuberculosis, 288, 289
mydriatic, 166
myelitis, 136
myelodysplasia, 136
myelography, 136
myelopathy, 136
myelotome, 136
myocardial infarction, 209
myocardium, 202
myofascial, 109
myolysis, 108
myomalacia, 109
myomelanosis, 109
myometritis, 320
myometrium, 320
myopia, 161
myosarcoma, 109
myositis, 105
myringectomy, 154
myringoplasty, 154
myringoscope, 154
myringotome, 154
myringotomy, 154
myxedema, 184, 191

N

Na, 308
nail, 24, 41, 49, 49–51, 49*f*
nail biting, 50
narcolepsy, 140
nasal cavity, 278*f*, 279*f*
nasomental, 277
nasopharyngitis, 277
navel, 24
nearsightedness, 161
neck, 24
necrosis, 14
Neisseria gonorrhoeae, 359
neonatal, 327
nephrectomy, 298
nephritis, 298
nephroma, 298
nephromalacia, 298
nephromegaly, 298
nephron, 299*f*, 302
nephropathy, 298
nephropexy, 298
nephroptosis, 298
nerve, 24, 125
nerve, efferent, 123
nerve fibers, 125
nerve tracts, 125
nervous system, 28, 29*f*, 123
  divisions of, 124*f*
  drugs for, 141
neuralgia, 129
neurasthenia, 129
neurectomy, 129
neuritis, 129
neurofibromatosis, 129
neuroglia, 123
neurohypophysis, 183
neurological diseases, 362
neurologist, 127
neurology, 127
neuroma, 129
neuron, 123
neuropathy, 129
neurosis, 129
neurosurgery, 127
neutron, 25
neutrophil, 233
nevus, 59, 59*f*
NIDDM, 186, 191
night
night blindness, 161

night sweats, 288
night vision, 164
NIH, 362
nitrate, 219
nitrite, 306
nitrogen, 21, 23*f*
nocturia, 305
nodule, 52, 53, 54*f*
noninsertional tendinitis, 117
noninsulin-dependent diabetes mellitus (NIDDM), 186, 191
norepinephrine, 189
normal-tension glaucoma, 168
nose, 24, 275, 277, 279*f*
nosebleed, 285
NPT, 361
NSAIDs, 91, 92, 116
nucleus, 13, 25
nullipara, 327
numbers, prefixes pertaining to, 5
nutritional cirrhosis, 262
NVA, 167
nyctalopia, 161

O

O_2, 287
OA, 92
occipital lobe, 134
ocular, 159
oculomoter nerve (III), 129
OD, 167
oily, 62
olfactory nerve (I), 129
oligospermia, 354
oliguria, 305
OM, 158
oncology, 9, 14
onychomycosis, 50, 50*f*
onychophagia, 50
oogenesis, 326
oophorectomy, 325
oophoritis, 325
oophorohysterectomy, 325
oosperm, 326
opacity, 164
open fracture, 85
ophthalmologist, 159
ophthalmology, 159
ophthalmopathy, 159
ophthalmoscope, 159
optic, 159
optic nerve (II), 129
optomyometer, 159
oral cavity, 254, 256*f*
oral contraceptive, 336
orbit, 159
orchidectomy, 350
orchidopexy, 351
orchidoplasty, 351
orchidotomy, 351
orchiectomy, 350, 351
orchiopexy, 351
orchioplasty, 351
orchitis, 351
organ, 28
organ system, 28, 29*f*
organelle, 21, 23*f*
origin, 108
orthopedics, 76
orthopedist, 76
orthopnea, 285
OS, 167
ossicle, 154
osteoarthritis, 76
osteoblast, 76
osteocarcinoma, 76
osteochondritis, 76
osteomalacia, 76
osteomyelitis, 76
osteoporosis, 84, 92, 336
osteotome, 76
ostium, 324
otalgia, 153
otitis, 153
otitis media, 169
oto, 158
otodynia, 153, 169
otolith, 153
otomycosis, 153
otoneurology, 153
otopharyngeal, 153
otoplasty, 153
otopyorrhea, 153
otorhinolaryngologist, 151
otorhinolaryngology, 151
otosclerosis, 153
otoscope, 153
OU, 167
ova, 12
ovarian, 325
ovarian cyst, 325
ovariectomy, 325
ovariocele, 325
ovariocentesis, 325
ovariohysterectomy, 325
ovariopathy, 325
ovaritis, 325
ovary, 315, 316, 318*f*, 319*f*, 324–325
oviduct, 324
ovulation, 323
ovum, 12, 21, 326
oxygen, 106, 275
oxytocin, 183

P

P wave, 217
pacemaker, 202, 213
pachyderm, 58
pain, 207
palate, 254
palsy, 140
pancreas, 176, 185, 254, 264
pancreatitis, 264
panhysterectomy, 320
Pap, 337
Papanicolaou smear, 322
papillae, 42
papule, 52, 53, 54*f*
paraplegia, 137
parathormone (PTH), 185
parathyroid gland, 185
parietal lobe, 133
Parkinson's disease, 140
paronychia, 50
passive exercise, 113
passive immunization, 244
patella, 24
pause, 323
pc, 268
PCP, 244
PD, 308
pectoralis major, 100
pediculosis, 55
pediculosis capitis, 55*f*
pelvic cavity, 32
pelvis, 90*f*, 91
female, 328*f*
male, 349*f*
penicillin, 309, 358
penile, 297, 350
penile prosthesis, 350
penis, 345, 346–350
structures of, 355*f*
penitis, 350
peptic ulcer disease, 269, 269*f*
pericardium, 202
perilymph, 156
perineum, 330
periosteum, 77, 78*f*
periphereal nervous system (PNS), 123, 124*f*
peristalsis, 257
pernicious anemia, 233
pertussis, 244, 286
pes planus, 89
PET, 142
petechiae, 59
PH, 63
phacolysis, 165
phacosclerosis, 165
phagocytosis, 240
phalanges, 12, 89
phalanx, 12
pharyngalgia, 280
pharyngitis, 280
pharynx, 24, 251, 254, 257, 275, 277, 278–280, 279*f*
phimosis, 350
phlebitis, 216
phlebotomy, 215

phosphorus, 21, 23*f*
physiology, 25
pia mater, 130
PID, 337
pigment, 43, 47
pilonidal cyst, 53
pilose, 53
pilosebaceous,53
pimple, 53
pineal gland, 183
pinealectomy, 183
"pinkeye," 162
pituitarism, 182
pituitary gland, 180, 182
  anterior lobe, 182
  posterior lobe, 183
placement, prefixes pertaining to, 5
plasma, 236
platelet, 231, 233, 234
pleurisy, 286
PMP, 337
PMS, 337
PND, 287
pneumatothorax, 283
pneumococcal disease, 245
pneumoconiosis, 283
Pneumocystis carinii, 242
pneumonectomy, 283
pneumonia, 283
pneumonitis, 283
pneumothorax, 283
PNS, 142
point, 87
poliomyelitis, 136, 244, 245
pollinosis, 286
polycythemia, 234
polycythemia vera, 143
polydipsia, 187
polymyoclonus, 10
polyphagia, 187
polyuria, 187, 305
pons, 131, 132
position, prefixes pertaining to, 5
posterior, 30
postnecrotic cirrhosis, 262
postpartum, 327
postprandial, 264
potassium, 21, 23*f*
Pott's fracture, 85
PP, 268
PPD, 288
prefix, 4
  descriptive/used in general, 5
  pertaining to numbers/amounts, 5
  pertaining to position/placement, 5
pregnancy, 316, 326
prenatal, 326
prepuce, 347
presbycusis, 156
presbyopia, 161
prescription drugs, 429
pressure, 207
primary open-angle glaucoma (POAG), 168
primary organ, 254
primary pulse point, 204*f*, 205
prime mover, 108
primigravida, 327
primipara, 327
proctologist, 261
progeria, 190
progesterone, 315, 324
progestin, 336
prolactin hormone (PRL), 177
pronation, 83
prone, 30
pronunciation, 13
Proscar, 360, 363
prostatalgia, 356
prostate, 356
prostate cancer, 356
prostate gland, 345, 348*f*, 354, 355*f*
  enlarged, 356
  structures of, 355*f*
prostate-specific antigen (PSA), 420, 426
prostatectomy, 356
prostatic, 355
prostatitis, 356
prostatism, 356
prostatocystitis, 357
prostatomegaly, 357
protection, 41
prothrombin, 361
proton, 25
protoplasm, 27
protraction, 83
proximal, 30
pruritus, 59
PSA, 356, 361
psoriasis, 55, 56*f*
psychiatrist, 141
psychiatry, 141
psychoanalysis, 141
psychological problems, 362
psychology, 141
psychopath, 141
psychosis, 141
psychosomatic, 141
psychotropic, 141
PTH, 191
pudendum, 239
pulmometer, 283
pulmonary, 277, 283
pulmonary medicine, 274
pulmonary surfactant, 284
pulmonary tuberculosis, 289–290
pulmonectomy, 283
pulmonitis, 283
pulmonologist, 277
pulse, 204, 205
pupil, 164
purpura, 14
pustule, 52, 53, 54*f*
pyelocystitis, 301
pyelocystostomosis, 301
pyelolithotomy, 302
pyelonephritis, 302
Pyridium, 309
pyrosis, 266
pyuria, 305

Q

Q wave, 217
quadrant, 34*f*, 35
quadriceps, 111
quadriplegia, 137

R

R, 288
R wave, 217
RA, 92
rabies, 245
radial keratotomy, 161
radial pulse point, 204, 205
radius, 68
range of motion, 113
RBC, 244
RD, 288
RE, 167
rectum, 251, 260
rectus abdominis, 100
rectus femoris, 100
red blood cell (RBC), 231, 232
regional enteritis, 259
regulation, 42
relaxant, 115
relief of tension, 113
renal, 298
renal calculus, 298
renal colic, 298
renal failure, 298
renal pelvis, 302
renal transplant, 298
replacement therapy, 336
reproductive system, 28, 29*f*
  female. *See* female reproductive system
  male. *See* male reproductive system
respiration, 275, 284
respiratory distress syndrome, 284
respiratory rate, 283
respiratory system, 28, 29*f*, 274–292, 278*f*
  drugs for, 286–287
Retin-A, 63
retina, 163
retraction, 83, 334
retroflexion, 321
retroversion, 321
Reye's syndrome, 140

Rh, 244
Rh factor, 236
rhabdomyoma, 106
rheumatism, 104
rheumatologist, 105
rheumatology, 104
Rheumatrex, 91
rhinitis, 277
rhinoplasty, 277
rhinorrhagia, 277
rhinorrhea, 277
rhinostenosis, 277
rhinotomy, 277
rhodopsin, 164
rhytidectomy, 59
rhytidoplasty, 58
rib, 24
RICE, 114, 115
rifampin, 288
right hypochondriac region, 34
right iliac region, 34
right inguinal region, 34
right lower quadrant (RLQ), 35
right lumbar region, 34
right upper quadrant (RUQ), 35
ringworm, 47
rod, 164
Rogaine, 63
root, 7
rotation, 83
rotator cuff, 113
rrhythm, 213
rubella, 244, 245
rubeola, 61

S

S wave, 217
S-A, 220
SA, 220
SAC, 92
sacral, 87
sagittal plane, 30
saliva, 251, 254
salivary gland, 293, 251, 254
salpingectomy, 324
salpingitis, 324
salpingo-oophorectomy, 324
sarcolemma, 106
sartorius, 100
scale, 53
scar, 57
sciatica, 140
sclera, 163
scoliosis, 84, 84*f*, 85
scrotum, 345, 346, 350
sebaceous gland, 42, 51
seborrhea, 51
secretin, 178
secretion, 42
sedative, 141
semen, 346, 352, 353
semicircular canals, 152
seminal vesicle, 245, 348*f*, 352
seminiferous tubule, 345, 350
semitendinosus, 101
sensation, 42
sensory neuron, 125
sepsis, 241
septum, 202
sera, 13
serotonin, 183
sex therapy, 362
sexually transmitted diseases (STDs), 358
shingles, 57, 139
sickle cell anemia, 233
sickle cell disease, 143
SIDS, 288
sigmoid colon, 270
sigmoidoscope, 260
sigmoidoscopy, 260
sildenafil citrate, 362
Simmond's disease, 182
sinoatrial node, 202
sinus, 78, 279*f*, 286
sinusitis, 286
skeletal muscles (anterior view), 100, 102*f*
skeletal muscles (posterior view), 101, 103*f*
skeletal muscle, 99, 100, 100f, 107*f*
skeleton. *See* appendicular skeleton; axial skeleton.
skeltetal system, 28, 29*f*, 70–97
skin, 24, 28, 41, 42, 45, 51
skin cancer, 64
skin signs, 53, 54*f*
skull, 24, 87, 89, 133
sleep apnea, 284
small intestine, 251, 254, 258, 259
smegma, 347
smoking, 221
smooth muscle, 101, 111
Snellen eye chart, 164, 165*f*
SOB, 288
sodium, 21, 23*f*
soleus, 100
SOM, 158
somatostatin, 185
somatotropin, 182
spadias, 347, 357
special senses, 149–172
specialized language, 4
sperm, 347, 353, 354
sperm duct, 348*f*
spermatoblast, 353
spermatocyst, 353
spermatogenesis, 354
spermatozoon, 12, 326, 345, 353*f*, 354
structures of, 353*f*
spermaturia, 354
spermicide, 354
sphygmomanometer, 210, 211*f*
spinal cavity, 32, 33
spinal cord, 33, 123, 135*f*, 136
spinal cord injury, 136
spinal injury, 362
spinal nerve, 129, 135*f*
spine, 24, 79
  abnormal curvature of, 84, 84*f*
  curves of, 87, 88*f*
spleen, 239*f*, 240
splenemia, 240
splenomegaly, 240
splenopexy, 240
SPP, 361
sprain, 114
sputum, 286
sputum culture, 288, 289
ST, 167
stapes, 154
Staphylococcus aureus, 323
starch, 265
STD, 358, 361
stem cells, 338
stem-cell line, 338
stem-cell transplantation, 338
sternocleidomastoid, 100
stethoscope, 210
STH, 191
stirrup, 154
stomach, 24, 251, 252, 254, 258
Stoxil, 166
strabismus, 166
strain, 114
stratum corneum, 42
stratum germinativum, 42
stratum granulosum, 42
stratum lucidum, 42
stress fractures, 93
stress test, 217
striated muscle, 99
stroke, 137, 142
  warning signs for, 137
stroke, hemorrhagic, 143
stroke, ischemic, 143
STS, 361
stye, 162
subcutaneous, 46
subcutaneous tissue, 42, 44*f*
sublingual, 257
substance abuse, 362
subungual, 51
sucralfate, 267
sudoriferous glands, 42
suffix, 4, 8, 13
  pertaining to pathologic conditions, 9
  used in diagnostic/surgical procedures, 9
  used in general, 9
sulfa drugs, 309

sulfonamide, 307, 309
sulfur, 21, 23*f*
superficial, 30
superior, 30
supination, 83
supine, 30
surgery, 362
surgical, 214
surgical procedures, suffixes used in, 9
sweat, 51
sweat gland, 42, 51
Sx, 63
syllable, 4
synarthrosis, 81
syncope, 139
synergist, 108
synovia, 110
syphilis, 309, 358
system, 23
systolic, 210

T

T lymphocyte, 189, 233
T wave, 217
T_3, 191
T_4, 191
tachycardia, 213
tachypnea, 285
tailbone, 24
tarsal, 89
TB, 288
teeth, 24, 254, 257
temple, 24
temporal lobe, 133
temporal pulse point, 204
tendinitis, 110
tendinitis, insertional, 117
tendinitis, noninsertional, 117
tendon, 110
tendonitis, 114
tenodynia, 110
tenorrhaphy, 110
tenosynovitis, 110
tenotomy, 110
testes, 345
testicular, 351
testicular cancer, 351
testis, 345, 350–351
testosterone, 188, 345, 350, 360
tetanus, 244, 245
tetany, 185
tetracycline, 309, 358
thermotherapy, 115
thoracic, 87
thoracic cavity, 32
throat, 24, 278
thrombectomy, 234
thrombocyte, 231, 234–235
thrombogenic, 235
thrombolysis, 235
thrombosis, 209, 235
thrombus, 13, 137
thymectomy, 190
thymitis, 190, 240
thymocyte, 240
thymopexy, 190
thymopoietin, 189
thymosin, 189
thymus gland, 189, 190*f*, 239*f*, 240
thyrocalcitonin, 185
thyroid, 184
thyroid cartilage, 280
thyroid gland, 184–185
thyroid hormone, 191
thyroid-stimulating hormone (TSH), 178
thyroidectomy, 184
thyroiditis, 184
thyroptosis, 184
thyrosis, 184
thyrotoxicosis, 184
thyroxine, 184
TIA, 142
tibia, 77
tibialis anterior, 100
tinea, 47
tinea capitis, 47
tinea cruris, 47
tinnitus, 157
tissue, 27
tissue plasminogen activator, 209
toe, 24
toenail. *See* nail
tongue, 24, 254, 257
tonicity, 108
tonometer, 166
tonsil, 228, 239*f*
tonsillitis, 240
torticollis, 105
toxic goiter, 184
toxic shock syndrome (TSS), 323
TPA, 220
tPA, 220
trachea, 275, 277, 278*f*, 281, 282*f*
tracheal, 281
trachealgia, 281
tracheitis, 281
tracheolaryngotomy, 281
tracheostomy, 281
transverse colon, 260
transverse plane, 30
trapezius, 101
Treponema pallidum, 358
tretinoin, 63
triceps, 101, 111
triceps brachii, 111
Trichomonas, 358
trichomoniasis, 358
trichomycosis, 52
trigeminal nerve (V), 129
trigone, 302
triiodothyronine, 184
trochanter, 78
trochlear nerve (IV), 129
TSS, 323, 337
tubal ligation, 326
tubercle, 79
tuberculin test, 288
tuberculosis, 288–289
tuberculosis, multidrug-resistant, 288
tuberosity, 79
tumor, 8
TUR, 361
TURP, 361
Tx, 92
tympanic, 154
tympanic membrane, 154
tympanectomy, 154
tympanitis, 154
tympanoplasty, 154

U

UA, 308
UG, 361
ulcer, 53, 54*f*
  gastric, 258, 269, 270
  peptic, 269*f*
ultrasonogram, male fetus, 327*f*
umbilical region, 34
unstriated muscle, 111
upper GI series, 269, 270*f*
uremia, 306
ureter, 295, 296*f*, 300–302
ureterocolostomy, 300
ureteronephrectomy, 300
ureteroplasty, 300
ureterorrhaphy, 301
ureterostenosis, 301
ureterovesical, 301
urethra, 295, 296*f*, 303, 304, 345, 348*f*
urethral, 357
urethralgia, 303, 357
urethrectomy, 357
urethrism, 357
urethritis, 357
urethropenile, 303
urethropexy, 303
urethrophraxis, 303, 357
urethrospasm, 303
urethrovaginal, 303
URI, 288
urinalysis, 305
urinary bladder. *See* bladder
urinary meatus, 303
urinary system, 28, 29*f*, 294–313, 296*f*
  drugs for, 307
  organs of, 301*f*
urinary tract infection, incidence of, 309
urination, 304
urine, 295, 304

urinometer, 306
urobilinogen, 306
urogenital system, 295
urologist, 298
urology, 298
urticaria, 61, 61*f*
uterine, 321
uterine adnexa, 321
uterine fibroid tumor, 321
uterine tube, 318*f*, 324
uterocele, 321
uteroplasty, 321
uteroscope, 321
uterotomy, 321
uterus, 315, 316–321, 318*f*, 319*f*
UTI, 308
uvea, 163

V

VA, 167
vaccine-preventable diseases, 245
vagina, 315, 316, 318*f*, 328–329
vaginitis, 328
vagus nerve (X), 129
valacyclovir, 359
Valtrex, 359
varicella, 56, 57*f*
varicella-zoster virus, 57
variocele, 352
vas deferens, 352
vascular diseases, 362
vasectomy, 352
vasitis, 352
vasoconstriction, 217
vasodilation, 217
vasopressin (VP), 183
vasopressor, 219
vasotripsy, 216
VD, 361
vein, 200, 214
venereal, 358
venipuncture, 216
ventral, 30
ventral cavity, 32
ventricle, 202
verruca, 60
verrucae (warts), 60*f*
vertebrae, 13, 87
regions of, 88
vertex, 30
vertigo, 157
vesicle, 53, 54*f*
vestibule, 254
VF, 167
Viagra, 362
visceral, 111
visceral muscle, 111
visual acuity, 164
vitamin, 262
vitamin B_{12}, 243
VLDL, 207, 220
voice box, 24, 280
void, 304
Volkmann's contracture, 111
voluntary, 99
volvulus, 265, 265*f*
vomiting, 264, 360
vowel, 4, 8, 13
VP, 191
vulgaris, 63
vulva, 315, 316, 329

W

wart, 60, 60*f*, 358
water, 25, 35
wave, 202
WBC, 244
weight, 6, 13
wheal, 53, 54*f*
white blood cell (WBC), 233, 235
whooping cough, 286
windpipe, 281
word elements pertaining to color, 14
word root, 4, 7
WR, 361
wrist, 24
wt, 116

X

xeroderma, 46
XT, 167

Z

Zantac, 270
zidovudine, 245
zinc 21, 23*f*
Zovirax, 62
zygote, 326